COMPLEMENTARY THERAPIES FOR THE CONTEMPORARY HEALTHCARE

Edited by **Marcelo Saad**
and **Roberta de Medeiros**

Complementary Therapies for the Contemporary Healthcare
http://dx.doi.org/10.5772/3307
Edited by Marcelo Saad and Roberta de Medeiros

Contributors

Roberta de Medeiros, Marcelo Saad, Trisha Dunning, Vilelmine Carayanni, Anson Chui Yan Tang, Graham Wilfred Ewing, Vitor Engrácia Valenti, Luiz Carlos de Abreu, Heraldo L. Guida, Luiz Carlos M. Vanderlei, Lucas Lima Ferreira, Celso Ferreira, Maria Franco Trindade Medeiros, Luci de Senna-Valle, Regina Helena Potsch Andreata, Kalavathy Ramasamy, Zuhailah Mohd Shafawi, Vasudevan Mani, Ho Yin Wan, Abu Bakar Abdul Majeed, Bowirrat Abdalla, Mustafa Yassin, Menachem Abir, Bishara Bisharat, Zaher Armaly

Published by InTech
Janeza Trdine 9, 51000 Rijeka, Croatia

Publishing Process Manager Dragana Manestar
Technical Editor InTech DTP team
Cover InTech Design team

Additional hard copies can be obtained from orders@intechopen.com

Complementary Therapies for the Contemporary Healthcare,
Edited by Marcelo Saad and Roberta de Medeiros
p. cm.
ISBN 978-953-51-0801-6

For EU product safety concerns:
IN TECH d.o.o., Prolaz Marije Krucifikse Kozulić 3, 51000 Rijeka, Croatia,
info@intechopen.com or visit our website at intechopen.com.

Meet the editors

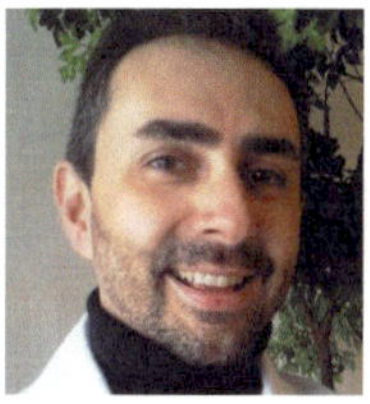

Marcelo Saad graduated Medicine at Federal University of S. Paulo, Brazil. At the same University, he achieved the degrees of MSc and PhD in Rehabilitation Sciences. Currently, he is Director Member at Medical College of Acupuncture of S. Paulo, Board Certified in Physiatry and Acupuncture and coordinates projects for inpatients spiritual support at Medical Spiritist Association of S. Paulo. He is also a Physiatrist and Acupuncturist for the clinical staff at the Hospital Israelita Albert Einstein, one of Latin America's most advanced hospitals. Besides his work as a physician, he is actively involved in scientific publishing, giving lectures and serving as an editorial board member for several medical journals.

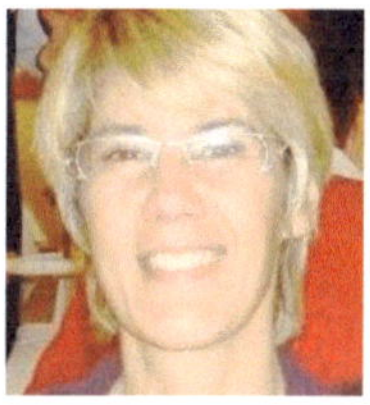

Roberta de Medeiros graduated in Biology at the State University of S. Paulo, Brazil, where she also obtained the PhD in Neurophysiology. Currently she is a Full Professor of Physiology at Centro Universitario S. Camilo (S. Paulo, Brazil), participating in scholar and scientific activities with students of Medicine, Physiotherapy, Nursing, Nutrition, Occupational Therapy and Speech Therapy. She is also an editorial board member for the Journal of Naturology and Complementary Therapies and she has published many papers and book chapters in this filed.

Contents

Preface

The concepts of health, illness and healing have evolved over the centuries. But it was always a concern of humanity to eliminate suffering and prevent death. The resources used for these purposes were evolving as knowledge about the nature of the diseases improved. Modern medicine achieved amazing progresses but, in recent years, many patients have expressed their dissatisfaction with the conventional healthcare because of its increasingly technical approach, morbidity by the side effects of treatment and the absence of cure for certain diseases.

Complementary therapies (CTs) are practices, products or systems for health that are outside the domain of conventional medicine (also called Western or allopathic medicine), used either to treat illnesses or to promote health and well-being. Defining CTs is difficult, because the field is very broad and constantly changing. The list of what is considered CT changes continually, and therapies whose safety and effectiveness are demonstrated may become part of conventional medicine.

The number of patients who question their general practitioners about CTs increases continuously. These therapies complement the conventional medicine by fulfill demands not attended by the standard approach and by diversify the conceptual chart of medicine. An approach oriented for a broader meaning of cure (physical, mental, emotional, social and spiritual) should combine in a coordinated way treatments from conventional medicine and CTs for which there is some high-quality evidence of safety and effectiveness.

Modernly, this is achieved by the "Integrative Medicine" approach. This is aligned to the concept of patient-centered healthcare, which is the provision of what an individual needs particularly. It is a model of care that promotes patient recovery at all levels. However, there are several issues still unanswered in the field of CTs, that include: How does it work? Will it interact with conventional medical treatments already in use? What objective benefits can be expected? Do the potential benefits outweigh the potential risks? How long must the treatment last?

In order to walk towards a balanced situation in the field of CTs, we need to ask and answer questions that generate useful directions. Using a SWOT analysis (Strengths, Weaknesses, Opportunities, Threats), we may risk to frame the current scenario and to project the possible future of CTs. Besides the here listed strengths, opportunities, weaknesses and threats, there must be many others.

1. STRENGTHS are characteristics that give to the issue an advantage. This item has to do with survival. Key questions for this issue include: What are our advantages? What other people see as our strengths? What we do exceptionally well? What valuable assets do we have? We may identify at least two major Strengths of CTs: the public preference and the ancient tradition.

1.1. Public Preference. The interest in CTs among patients is increasing worldwide. One of the main reasons is a growing trend for patients to take a more proactive approach to their own health. Patients also focus self-care to prevent diseases and improve quality of life. Also, some individuals feel some frustration with the dominant health care system. The patients expect that the health services respect and support their willing about CTs, following the model of patient-centered care. Many people are prone to pay for CTs out-of-pocket to be treated in a more holistic way.

1.2. Ancient Tradition. Many CTs have originated hundreds or thousands years ago, and have successfully survived till our days. This only fact may be viewed as a proof of value of these techniques, which deserves the due respect. The ancestral root of many CTs produces a great appeal for the ancient knowledge they save.

2. WEAKNESSES (or Limitations) are characteristics that place the issue at a disadvantage. This item has to do with maintenance. Key questions for this issue include: What do we do badly? What should we avoid? There are weak links in the chain? What could we do better? From what we are criticized? Where are we vulnerable? We may identify at least two major Weaknesses of CTs: the "mystique" language and the unpredictability of outcomes.

2.1. "Mystique" language. Communication is a weak point in CTs. The concepts of the techniques are often elaborate, transcending biophysical models and employing the principles of salutogenesis. Terms as "prana" and "chi", among many others, don't correlate to modern biologic concepts. This gap reinforces the skepticism among scientists. Also there are some misunderstandings, such thinking that "every natural product must be healthy", hiding the fact that, as with any medical treatment, there can be risks with some CT.

2.2. Unpredictability of Outcomes. The lack of uniformity on the patients' responses to CTs is responsible for many reports of bad results on researches. Many CTs work well for some patients while don't work at all for others. There may be factors determining these differences, which remain still unknown because these factors must be beyond the data obtained from randomized double-blind clinical trials.

3. OPPORTUNITIES are external chances to improve performance. This item has to do with growth. Key questions for this issue include: What are the good opportunities ahead? In which emerging trends can we capitalize? What are the opportunities not still addressed? We may identify at least two major Opportunities of CTs: better general acceptance and the need for low-cost healthcare.

3.1. Better General Acceptance. The interest in CTs arrived to universities, which encourages high level academic studies in this field. Currently, there are many valuable scientific journals dedicated to publish articles about CTs. Some respected healthcare institutions started to offer many CTs techniques besides conventional treatments.

3.2. Need for Low-Cost Healthcare. All over the world, governments face difficulties to maintain the current financial investment in healthcare. At same time, there is a growing body of evidence indicating that CTs are making a significant and cost effective contribution to the health of the community, especially in chronic disease management and prevention of diseases.

4. THREATS are external elements that could cause trouble. This item has to do with development. Key questions for this issue include: Do we have all the necessary skills? Deficiencies can make us critically vulnerable? What obstacles ahead can block progress? There are changes coming in our field? We may identify at least two major Strengths of CTs: the charlatanism by some practitioners and the prejudice and disinterest from health professionals.

4.1. Charlatanism by Some Practitioners. Charlatans may be motivated either by greed or ignorance. Anyway, some practitioners of CTs make exaggerated claims about curing diseases, and some ask their patients to abandon the conventional treatment. For these reasons, many doctors are conservative about recommending CTs. Challenges include also the user behavior. Patient may seek CTs for wrong motivations, as a shortcut to resolve problems. The results may include from disappointment to retardation of clinical investigation, with serious consequences.

4.2. Prejudice and Disinterest from Health Professionals. Many people ridicule CTs even before to collect all information for a critical analysis. The attachment to conventions results from the sloth to remain in a comfort zone. As a rule, health professionals don't receive training in CTs, so they may not feel comfortable making recommendations or addressing questions in this area. Many physicians are familiar with acupuncture or chiropractic, but are not quite sure how to respond to patients who ask for music therapy or Reiki.

Based on the above facts, we could propose some actions to support the development of CTs and their integration to conventional care. Figure 1 represents the framing of the CTs question and illustrates the actions to support a full integration with conventional healthcare.

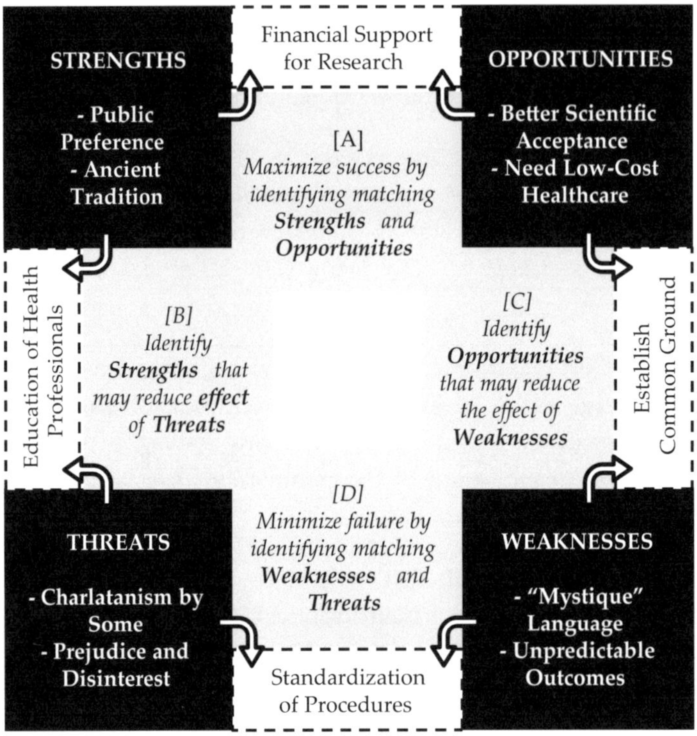
Financial Support for Research
STRENGTHS
- Public Preference
- Ancient Tradition
OPPORTUNITIES
- Better Scientific Acceptance
- Need Low-Cost Healthcare
[A]
Maximize success by identifying matching Strengths and Opportunities
Education of Health Professionals
[B]
Identify Strengths that may reduce effect of Threats
[C]
Identify Opportunities that may reduce the effect of Weaknesses
Establish Common Ground
[D]
Minimize failure by identifying matching Weaknesses and Threats
THREATS
- Charlatanism by Some
- Prejudice and Disinterest
WEAKNESSES
- "Mystique" Language
- Unpredictable Outcomes
Standardization of Procedures

Figure 1. SWOT representation for CTs (black squares), strategies for improvement (grey arrows) and actions required (dotted squares).

Strategy A - Maximize success by identifying matching Strengths and Opportunities. The main action for this purpose is **financial support for research**. One reason for the lack of research in CTs is that large, carefully controlled medical studies are costly. Trials for conventional therapies are often funded by large companies that develop and sell drugs. Fewer resources are available to support trials of CTs. Governments, universities, independent institutions and professional associations must join resources to solve this gap.

Strategy B - Identify Strengths that may reduce the effect of Threats. The main action for this purpose is **education of healthcare professionals**. Because of the increased use of CTs, all health professionals need to be familiar with this subject so they can assist clients to make informed decisions in the use of these therapies. Although many health professionals are developing a favorable opinion toward CTs, they commonly have difficulty to supply orientation for patients about benefits and risks, limitations and characteristics of the techniques, due to lack of training. The body of evidences about the efficacy and the security of the diverse modalities of CTs is dynamic and request constant updating by the health professionals.

Strategy C - Identify Opportunities that may reduce the effect of Weaknesses. The main action for this purpose is **establishing common ground**. CTs must be integrated to conventional healthcare in a cooperative, non-competitive way. Advances in physiologic knowledge will act as a bridge linking the biologic facts with the proposals of CTs. For many complementary therapies is almost impossible to conduct this type of study, due to the difficulty in creating a control group. Alternative ways to validate CTs must be explored.

Strategy D - Minimize failure by identifying matching Weaknesses and Threats. The main action for this purpose is **standardization of procedures**. There is no standardized system for credentialing CTs practitioners, as a whole, to provide services. The extent and type of credentialing vary greatly among regions and from one CT profession to another. In different countries, a same product may be labeled as food supplement or as medication. A safe, ethical, efficacious treatment with CTs can only be offered when fully incorporated into conventional healthcare. An orthodox clinical diagnosis must be established, to make sure that not only the symptoms are being treated, but also their causes.

To conclude, we foresee an epoch when CTs may complete the definition of health adopted by the World Health Organization (WHO): "a state of complete physical, mental and social well-being, and not merely the absence of disease or infirmity." This definition was adopted during the founding of this entity in 1948, and has not been modified since then. In the late 1970s, the WHO created the Traditional Medicine Program. Since then, the WHO expressed its commitment to encourage Member States to formulate and implement public policies for integrated and rational use of traditional medicine and CTs in the national health care as well as the development of scientific studies.

We hope the information from the present book can collaborate in some manner with the ongoing process of evolution of the paradigms related to concepts of health, disease and healing.

Marcelo Saad, MD, PhD
Acupuncturist at Hospital Israelita Albert Einstein
Director of S. Paulo Medical College of Acupuncture,
S. Paulo
Brazil

Roberta de Medeiros, Biologist, PhD
Full Professor of Physiology at Centro Universitario S. Camilo
S. Paulo
Brazil

Section 1

Current Scenario

Chapter 1

Complementary Therapies – Considerations Before Recommend, Tolerate or Proscribe Them

Roberta de Medeiros and Marcelo Saad

Additional information is available at the end of the chapter

http://dx.doi.org/10.5772/50446

1. Introduction

According to the World Health Organization, "health is a state of complete physical, mental and social wellbeing, not merely the absence of disease or infirmity." This definition was adopted at the founding of this organization in 1948 and has not been modified since then [1]. By this definition, clinical and conventional surgical treatment, in their strict sense, would not encompass everything the patient needs to balance your health. When applied alone, conventional health treatment may bring limited results, adverse effects from the interventions, and the high inherent cost. Many symptoms are multi-factorial and the role of the psyche is crucial. In such cases, many complementary interventions have great potential to alleviate these symptoms.

In recent years, many patients have shown dissatisfaction with conventional medicine due to its more technical approach, the morbidity by side effects of the treatment, and absence of cure for some diseases. In this scenario, complementary therapies have become an attractive option for many patients. The growing interest of patients by complementary therapies is due to [2]: evidences linking many diseases to some lifestyle; patients focusing more their welfare; and their desire to consume fewer drugs. At the same time, physicians and health services are progressively having more positive attitudes about to complementary therapies. The CT aim to optimize physical symptoms, quality of life and emotional aspects, and to prevent or delay the onset of some diseases. There are many advantages resulting from the use of CT: it emphasizes the well-being and global healing (not just symptoms or diseases), encourages the patient to actively participate in their healing process, and supports the concept that treatment is possible even when the cure is not.

An estimated 30 to 62 percent of adults in the United States use CT [3]. A lack of consensus on the definition of CT has led to inconsistencies among the reports of various surveys on CT prevalence and patterns of use. Educated individuals tend to use CT more than poorly educated individuals [3]. This goes against the idea that using CT is a non informed choice resulted from ignorance. This chapter will discuss controversies related to complementary therapies and the ways to increase their integration to the present biomedical model. The following topics will be addressed:

- Concepts
- Elements that may limitate the use of ct
- A special word on the placebo effect
- A special word on herbal treatment
- Roles of the involved personages
- Integrating conventional and complementary healthcare
- A framework for rational decision
- Conclusions

2. Concepts

In this field, the most used term is Complementary and Alternative Medicine (CAM). We instead prefer the term Complementary Therapies (CT), not only because it is simpler, but also because the adjectives "complementary" and "alternative" should not be used together in one expression. "Complementary" therapies are used together with conventional medicine, unlike "alternative" therapies, which are used in place of conventional medicine. In addition, the "medicine" from CAM is compromising, suggesting a parallel model. However, in practice, CT and CAM are used almost as synonyms, without harm for the overall comprehension.

These terms refer to a broad range of healing philosophies (schools of thought), approaches and therapies that mainstream Western (conventional) medicine does not commonly use, accept, study, understand, or make available [3]. CT are therapeutic products or practices which are not currently part of the conventional curative approach, but whose safety and efficacy have been scientifically studied. CT compose a group of diverse health care systems, practices, and products [4]. Many CT are also called holistic, because generally they consider the whole person, including physical, mental, emotional and spiritual aspects.

There are many definitions of CT, none of them perfect. The National Center for Complementary and Alternative Medicine (NCCAM, a department from National Institutes of Health, from USA) defines them simply as a group of diverse medical and health care interventions, practices, products, or disciplines that are not generally considered part of conventional medicine [5]. Broadly, CT are practices and ideas that are outside the domain of conventional medicine in several countries and defined by its users as preventing or treating illness, or promoting health and well-being. These practices complement mainstream medicine by satisfying a demand not met by conventional practices and diversifying the conceptual framework of medicine [6].

Defining CT is difficult, because the field is very broad and constantly changing. There is much debate over accurately defining CT and as more therapies and practices appear (or re-emerge) in popular culture, and as more gain scientific merit and become conventional treatments, definitions continue to evolve [7]. The list of what's considered CT changes continually and therapies whose safety and effectiveness are demonstrated will become part of conventional medicine. For instance, several orthodox pharmaceuticals including anti-inflammatories and diuretics have been found from traditional herbal medicines.

3. Elements that may limitate the use of CT

Efficacy: Three concepts related to testing healthcare interventions must be differentiated [8]:

- Efficacy is the extent to which an intervention does good in ideal circumstances. The question is: "Can it work?" The answer is given by explanatory trials
- Effectiveness refers to whether an intervention does good under usual healthcare practice. The question is: "Does it work in practice?" The answer is given by management trials
- Efficiency refers to the effect of an intervention in relation to the resources it consumes. The question is: "Is it worth it?" The answer is given by cost benefit trials

Studies in complementary therapies follow a different dynamic from that of studies with drugs. Figure 1 (adapted from Kienle [9]) illustrates this reality. Some characteristics of CT treatments and modalities make it difficult to apply the traditional RCTs or treatment effectiveness studies used in conventional medicine. Some study designs that might be used to address some of these characteristics including [3]: N-of-1 trials, preference RCTs, observational and cohort studies, case control studies, studies of bundles or combinations of therapies, attribute-treatment interaction analyses, and qualitative research. It is difficult or impossible to conduct double-blind trials with some modalities. The concept of blinding in which the patients and the treating clinicians participating in clinical trials do not know what treatment the patient is receiving is an important way to minimize expectation effects and biases on the part of both the patient and the clinician. For most CT modalities, however, blinding is very difficult or impossible.

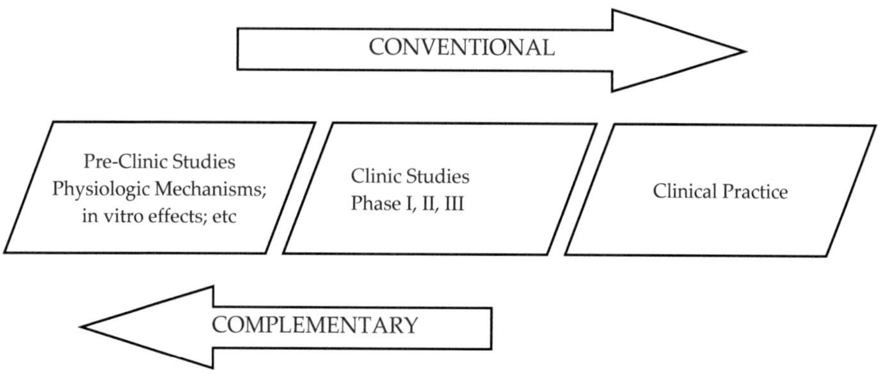

Figure 1. In the model proposed by Kienle [9], the investigation of complementary therapies follow the opposite flux of that one followed by the investigation of conventional pharmacotherapy.

Finally, when considering scientific evidence about the efficacy of any treatment, one must remember that "absence of evidence" (meaning that currently there are no adequate studies) is different from "absence of effect" (meaning that studies have failed to show adequate improvement). This classification is dynamic, as new studies being published periodically and bringing new information.

Safety: It is always important to remember that natural therapy is not synonymous of safe therapy. The general opinion that CT are harmless, healthy, pure, biological and without adverse events is a myth. There are varying degrees of potential patient harm that can result from either conventional medical practices or CT [3]:

- Economic harm, which results in monetary loss but presents no health hazard;
- Indirect harm, which results in a delay of appropriate treatment, or in unreasonable expectations that discourage patients and their families from accepting and dealing effectively with their medical conditions;
- Direct harm, which results in adverse patient outcome.

Legislation: CT are unregulated in most countries, and there is an urgent need to develop policies in order to minimize the risks and maximize the benefits of CT use [10]. CT must ideally be provided by a qualified practitioner, preferably registered and certified, with adequate training background, good skills and knowledge. The provider must be competent to provide CT services of quality. A surveillance system for malpractice must be established. In different countries, the same product can be labeled as a dietary supplement (available in stores) or medication (available at drugstores).

Cost-Benefit: CT have a potential for reducing costs in health because they are relatively non-expensive and avoid high technology, among other motives. Obviously, immediately after their introduction, there is a small increase in cost, which is added to the sum of treatments. The cost-benefit may appear later, by saving money with further healthcare. A number of systematic reviews of economic evaluations of CT have been published. These reviews almost universally conclude that the economic outcomes of some CT therapies are encouraging, but that more and better quality studies are needed. A recent study [11] showed that patients whose general practitioner has additional CT training have 0–30% lower healthcare costs and mortality rates, depending on age groups and type of CT. The lower costs result from fewer hospital stays and fewer prescription drugs.

Risk-Benefit Analysis: There is also little research on how the public understands the information in terms of risks and benefits and how such perceptions support decision making process. Considerable misinformation is dispersed by vendors and on the Internet. A significant percentage of CT use is unsupervised and engaged in as self-care [3]. A majority of patients who use CT do not disclose such use to their physicians.

Adams et al [12] tracing some guidelines for risk-benefit analysis, invites us to consider:

- Severity and acuteness of illness
- Curability with conventional treatment
- Degree of invasiveness, associated toxicities, and side effects of the CT

- Quality of evidence of safety and efficacy of the desired CT treatment
- Degree of understanding of the risks and benefits of CT treatment
- Knowledge and voluntary acceptance of those risks by the patient
- Persistence of the patient's intention to use CT treatment

So, the efficacy is just one of the factors that must be considerate. CT would be used even without solid evidence of efficacy if:

- The condition is highly prevalent (e.g., diabetes mellitus).
- The condition causes a heavy burden of suffering.
- The potential benefit is great.
- Some evidence that the intervention is effective already exists.
- Some evidence that there are safety concerns exists.

Physician must also consider a balance between efficacy and safety, classifying treatments as:

- effective and safe (having adequate scientific evidence of efficacy and/or safety or greater safety than other established treatment models for the same condition). CT belonging to this group surely must always be used.
- effective, but with some real or potential danger (having evidence of efficacy, but also of adverse side effects). CT belonging to this group may sometimes be used, under close supervision.
- unknown effectiveness, but safe (having insufficient evidence of clinical efficacy, but reasonable evidence to suggest relative safety). CT belonging to this group may sometimes be used, under close supervision.
- ineffective and dangerous (proven to be ineffective or unsafe through controlled trials or documented evidence or as measured by a risk/benefit assessment). CT belonging to this group may never be used.

4. A special word on placebo effect

The placebo effect is the therapeutic effect produced by something that objectively has no activity on thetreated condition [13]. It corresponds to a physical or psychological benefical change that occurs in response to factors that can be considered a placebo, such as an inactive substance made to resemble a drug (as a flour tablet), a false equipment or procedure (as acupuncture needle which does not penetrate effectively into the skin) or a therapeutic experience or a symbol (such as doctor-patient relationship in the "white-coat effect").

In any health treatment, the following factors are at stake: (a) specific elements (such as acupuncture needling); (b) undetectable and incidental elements (such as patient's beliefs, contextual factors and meaning, the listening and speech process); and (c) items not related to treatment (such as the natural course of disease or spontaneous regression). The placebo effect is in the second group, comprising the non-specific effects present in any doctor-patient relationship, including: attention, empathic concern, examinations, qualifications of health status and monitoring.

The dynamic set of all these treatment elements impacts over the patient's anxiety and the relationship he makes with the disease. As each therapy has these elements, even surgery is a field in which the placebo effect may be present in some degree [13]. So, to say that a CT "is no better than placebo" does not mean that this therapy is ineffective.

All facets of the placebo effect can not be explained by a single theory. Several explanations take into account the inter-relations between mental processes (expectations) and brain (neurophysiology). Currently, two theories have been more involved: the classical theories of conditioning and expectation [14]. Studies on the placebo effect have assisted in understanding the influence of mind over body. Placebo analgesia (caused by the injection of saline solution) elicits the production of endogenous opioids. It can be reversed by opioid antagonists such as naloxone. [13].

The randomized controlled trial was designed to test new drugs and it is based on physiological biomedical assumptions. In an essay on drugs, some elements such as speaking and listening are taken as incidental factors separate of the objective effect of pharmacological treatment. On CT, both incidental and biological phenomena are intertwined and can be equally important (Figure 2). A factor that is also at stake is the performative efficacy. This is based on the power of belief, mentalizing, the expectation of the symbols and their meanings. Complementary therapies, therapeutic rituals tend to have an especially powerful performative efficacy. This could amplify the extension of the non-biological effects.

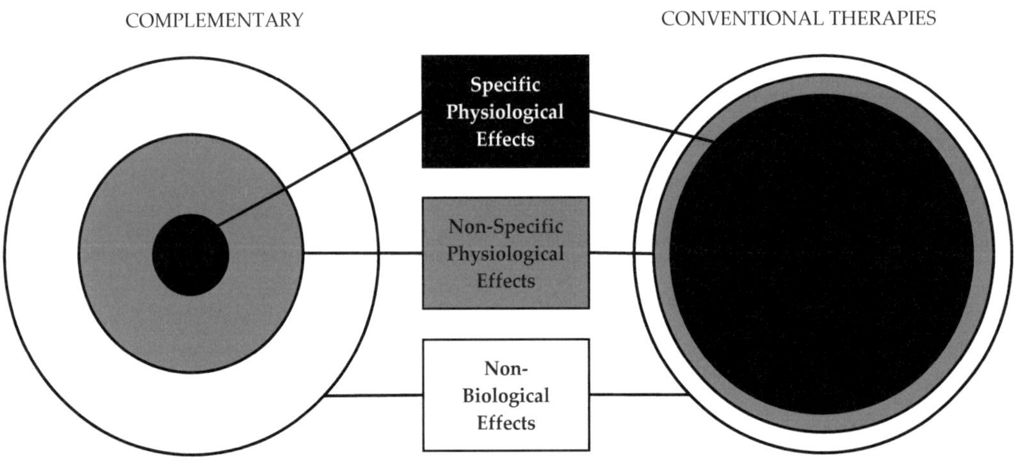

Figure 2. Representation of the importance of specific physiological effects, non-specific effects and non-biological effects on conventional and on complementary therapies.

The use of placebo-controlled trial to study unconventional interventions can lead to false-negative results. A recurrent paradox related to clinical trials with acupuncture is the fact that both the false and real acupuncture have good therapeutic effects [15]. This could lead to the belief that acupuncture acts exclusively via the placebo effect. However, this belief would be inappropriate. The classic design of a trial controlled by false acupuncture is based on the assumption that only the needling is effective treatment in acupuncture. Thus, patients in the control group receive almost everything except the real needling. As other elements of treatment (such the diagnostic process of Chinese medicine that involves listening and speaking) also have practical effect, this design is inappropriate because the two groups are getting these other elements. Consequently, the difference between the groups may underestimate the total therapeutic effect of acupuncture [15].

By studying the placebo effect in complementary therapies, Kaptchuk [16] divided the factors that may modulate this effect in groups: (a) patient characteristics (expectations, preference for participatory interventions); (b) the therapist characteristics (the image of "savior" that he can pass to the patient by an enthusiastic attitude); (c) therapist-patient interaction (when both share beliefs, generating empathy in clinical consultation); and (d) the nature of the disease (good results in situations with subjective symptoms, chronic conditions with variable course influenced by selective attention and affective disorders. Examples include chronic pain, fatigue, headache, arthritis, allergies, hypertension, insomnia, asthma, digestive disorders, depression and anxiety).

5. A special word on herbal treatment

CT are perceived by general population as more "natural" and less aggressive. Although the side effects of CT are generally smaller, they are not negligible. For example, many botanical products contain active ingredients potentially harmful [17]. Herbal medicines may have adverse events, which are attributable to irregular quality of the products, as well as unwanted interactions (with drugs or other supplements). As many supplements are not categorized as drugs, their manufacturers are not required to prove they are safe and effective (although supplements must have a safety record). The lack of reliable and consistent products is a challenge to the research and clinical practice.

- The main problems regarding use of herbal treatment is listed below [18]:
- Contamination with heavy metals: mercury, arsenic and lead are the most commonly detected
- Contamination with agriculture inputs: insecticides, fungicides and herbicides.
- Contamination with pathogenic microbes and poisonous mycotoxins
- Absence of laws to regulate and commercialize with proof of efficacy and safety.
- Variation in the amount of active ingredients (related to purity and standardization).
- Variation on the origin (local harvest, harvest, plant species, etc.).
- Unlike vitamins and minerals, herbal supplements are composed of many active compounds

Health professionals and providers of CT involving herbal medication should follow the national pharmacovigilance legislation [10]. At other side, manufacturers and importers/distributors of CT medication products could be a source of information on adverse events involving their products. Some countries have included this source of information as part of their regulatory framework. Manufacturers should report directly to the national pharmacovigilance centre or to the regulatory authority.

Herbal medications must bring wrote information equivalent to conventional remedies, such as precise therapeutic claims and corresponding level of evidence, quality control on production, precautions and adverse events, interactions and contraindications, posology and methods of administration, and considerations for children, pregnant or lactating women and the elderly [10].

6. Roles of the involved personages

There is a challenge to provide ethical, medically responsible counseling and provision of CT that respects and acknowledges the patient's values. For the proper use of a CT is necessary for the physician, the patient, the therapist and the health services to play their expected roles. Table 1 provides a description of these expected obligations.

Role of the Health Care Service	- Focus on the patient's interest, according to a humanized care giving. - Allow and encourage the use of CT in an open and evidence-based way. - Disseminate guidance on the nature of these treatments and their features. - Inform the patient about potential risks and benefits, on realistic expectations.
Role of the physician	- Actively ask the patient about past and current use of CT. - Educate and encourage patients to use CT when indicated. - Help the patient to interpret texts found on CT elsewhere. - Respect and support the wishes and values of the patient.
Role of the CT therapist	- Have written policy and procedures in place to avoid any misunderstandings. - Contact local council to check out health and safety requirements. - Ensure adequate data storage and protection when retaining client information. - Check about professional indemnity insurance with your professional body.
Role of the patient	- Do not stop conventional treatments on your own. - Inform your assistent physician which CT is being used. - Request information from reliable sources. - Find the indication of a therapist of confidence. - Supplements should be from a reliable source. - Be aware that different patients respond in different ways .

Table 1. Description of the expected roles for the proper use of CT in health services.

Patients as informed clients: Clients may identify reliable information by their purpose, relevance/accuracy, sources, updated information, and objectivity [10]. For example, is the information intended to educate the consumer or sell a product? Also, good information meets the needs of the consumer and is relevant to his/her lifestyle and situation. It should not give unrealistic recommendations and should be written in a language that is easy to understand and does not contain obvious errors such as misspellings and grammatical mistakes. Credible information states clearly who is responsible for the information, who is financially supporting the information and where the information comes from (i.e. the original source). It should be clear whether the information is opinion-based or factual. A good source of information provides unbiased and balanced information. Such information should be honest about areas of uncertainty and enable consumers to make therapy choices that are in his/her best interest. In case of commercial information, relationships to product manufacturers, for example, should be clearly stated.

Motivations to use CT: The motivations for using CT are numerous, but a major contributor appears to be the pursuit of wellness. Many patients appear to use CT for this goal and not just the treatment of disease. Besides well-being, patient may be seeking cure for a disease, symptom control. It is important that patient expectations be realistic about the results under the current knowledge. Certainly it will be always a wrong motivation to search a CT only based on "fashion". There is a natural selection that leads people to use CT. People with a low taste for medical interventions might be more likely to choose CT. Also patient may seek better practices (less overtreatment, more focus on preventive and curative health promotion).

7. Integrating conventional and complementary healthcare

An unconventional therapy may be used alone, as an alternative to conventional therapies, or in addition to conventional therapies. This third trend is referred to as an integrative approach. Health care that integrates CT therapies with conventional medicine has been termed "integrative medicine" by many. Whatever term is used, the goal should be the provision of comprehensive care that is safe and effective, care that is collaborative and interdisciplinary, and care that respects and joins effective interventions from all sources. This comprehensive approach should be based on customization based on patient needs and values, being the patient as the source of control.

The boundaries between CT and conventional medicine are constantly evolving, since interventions such as hospice care or relaxation and breathing techniques in childbirth that were once considered unconventional are now widely accepted. CT interventions are being incorporated into integrative medicine practices located in conventional medical care settings.

As the quantity and quality of research in CT is growing, there is a more open attitude to CT among conventional health professionals. Guidelines and consensus statements issued by conventional medical organizations have recommended some CT, which are increasingly practiced in conventional medical settings, particularly acupuncture for pain, and massage, music therapy, and relaxation techniques for mild anxiety and depression. Some forms of CT are being incorporated into services provided by hospitals; covered by health maintenance organizations; delivered in conventional medical practitioners' offices; and taught in medical, nursing, and other health professions schools. Insurance coverage of CT therapies is increasing and integrative medicine centers and clinics are being established.

Comprehensive health care must go beyond the conventional clinical and surgical treatment. Ideally, it should also involve changes in the patient's lifestyle (nutrition, exercise, stress management, etc..), associated with multidisciplinary treatments (physiotherapy, psychotherapy, etc..) and complementary therapies (CT) (Figure 3). This ideal model should include both conventional medical and CT approaches to health promotion, disease prevention, and the treatment of illness that have been shown to be safe and effective.

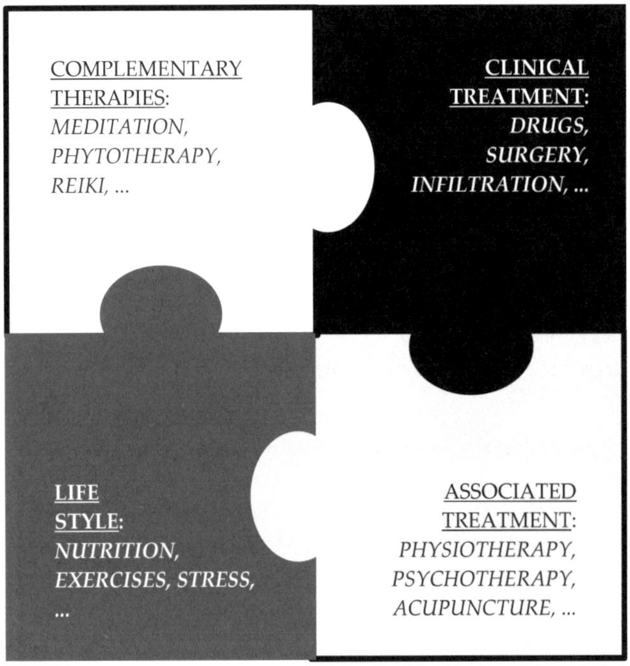

Figure 3. Illustration of an ideal model of integrative health approach

An example of successful use of CT in a general hospital was published by Dusek [19]. The adoption of CT had a significant impact in promoting analgesia with a reduction in pain score by an average of 50%. The techniques used were relaxation, acupuncture, acupressure, massage, therapeutic touch, music therapy, aromatherapy and reflexology.

Education in CT is an important field for all health professionals. Although many non-conventional therapeutic modalities have already passed through scientific analysis, there is still much ignorance and prejudice from health professionals. For those in conventional practice, it is important to learn about CT to appropriately interact with and advise patients in a manner that contributes to high-quality, comprehensive care. Health profession schools (e.g., schools of medicine, nursing, pharmacy, and allied health) incorporate sufficient information about CT into the standard curriculum at the undergraduate, graduate, and postgraduate levels to enable licensed professionals to competently advise their patients about CT.

Education is also important because patient prone to use CT may search it independently of approval of the physician. Patient must feel safe and comfortable to bring this discussion to the clinical visit. Otherwise, there is the risk of seeking a non-orthodox treatment without the knowledge of the assistant physician. The lack of guidance by the physician may lead to harming results. Physician and patient, in joint decision, may choose CT that are safe and have some potential benefit.

8. Future steps

The NCCAM (already cited) proposed these 3 goals for the period 2011–2015: advance the science and practice of symptom management; develop effective, practical, personalized strategies for promoting health and well-being; and enable better evidence-based decision making regarding CT use and its integration into health care and health promotion. To achieve it, the institution stated these strategic objectives [5]:

- Advance research on mind and body interventions, practices, and disciplines.
- Advance research on CT natural products.
- Increase understanding of "real world" patterns and outcomes of CT use and its integration into health care and health promotion.
- Improve the capacity of the field to carry out rigorous research.
- Develop and disseminate objective, evidence-based information on CT interventions.

It will be important to understand how CT and conventional treatments interact with each other and to study models of how CT and conventional medical treatments can be provided in integrated and coordinated ways. Unfortunately, little information is available about the outcomes and the effectiveness of various models of integration.

Many critics of CT argue that some of them are explained by theories that do not follow the current biomedical model. The fact is these CT were born in the past and reflect the worldview of that time. But a model is just a way to explain a phenomenon and make it teachable. This model might make sense in that epoch, and we must understand the theory of CT under the light of this sense. If it does not fit the current model, there should not be immediately discarded. In the past, conclusions were drawn from the intensive observation of nature, and they have insights we could not draw today.

Thus, old theories have considerable value, although they may have gross errors (for example, on anatomy and physiology). One way to reconcile this dilemma could be the realization that current conventional model best explains mechanical (materials) problems, while CT best explain functional disorders (which are actually related to most of the medical appointments). An allegory for this would imagine that if human beings were a computer, the current biomedical model would better take care of the hardware, whereas CT better fix the software.

9. A framework for rational decision

The increasing use of CT by patients, health care providers, and institutions makes it imperative that physicians consider their ethical obligations when recommending, tolerating, or proscribing these therapies. Table 2 proposes a framework for rational decisions about CT based on different scenarios. Note that no isolated factor (such as efficacy) is the only one to be scaled. The decision about a CT will be based ultimately on the judgment of the components of this matrix. For example: when a technique has not proven efficacy, but it can improve the quality of life of patient, it should not be discarded immediately. It could not be used for therapeutic purposes, but to enhance well-being. For such, it is necessary the technique be not harmful and be aligned to the values of the patient. This is the case of techniques such Reiki and Bach Flower Remedies.

	Use broadly this CT without major concerns	**Use this CT in some cases with close supervision**	**Avoid use this CT and counter-indicate it**
Efficacy (mechanisms of action)	Totally known	Partially known	Totally unknown
Effectiveness (effect in practice)	Well documented for the condition treated	Some evidences for the condition treated	Unknown results for the condition treated
Efficiency (cost-benefit ratio)	Certainly worthy	Potentially worthy	Not worthy at all
Safety	No possible direct harm	Potential harm	Documented major harm
Risk-benefit ratio	Patient has incurable burdened disease	Patient has chronic burdened disease	Patient has mild self-limited disease
Legislation	Board or council regulations	Acknowledged by some agencies	Marginal situation before health agencies
Patient characteristics	Adequately informed, motivated and/or expectant	Moderately informed, motivated and/or expectant	Badly informed, motivated and/or expectant
Physician characteristics	Partnership on a real patient-centered care	Respect to the will of patient, but suspicious about CT	Very uncomfortable with these patients values
Healthcare service (HS) characteristics	CT offered inside HS	CT referred from HS	CT not linked at all with a HS
Practitioner characteristics	Well trained, board certified, good experience	Some training , informal certification, some experience	Self trained, no certification, unknown experience
Objective (Purpose)	Realistic (e.g. searching for wellbeing)	Unrealistic (e.g. stop all conventional remedies)	Impossible (e.g. to cure advanced cancer)
Combination with conventional treatment	Full compatibility, no conflict if used simultaneously	Some paradigm conflict between conventional and complementary	Use of CT demands abandonment of conventional treatment

Table 2. A framework for rational decisions when recommending, tolerating or proscribing a CT

10. Conclusions

There is a growing interest of patients by complementary therapies (CT), the therapeutic products or practices which are not currently part of the conventional curative approach, but whose safety and efficacy have been scientifically studied. Defining CT is difficult, because the field is very broad and constantly changing. Health care that integrates CT therapies with conventional medicine has been termed "integrative medicine". There is a challenge to provide ethical, medically responsible counseling and provision of CT that respects and acknowledges the patient's values. For the proper use of a CT is necessary for the physician, the patient, the therapist and the health services to play their expected roles.

This chapter proposes a framework for rational decisions when recommending, tolerating or proscribing a CT, based on different scenarios. A matrix of factors that must be considered includes efficacy (mechanisms of action); effectiveness (effect in practice); efficiency (cost-benefit ratio); safety; risk-benefit ratio; legislation; patient characteristics; physician characteristics; healthcare service characteristics; practitioner characteristics; objective (purpose); and potential of combination with conventional treatment. Based on these elements, the decision may be: (a) Use broadly this CT without major concerns; (b) Use this CT in some cases with close supervision; or (c) Avoid use this CT and counter-indicate it.

Author details

Roberta de Medeiros
Centro Universitario S. Camilo, S. Paulo, SP, Brazil

Marcelo Saad*
Physiatrist and Acupuncturist at Hospital Israelita Albert Einstein, S. Paulo, SP, Brazil

11. References

[1] WHO. Constitution of the World Health Organization as adopted by the International Health Conference, New York, 19-22 June, 1946; signed on 22 July 1946 by the representatives of 61 States (Offi cial Records of the World Health Organization, no. 2, p. 100) and entered into force on 7 April 1948. Preamble.
[2] Santa Ana CF. The adoption of complementary and alternative medicine by hospitals: A framework for decision making. J Healthc Manag. 2001;46(4):250-60.
[3] IOM (Institute of Medicine of the National Academies). Complementary and Alternative Medicine in the United States. ISBN 0-309-09270-1, USA, 2005
[4] Filshie J, Rubens CNJ. Complementary and Alternative Medicine. Anesthesiol Clin N Am. 2006;24(1): 81-111.
[5] NCCAM (National Center for Complementary and Alternative Medicine). Exploring the Science of Complementary and Alternative Medicine - Third Strategic Plan 2011–2015. NIH Publication No. 11-7643. USA, February 2011

* Corresponding Author

[6] Manheimer E, Berman B. Cochrane Complementary Medicine Field. 2008; 2011(12)
[7] Whitford HS, Olver IN. PRAYER AS A COMPLEMENTARY THERAPY. Cancer Forum Volume 35 Number 1 March 2011
[8] Haynes B. Can it work? Does it work? Is it worth it? BMJ 1999;319:652–3
[9] Kienle GS, Albonico HU, Fischer L, Frei-Erb M, Hamre HJ, Heusser P, Matthiessen PF, Renfer A, Kiene H. Complementary therapy systems and their integrative evaluation. Explore (NY). 2011 May-Jun;7(3):175-87.
[10] WHO. World Health Organization guidelines on developing consumer information on proper use of traditional, complementary and alternative medicine. ISBN 92 4 159170 6. Printed in Italy. 2004
[11] Kooreman P, Baars EW. Patients whose GP knows complementary medicine tend to have lower costs and live longer. The European Journal of Health Economics. Published online: 22 June 2011. DOI 10.1007/s10198-011-0330-2
[12] Adams KE, Cohen MH, Eisenberg D, Jonsen AR. Ethical considerations of complementary and alternative medical therapies in conventional medical settings. Ann Intern Med 2002;137:660-4.
[13] Moerman DE, Jonas WB. Deconstructing the placebo effect and finding the meaning response. Ann Intern Med. 2002;136(6):471-6.
[14] Stewart-Williams S, Podd J. The placebo effect: dissolving the expectancy versus conditioning debate. Psychol Bull. 2004;130(2):324-40.
[15] Paterson C, Dieppe P. Characteristic and incidental (placebo) effects in complex interventions such as acupuncture. BMJ. 2005;330(7501):1202-5.
[16] Kaptchuk TJ. The placebo effect in alternative medicine: can the performance of a healing ritual have clinical significance? Ann Intern Med. 2002;136(11):817-25.
[17] Niggemann B, Grüber C. Side-effects of complementary and alternative medicine. Allergy. 2003;58(8):707-16.
[18] Zhang J, Wider B, Shang H, Li X, Ernst E. Quality of herbal medicines: challenges and solutions. Complement Ther Med. 2012 Feb-Apr;20(1-2):100-6. Epub 2011 Nov 1.
[19] Dusek JA, Finch M, Plotnikoff G, Knutson L. The impact of integrative medicine on pain management in a tertiary care hospital. J Pat Safety. 2010;6(1):48-51.

Chapter 2

Integrating Complementary and Conventional Care Using Quality Use of Medicines as a Framework

Trisha Dunning

Additional information is available at the end of the chapter

http://dx.doi.org/10.5772/50445

1. Introduction

"Tis impossible to separate the chance of good from the risk of ill."

(Hume 1998).

Complementary and Alternative Therapy (CAM) use is increasing: prevalence of use in the general population ranges between 50 and 80% globally (World Health Organisation (WHO) 2002). High CAM users include people with chronic diseases, women educated to high school level or higher, people with poor health, those who are employed and people interested in self-care (Lloyd *et al.* 1993; Eisenberg 1998; Egede *et al.* 2002; MacLennan *et al.* 2002).

Many people regard CAM as a solution to modern health and social problems such as chronic lifestyle diseases, obesity and depression. Significantly, people consider their health care options and make choices that are congruent with their life philosophy, knowledge, experience, societal norms, and culture. Depending on these factors, they may or may not choose to be actively involved in their care and/or incorporate CAM in their health care regimen.

Understanding these factors can help health professionals understand people's health care choices, self-care behaviours, adherence to management recommendations and their capacity to be empowered. For example, there is a strong association among health beliefs, spirituality and CAM use (Hildreth & Elman 2007). In addition, there is good evidence that CAM users adopt health-promoting self-care behaviours, undertake preventative health care and believe they are ultimately responsible for their health (Kelner & Welman 1997; Garrow *et al.* 2006; Parsian & Dunning 2009).

People using CAM are largely satisfied with their CAM choices and outcomes even if it 'did not work' (House of Lords Select Committee on Science and Technology 2000). Significantly, satisfaction with treatment improves well being. However, 'satisfaction' is an elusive concept and there are many ways to define and measure 'satisfaction:' not all are objective, and some are more useful in research than for determining individual satisfaction, including with CAM.

Rittenbaug et al. (2011) developed an 18-item patient-centred CAM outcome measure to determine the multidimensional impact of CAM. The items encompass physical, emotional, cognitive, social and spiritual domains, which is consistent with holistic CAM philosophy. The psychometric properties of the tool were not reported but it is currently undergoing further testing. If it is valid and reliable, the tool could be useful in clinical care and research. It could enable meaningful comparisons to be made and might go some way towards developing a common language.

2. Integrative medicine

Some experts regard integrative medicine (IM) as a new evolving care paradigm; however, it could reflect a rebalancing process towards the system that operated before the rise of 'scientific medicine' in the early twentieth century. Research suggests most CAM users combine conventional and CAM therapies: often several CAM). Likewise, health professionals, especially general practitioners (GP) and nurses, combine both types of therapies to provide holistic care (Braun & Cohen 2010). The combination of CAM and conventional therapies is increasingly known as Integrative Medicine.

IM focuses on wellness, and the spiritual, environmental, social and lifestyle factors that enhance or compromise wellness. IM aims to provide individualised 'effective and compassionate care on many levels' (Cohen 2005). Researchers and clinicians use a variety of definitions of IM, which makes it difficult to compare and apply research findings. The definition of IM developed by the Royal Australian College of General Practitioners (RACGP) and the Australasian Integrative Medicine Association (AIMA) (2009) was adopted for this chapter because it encompasses evidence-based care, practitioner responsibility, holistic person-centred care and, is self-explanatory and practical. IM is:

> *The blending of conventional and complementary medicines and therapies with the aim of using the most appropriate of either or both modalities to care for the person as a whole.*

Although not specifically listed in the RACGP/AIMA definition, health promotion and encouraging self-care are central to IM, as they are to CAM philosophy, and increasingly to conventional care. Significantly, IM is essentially a transformative process that has four main dimensions (Bell et al. 2002; Mulkins & Verhoef 2004):

1. Access to and availability of a range of therapies to support the individual's lifelong health journey.
2. Care that considers the individual's overall health and well being.
3. Involving the individual in decisions about their health goals and care plan.

4. A healing or therapeutic relationship between health professionals and individuals, which is essential to achieving optimal outcomes.

Bell et al. and Mulkins & Verhoef might have intended to include timely communication among health professionals and between health professionals and individuals in the fourth dimension; however, 'effective communication' could be regarded as an essential fifth dimension.

These IM definitions and dimensions reinforce the fact that IM does not aim to reject or replace either CAM or conventional therapies: it advocates combining both types of therapies when the combination is relevant to the individual's needs and is safe and evidence-based (Kotsirilos et al. 2010). Khorsan et al. (2011) undertook a systematic review of IM and identified an extensive and increasing body of literature on the subject that can be used to support practice. However, because IM is an emerging field in many countries, there may be less evidence for IM than for individual CAM.

Marshall et al. (2004) used the acronym BEECH to describe IM care:

- B: Balance between CAM modalities and/or CAM and conventional modalities.
- E: Empowerment and self-healing.
- E: Evidence-based care based following the concept 'first do no harm.'
- C: Collaboration between the health professional and the individual and among professionals, and respect for the individual's choices.
- H: Holistic multidimensional care including promoting optimal healing environments, consistent with holistic care.

Some elements of BEECH are similar to Bell et al. and Mulkins & Verhoef's IM dimensions.

3. Does integrative care exist?

The WHO (2002) described three main levels of CAM integration:

1. Integrative level where CAM is officially recognised at Government level and incorporated into health systems for example, in national medicine policies, product regulatory procedures, hospital and community guidelines and is reimbursed under health insurance systems.
2. Inclusive level where CAM is recognised and largely accepted but not fully integrated into health systems.
3. Tolerance level where CAM is not officially part of the national health system.

Level one integration is rare. For example, CAM is not formally integrated in most hospitals in Australia, although IM is becoming more acceptable/common in general practice, aged care facilities and some specialist services such as cardiology and cancer. CAM medicines are regulated under the same regulatory processes as conventional medicines in Australia but they are not funded by the government Pharmaceutical Benefits Scheme, as many conventional medicines are. However, some health benefit schemes reimburse members for some CAM therapies.

As indicated, there is a professional association for IM practitioners in Australia, AIMA, and at least two evidence-based Australian IM textbooks were published in 2011 (Phelps & Hassed 2011; Kotsirilos et al. 2011). These initiatives demonstrate a response to public demand for CAM and increasing health professional acceptance, or at least tolerance, of IM. Thus, CAM in Australia, like Canada, the USA and the UK, probably fits into the WHO integration levels two or three.

However, CAM use and IM is more structured and integrated in countries such as China, Taiwan, India, and Germany. Some developing countries include CAM within the dominant health system, but it is not necessarily systematically integrated. Many people in developing countries rely on CAM as first line treatment because conventional care is costly, inaccessible, unavailable, or all three.

In reality, many individuals self-diagnose and select management options to suit their needs and many combine CAM and conventional care. They often do not consult or inform CAM and/or conventional health professionals about their care decisions. While these behaviours are consistent with personal empowerment and choice, they can delay diagnosis or mask important symptoms and have adverse outcomes.

4. Safety, quality and IM

Safety and quality are key health care issues and need to be considered in all countries and at all levels: regulatory bodies, service providers, health professionals and individuals. The evidence-base for IM and the way it is delivered and evaluated (outcome measures) are important issues to help professionals decide what CAM/IM could meet the public demand, respect individual's choices and people's right to appropriate information to help them make informed health care decisions, but still meet quality and safety standards.

A consistent approach to delivering health care and standards of care that encompass product and professional regulation, professional self-regulation, public and professional education, and all types of rigorous research, quantitative, qualitative, evaluation, audit and translational, to generate and translate knowledge is needed (Commonwealth of Australia 2003). Table 1 provides an overview of some of the inter-related factors that affect safety.

There appear to be four key areas that need to be addressed to ensure CAM is systematically and safely integrated:

1. National policies and regulatory processes including professional regulation.
2. Processes for defining and monitoring safety and efficacy including pharmacovigilence.
3. Equitable access to CAM and conventional modalities and IM.
4. Rational use of CAM and conventional modalities (Bodeker et al. 2005).

Stakeholder collaboration/engagement is inherent in all four areas and is essential to systematically implement IM. Stakeholder consultation/engagement could include determining the priorities for action and/or for research concerning CAM and IM in relevant countries, willingness to share and learn from each other, and willingness to undertake rigorous research to determine the benefits, risks and cost implications of IM for individuals and health systems. However, it is often difficult to assess benefit and risks from a great deal of existing research due to a multiplicity of factors such as methodological flaws, different definitions of terms and other confounding factors. Thus, it is difficult to generalise findings and/or translate them into clinical guidelines.

Inter-related factor	Factors that enhance safety
Therapies	Regulatory processes: government, professional and self. Evidence base for safety, quality and efficacy. Quality control safety monitoring processes including international monitoring bodies such as the Uppsala Centre. Manufacturing processes including product labeling. The label must be readable. Appropriate storage and transport and disposal procedures. Adherence to conventions such as The Convention on International Trade of Endangered Wild Flora and Fauna.
Health professional	Education and competence to provide and/or offer advice about CAM and IM. Duty of care to practice within their level of knowledge and competence and regulatory framework. Access to relevant, accurate information Managing conflict of interest such as the professional prescribing/recommending and selling products at the point of care. Ability to reflect on attitudes to CAM, conventional and or IM. Ability to communicate effectively and develop therapeutic relationships with the people they care for and collegiate relationships with other professionals. Access to qualified health professional from a range of CAM and conventional disciplines. Ability to critically review research publications and determine how rigor was demonstrated in order to make informed judgments about the applicably to practice.

Inter-related factor	Factors that enhance safety
Environment in which care is provided	Infection control procedures. Accessible relevant policies and guidelines. Able to ensure privacy and confidentiality of consultations. Overall staff attitudes to CAM, conventional care and IM. Well signposted. Disabled access. Meets safety standards and is visually appealing and welcoming
Individual receiving care and/or advice	Health status. Reasons/goals for using CAM or IM. Access to relevant, accurate information. Self-care capability and practices. Conventional management. Relationship with health professional. Support base. Disclosure of CAM/IM use. Health and literacy level. Access to relevant, objective information
The quality of the information provided	Relevant to the individual and their literacy level and culture. Objective Accurate. Available in a timely and accessible manner.

Table 1. Overview of some of the inter-related factors that affect safety of complementary, conventional and integrative health care.

Thus, more rigorous research to evaluate IM as well as individual CAM therapies is needed to determine safe, cost-effective models of IM and appropriate outcome measures in keeping with holistic care. In addition, individual countries may need to:

- Determine processes for funding and delivering IM services.
- Determine who could/should be responsible for coordinating IM care.
- Explore and describe health professional's roles and scopes of practice and the knowledge and competence they require to provide safe evidence based IM. Health professional's role and scope of practice influences the educational preparation required for safe practice.
- Ensure health professionals who provide CAM and/or combine CAM and conventional care are appropriately qualified. Although CAM is increasingly being included in conventional health professional education curricula, the information may not be at the level required to competently deliver CAM or IM care.

- Educate CAM users (the population) about IM so they can negotiate informed care decisions with health professionals.
- Establish and maintain effective shared documentation, communication and referral processes, including web-based and other electronic media. The social media plays an increasing role in education, communication and interdisciplinary collaboration.
- Systematically monitor outcomes including costs, benefits and adverse events.

5. Safety and risk

Many conventional practitioners believe CAM is 'not effective' and is 'risky business.' In addition, 90% of CAM users assume CAM is safe (Sharples 2003). All health care carries some risk. Currently more adverse events (AE) are reported for conventional care than CAM. Several factors could account for the difference, including different patterns of AE reporting. The same AE reporting system applies to both CAM and conventional therapies in Australia, but patients are more likely to report CAM AEs than health professionals.

Safety and risk are complex concepts and cannot be considered in isolation. Risk is inherent in everyday life: individuals determine whether they are willing to take/accept risk according to their situation and their perception of the degree of risk to *them* (Komesaroff 2003). People's perceptions of risk are subjective and are moderated or exacerbated by past experiences, current health status, mood, information including media reports, advertising, industry, health professionals, and their health beliefs and attitudes. People accept some risk as routine, but often underestimate their personal risk (optimistic bias) (Weinstein 1982; Sharot 2011).

Health professionals' perception of risk is usually more 'mathematical' than the general public because of their training. HP's perception of risk influences the information they provide to individuals, the language they use and the emphasis they place on the risks associated with health options. However, a health professional's perception of their *personal* risk is likely to be influenced by opportunistic bias. Significantly, individuals are unable to effectively estimate personal risk until they are in their late twenties.

6. What is risk?

Definitions and perceptions of risk change as society changes through research, technological advances and wealth, but are almost always concerned with harm to individuals (patients). The concept of health-related risk has been part of health care since it emerged in ancient cultures. For example, the Hippocratic Oath states doctors should 'first do no harm.' First do no harm is still encompassed in naturopathic philosophy. The 17th century *Code of Hammurabi* described punishments for 'harmful physician errors.' The punishment depended on to the social status of the patient.

Pliny the Elder (first century AD) suggested physicians should not learn their skills at the expense of the patient. He also introduced the concept of patient responsibility by suggesting patients were to blame if they sustained harm as a consequence of neglecting their treatment—

in modern terminology non-compliance or non-adherence. In the Middle Ages Paracelsus noted the dual nature of medicines—ability to cure and ability to kill. Paracelsus' observation could have influenced the decision to include product safety in the safety-risk matrix.

Modern concepts of risk are based on probability theory that calculates 'technical risk' objectively (Clarke 2004). Probability theory considers risk in terms of the probability of a loss and the degree and severity of the loss. Most modern definitions of risk encompass an estimation of the likelihood that an AE will occur and have negative consequences (loss) that are significant to the individual. These concepts are an important when considering informed consent and medico-legal issues.

Risk is reported as in several ways: absolute Risk (AR), relative Risk (RR), number needed to treat (NNT) or risk/benefit ratio. AR refers to the difference between the outcomes in a control group compared with an intervention group in a specified time period. RR refers to the absolute risk as a proportion of baseline. Benefits are often expressed as RR and harms as the AR. The NNT refers to the number of people who need to be treated for a specified period of time to obtain benefit.

The NNT to cause harm is the inverse of the absolute rate of adverse events occurring in a defined period of time. In order to estimate risk, the endpoints must be clearly stated. Surrogate endpoints might indicate potential benefit or potential harm.

7. Adverse events associated with CAM

The safety and risk profile differs according to the individual CAM therapy/ies, the IM combination used and the individual who uses them. Some therapies such as medicines are more likely to cause harm than others. Likewise, there is more evidence for some CAM than for others. However, it is important for health professionals to realise that lack of evidence does not mean there is no evidence, and understand that all of these issues apply equally to conventional therapies.

Estimates of safety and risk for many CAM medicines are based on a long history of safe traditional use. The term 'long traditional use' is open to interpretation: the European Directive on traditional herbal products regards use for at least 15 years within Europe and more than 30 years outside Europe as evidence of long traditional use. Most conventional medicine manufactures are not expected to fulfill such stringent duration of safe use criteria and AEs often emerge after conventional medicines are registered and used in clinical care.

In addition, modern technology and modern growing, harvesting and extraction techniques might mean modern CAM medicines have a different chemical makeup from medicines produced using traditional production processes and might be more safe or less safe, but such medicines are marketed under the 'long traditional use' mantra. These issues are rarely discussed but are worth considering and investigating systematically.

Many potential CAM/conventional interactions are theoretical (Braun 2006) and are hard to predict (Ulbricht 2012) but need to be considered as part of the overall care plan and monitoring process. People who use CAM often have several concomitant health conditions such as atopic conditions, diabetes and kidney and liver disease that increase the risk of AEs. Table 2 outlines key issues associated with pharmacovigiliance and table 3 depicts people most at risk of AEs.

Systems level	Pharmocovigilince-related processes
Health system	Degree of product regulation including manufacture and pre and post marketing surveillance processes. Affordability and accessibility of medicines and products. Equitable support for CAM, conventional and IM-related research. Availability of evidence based guidelines to support practice. Systems to schedule/register and monitor medicine use including adverse events. Process to learn from adverse events. Marketing processes: in some countries conventional medicines cannot be marketed directly to the public. Methods of communicating important medicine-related information to the public and health professionals.
Health professionals	Education and competence to perform role. Engagement in ongoing professional development. Licensing, regulatory and self-regulatory processes to protect the public. Professional liability insurance. Communication, documentation, and referral processes. Attitudes towards and beliefs about medicines CAM, conventional care and IM
Herbal medicines	All of the issues covered under health system section and: Manufacturing practices including whether the medicine was prepared according to the traditional method. Processes for identifying, handling, and storing herbs including using botanical names. Infection control procedures. Processes to detect and prevent adulteration and contamination of CAM medicines. Informative, honest labels. Prescribed in appropriate dose, dose intervals and for an appropriate time considering indications for use, precautions and contraindications and considering prescribing for people at high risk of adverse events. Produced considering sustainable agriculture methods and follow relevant conventions such as The Convention on International Trade of Endangered Wild Flora and Fauna.

Individual	Age. Physical and mental health status. Knowledge and health capabilities. Not disclosing herbal medicine use. Knows the consequences of polypharmacy. Self-diagnosis and self-treatment, which can delay treating serious problems. Method of storing and handling medicines and disposing of unused medicines appropriately. Inappropriate use of medicines and CAM e.g. sharing medicines with family members and friends. Know how to monitor defined outcomes Realistic expectations about curing or controlling diseases. Realises the cost implications of medicine use.

Table 2. Inter-related safety and quality issues related to pharmacovigilance.

Take conventional medicines with a narrow therapeutic index such as digoxin and warfarin.
Take high risk conventional medicines such as insulin.
Have renal disease or liver damage, which compromises medicine metabolism and excretion.
Has allergies such as dermatitis and asthma.
The elderly, children, and pregnant and lactating women.
Concomitantly using five or more medicines (polypharmacy).
Uses excess alcohol or illicit drugs.
Lacks sufficient knowledge/information to make appropriate decisions about CAM use or receives inadequate or inappropriate advice about CAM.
Do not advise all the health professionals they consult about their CAM and conventional medicine use.
Acquire CAM products from the Internet or overseas that are not subject to rigorous quality control and regulatory processes. Such products may be contaminated, inadequately labeled and/or the herbs may not be correctly identified.

Table 3. Individuals most at risk of herbal-conventional-food-interactions and other adverse events.

8. Standards and regulatory processes that aim to improve safety and reducing risk

Standards and regulatory processes are important to risk management strategies. They exist to protect the public (O'Keefe & Henderson 2012). In Australia, CAM, which includes herbal medicines, homeopathy, essential oils and vitamin and mineral supplements; and conventional medicines are regulated by the Therapeutic Goods Administration (TGA); The

Office of Complementary Medicines oversees the recall of faulty or dangerous CAM medicines.

All CAM medicines are assessed for safety and the quality of the ingredients but only CAM medicines deemed to be high risk are assessed for efficacy. The TGA critically analyses clinical trial data the manufacturer supplies to support their claims of safety and efficacy. If the TGA accepts the manufacturer's evidence, high risk medicines are registered and bear the words AUST R on the label.

Manufacturers of lower risk medicines must be able to substantiate their claims that the medicine is safe risk but are not required to submit evidence of safety when they apply to have the medicine listed. Manufacturers of low risk medicines are not permitted to use terms such as cure, treat, manage, and prevent on medicine labels or marketing strategies. Listed medicines are designated AUST L on the label. Ingredients included in listed and registered medicines must be included on the list of substances approved for use in Australia. Thus, medicine labels give some indication about the level of evidence available to support safety and efficacy. Other medicine-related quality control processes include labeling, manufacturing and advertising regulations and Acts and pre and post market surveillance.

Other countries have similar regulatory process although they might classify medicines differently. Many European countries require evidence to support manufacturer's claims in order for them to be registered. Other related processes include the The WHO International Terminologies on Traditional Medicine in the Western Pacific Region (WHO 2007) and the European Parliament and Council directive on the use of traditional products, which stipulated that herbal medicines must be produced according to good manufacturing practices from April 2011 (Efferth & Greten 2011).

The European Directive contains a number of other recommendations to provide guidance for retailers, wholesalers, manufacturers and importers about requirements for medication standards about their legal responsibilities. The WHO has produced many other informative guidelines and polices to communicate and support safe evidence-based herbal medicine use which can be sourced from the WHO website,

Contamination and adulteration of CAM medicines compromises safety in many countries. The Convention on International Trade of Endangered Wild Flora and Fauna (CITES), also known as the Washington Convention, was set up to protect vulnerable species form extinction. Over 150 countries are signatories to CITES.

Health professional knowledge and competence also influence safety and quality. CAM practitioners are self-regulated and/or regulated through professional association codes, standards, policies and continuing professional development processes in most countries but few are statutorily regulated. In Victoria, Australia Chinese Medicine practitioners, Chinese herbal practitioners and Acupuncturists are required be registered with the Chinese Medicine Registration Board: it is likely other states follow Victoria's lead.

A number of education providers in many countries, including universities and on-line education providers, offer a wide variety of CAM courses at all levels; certificates, diplomas and post graduate degrees. In some countries course providers must meet training standards but many people attend short courses that do not adequately prepare them to deliver safe informed CAM care.

9. Quality use of medicines

Quality use of medicines (QUM) is a useful framework for determining individual treatment options and assessing and monitoring risk at all levels of medicine use (Dunning 2004).

Australia's National Medicines Policy (NMP) incorporates QUM, which encompasses conventional, CAM and non-prescription medicines. Australia's QUM processes have been adapted and are used in many other countries such as Canada. QUM essentially puts the individual at the centre of care and refers to:

- Selecting management options wisely. Significantly, QUM and IM are not concerned with either/or choices: they espouse holistic care by recommending the best options for/with the individual, which may or may not include medicines
- Choosing suitable medicines if medicines are indicated. Not everybody requires medicines to maintain health, which is consistent with CAM philosophies. Wise medicine choice encompasses, prevention, lifestyle strategies, and risk management.
- Using medicines safely and effectively' (Commonwealth Department of Health and Aging 2002).

The extent to which QUM is applied to CAM is largely unknown. Dunning (2004) developed a QUM framework for using essential oils (aromatherapy) in nursing practice. It is not clear whether aromatherapists and other health professionals are aware of or use the aromatherapy QUM framework. The framework could be adapted for CAM generally.

Although not documented in current QUM policies, QUM encompasses sustainable agricultural and carbon reduction practices, which are important considerations, given the effects of climate change and the number of endangered plant an animal species, many of which are included in CAM medicines in some countries (Taylor 1996). CITES has made a major contribution to reducing the risk and saving many endangered plants and animals. In addition to its application to medicines use, QUM could serve as a research framework to evaluate IM and other CAM. .

10. Practical ways clinician health professionals can apply QUM

Health professionals have a responsibility to individualise care, respect people's choices and be non-judgmental about the choices they make. QUM can help health professionals realise these responsibilities:

Applying QUM at the individual patient level involves:

- Developing active partnerships with individuals, effective communication and collaboration processes and using evidence based policies and guidelines to deliver consistent care and enable benchmarking.

- Engaging the individual in setting care goals and making care decisions, which includes providing objective, ethical information about medicines and other care options in a language and format the individual can understand and that is culturally appropriate.
- Pharmacovigilence, which encompasses the entire medicine pathway as well as appropriate prescribing and monitoring.
- Monitoring outcomes including the individual's medicine self-management capability and adherence, and adverse event reporting.
- Documenting CAM use.

Developing a QUM philosophy

- Be sensitive to people's philosophical and cultural views and be aware that they probably perceive risks and benefits differently from health professionals.
- Follow guidelines for using CAM where they exist or seeking and using the best available evidence and being able to justify its use.
- Being appropriately qualified and competent to use, recommend or offer advice about CAM.
- Objectively communicating risks and benefits and management options to the individual and in some cases their families or carers. If the person chooses not to follow advice, documentation should outline what information was provided and the fact the individual elected not to follow the advice.
- Developing a 'portfolio of evidence' that can be used as a reference in clinical areas.
- Adopting the QUM approach to prescribing, administering, documenting and monitoring care. This includes asking about CAM use. One of the most common reasons people do not disclose CAM use is because Health professionals do not ask about it. Ask questions should be asked in a non-judgmental way. The patient has a responsibility to disclose: health professionals can make it easier for them to do so by using appreciate body and verbal language, and effective questioning skills. For every one problem missed by not knowing, nine others are missed by not looking.
- Valuing the therapeutic relationship and doing their utmost to develop and sustain relationships.
- Considering the effect of some CAM on other staff, visitors and other people when CAM is used in health care facilities for example, vaporising essential oils and playing music.
- Knowing how to report adverse events and reporting any that occur to add to the safety and risk profile of CAM and IM. The quality of the AE report is important rather than the source of the report.
- Having processes and policies in place to clean and maintain any equipment for example, vaporizers and infection control policies.
- Documenting the type, dose and duration of the therapy, reason for use, advice given, method to monitor outcomes and the expected and actual outcomes.
- Seeking advice or referring to an appropriate person when do not have the knowledge or competence to address the issue.

11. Chapter summary

Safety and health professional responsibility are not new concepts but notions of safety and regulatory processes have evolved over millennia. QUM is a useful framework for managing CAM and IM at all levels and exemplifies person-centred care, using non-medicine options where possible and pharmacovigilence

Author details

Trisha Dunning
Chair in Nursing and Director Centre for Nursing and Allied Health Research,
Deakin University and Barwon Health, Geelong, Australia

12. References

Australian Integrative Medicine Association. www.aima.net.au (accessed January 2012).

Bell I., Caspi O., Schwartz G. (2002) Integrative medicine and systematic outcomes research: issues in the emergence of a new model for primary care. *Archives of Internal Medicine* 162 (2):133–140.

Bodeker G., Ong C-K., Grundy C., Burford G., Shein K. (eds) (2005) *WHO Global Atlas of Traditional, Complementary and Alternative Medicine.* WHO, Geneva.

Braun L., Cohen M. (2010) H*erbs and Natural Supplements: an Evidenced Based Approach.* Elsevier, Sydney.

Clark R. (2004): *Health care and Notions of Risk.* Therapeutic Guidelines Limited, Melbourne pp 5–7.

Cohen M. (2005) Legal issues regarding complementary therapies www.camlawblog.com (accessed March 2012).

Commonwealth of Australia *Complementary Medicines in the Australian health System* (2003) Report to the Parliamentary Secretary to the Minister for Health and Aging, Commonwealth of Australia, Canberra.

Department of Health and Aging. (2002): *National Strategy for the Quality Use of Medicines.* Canberra http://www.health.gov.au/haf/nmp/advisory/pharm.htm (accessed April 2012)

Dunning T. (2004): Using a quality use of medicines framework for using essential oils in nursing practice. *Complementary Therapies in Clinical Practice*. 11: 172–181.

Efferth T., Greten H. (2012) The European directive on traditional herbal medicinal products: friend or foe fro plant-based therapies? *Journal of Chinese Integrative Medicine* 10 ($):357–361.

Egede L, Ye X, Zheng D, Silverstein M. (2002): The prevalence and pattern of alternative medicine use in individuals with diabetes. *Diabetes Care* 25: 324- 329.

Eisenberg D (1998) Advising patients who seek alternative medical therapies. *American Journal of Health Medicine* 127 (1):61–69.

Garrow D., Egede L (2006) association between complementary and alternative medicine use, preventive care practices, and use of conventional medical services among adults with diabetes. *Diabetes Care* 29:15–19.

Hildreth K, Elman C. (2007): Alternative worldviews and the utilization of conventional and complementary medicine. *Sociological Inquiry* 77(1): 76–103.

House of Lords Select Committee on Science and Technology Sixth Report (2000) chapter 3: patient satisfaction, the role of the therapist and the placebo response WWW.parliament UK (accessed May 2012)

Hume D in Sharpe V,. Faden A. (1998): *Medical Harm.* Cambridge University Press, Cambridge.

Kelner M, Wellman B. (1997): Health care and consumer choices: medical and alternative therapies. *Social Science and Medicine.* 45:203–212.

Khorsan R., Coulter I., Crawford C, Hsiao N-F. (2011) Systematic review of integrative health care research: randomized control trials, clinical controlled trials and meta-analysis. *Evidence Based Complementary and Alternative Medicine* doi.1155/2011/636134 (accessed April 2011).

Komesaroff P. (2003): Ethical perspectives on the communication of risk. *Australian Prescriber.* 26(2): 44–45.

Kotsirilos V., Singleton G., Warnecke E. (2010) Needs analysis for education in integrative and complementary medicine for general practitioners in Australia. Part 1. *Journal of Integrative Medicine* 15 (3): 12–16.

Kotsirilos V., Vitetta L., Sali A. (2011) *A Guide to Evidence-Based Integrative and Complementary Medicine.* Churchill Livingstone, Sydney.

MacLennan, A., Wilson, D. & Taylor, A. (2002) The escalating cost and prevalence of alternative medicine. *Preventative Medicine,* 35 (2), 166–173.

Marshall D.; Walizer E., Vernalis M. (2004) Optimal healing environments for chronic cardiovascular disease. *Journal of Alternative and Complementary Medicine* 10 (Suppl): S147–S155.

Mulkins A., Verhoef M. (2004) Supporting the transfromative process: experiences of cancer patients receiving integrative care. *Integrative Cancer Therapies* 3 (3):230–237.

O'Keefe M., Henderson A. (2012) Harmonising the layers of regulation. *Campus Review* 20 March www.campusreview.com.au.

Parsian N., Dunning T. (2009) Developing and validating a questionnaire to measure spirituality: a psychometric process. *Global Journal of Health Science* 1 (1): 2–11.

Phelps K., Hassed C. (2011) *General Practice: the Integrative Approach.* Churchill Livingstone, Sydney.

Ritenbaugh C., Nichter M., Nichter M., Kelly K., Sims C., Bell., Castaneda H., Elder C., Kiothan M., Sutherland E., Verhoef M., Warber S., Coons S. (2011) Developing a patient-centred outcome measure for complementary and alternative medicines therapies1: defining content and format. *BMC Complementary and Alternative Medicine* 11–135.

Royal Australian College of General Practitioners (RACGP) Australasian Integrative Medicine Association Joint Position Statement Complementary Medicine (2004) htpp://www.racgp.org.au/policy/complementary.medicine.pdf (accessed March 2011).

Sharot T. (2012) The optimism bias (2012). *Time Health* Sunday May 28 http://www.time.com/time/health/article/0,8599,2074067,00.html (accessed May 2012).

Sharples F., van Haselen R., Fisher P. (2003) NHS patients' perspective on complementary medicine: a survey. *Complementary Therapy Medicine*. 11(4):243–248.

Ulbricht C. (2012) What every clinician should know about herb-supplement-drug interactions. *Alternative and Complementary Therapies* 18 (2):67–70.

Weinstein N. (1982): Unrealistic optimism about susceptibility to health problems. *Journal of Behavioural medicine*. 5: 441–460.

World Health Organisation (WHO) (2007) *International Standard Terminologies on Traditional Medicine in the Western pacific Region*. WHO, Geneva.

World Health Organisation (WHO). (2002): Traditional Medicine Strategy 2002–2005. WHO, Geneva.

Chapter 3

Evaluating Homeopathic Therapies for Contemporary Health Care: An Evident Priority

Vilelmine Carayanni

Additional information is available at the end of the chapter

http://dx.doi.org/10.5772/53016

1. Introduction

Health spending continues to rise faster than economic growth in most OECD countries, maintaining a trend observed since the 1970s. Health expenditure reached 9.5% of GDP on the average in 2009 [1]. But the evolution of the health spending as a share of GDP is likely to stabilize or fall slightly in 2011. This is principally due to lowering health spending as governments seek to manage budget deficits. The economic evaluation has played a considerable role in this process in many countries such as the United Kingdom, the USA, Australia and Canada. Nevertheless, little attention has been given to the evaluation of complementary and alternative therapies, whereas their use has increased significantly in recent years: In the 2007 National Health Interview Survey (NHIS), in the USA, approximately 38 percent of adults reported using complementary and alternative medicine (CAM) in the previous 12 months. In the United States, patients are spending $34 billion dollars (a significant amount of expenditure) on contemporary and alternative medications [2].Among the forms of alternative medication that have been of interest to all parties in the health sector is homeopathic medication. Having started in Germany over two centuries ago, homeopathic therapy has grown and spread over the years across Europe, America and the rest of the world. In most countries the government authorises, registers and supervises the health professionals. Regulations vary depending on the country. In some countries, there are no specific legal regulations concerning the use of homeopathy, while in others, licenses or degrees in conventional medicine from accredited universities are required [3]. Doctors of all specializations may without interrupting or altering chemical or any other therapy they prescribe to the patient, provide at the same time the homeopathic medicine of their choice, while the patient's organism will be benefited especially with immediate time sequence between demand and offer of help.

In many ways, homeopathic therapy is different from conventional medicine [2]. Generally, homeopathic therapy is based on the principle that suggests as follows: Materials that cause a living organism to experience certain conditions can be used to treat those particular conditions for which they cause the given symptoms. This particular principle has an ancient origin in the research of Hippocrates [4]. For example, quinine can be used to treat the condition of malaria [4]. Here, it is worth mentioning that the above principle is not similar with the mechanism of immune response in a living organism. The differences concerning the traditions as well as the production and the use between homeopathic and conventional medicines have direct implications on the cost as we will see in the next paragraphs. Since homeopathy is emerging as a possible complementary or even alternative to contemporary medication for the treatment of various conditions, more and more resources will continue to be spent on homeopathic therapies and on homeopathic research. So, an economic evaluation of homeopathic practice is therefore useful in the direction of understanding the economical viability of homeopathic practice [2].

2. Homeopathic therapies: The beliefs of costs and effectiveness for homeopathic therapies

2.1. Efficacy: Does homeopathy work and how? Pre-clinical stage evidence

It needs to be mentioned that homeopathic therapies have no molecule of an active ingredient per volume. Since many scientists have had a materialistic training, their scepticism about effectiveness is understandable.

At pharmacology's rational level, in 1988, the INSERM's immunologist J. Benveniste claimed that IgE antibodies have an effect on certain cell type after being diluted by a factor of 10 120[6]. A simple experiment by scientists and professors at the renown Aerospace Institute of the University of Stuttgart in Germany is confirming Dr. Jacques Benveniste's 1988 assertion that water has an imprint of energies to which it has been exposed [7]. Also, electrochemical studies have shown that there is a structural difference in the chemical and physical nature of diluted homeopathic carriers from controls [8,9].Nevertheless, these results must be verified by other studies.

Botanical science has also been helpful in evaluating the potential of homeopathy in treating organisms. Just like in other studies of homeopathy, modern scientists have been reluctant to follow up on incomplete literature that had been done by older generation scientists. Recently, two important observations have been made [8]. First, homeopathic substances were shown to slightly impact the health of healthy plants by just over 2%. Here, although this particular impact was observed to be low, it was statistically consistent. In unhealthy plants, the impact of homeopathic substances rose to 20%. Such observations have been in agreement with the notion that homeopathic substances (which are usually highly diluted to levels of zero molecules per volume) are more effective in sickly organisms than in healthy ones [4].

The effectiveness of homeopathic treatment has also been applied to animals. Here, it has been observed that an intoxication of an animal can be reversed by the use of relevant homeopathic remedies [10]. A meta-analysis of 105 intoxication trials showed clear, clinically relevant and significantly positive effects for homeopathic treatment [11,112] . Also, studies have suggested that highly diluted homeopathic treatments can replace missing substances in animals [13-15].

Nevertheless, according to some authors, despite these encouraging observational studies, the effectiveness of the homeopathic prevention or therapy of infections in veterinary medicine is not sufficiently supported by randomized and controlled trials [16]. There has also been a number of experiments which have suggested against the effectiveness of homeopathic treatments. For example, some rat experiments have brought to doubt the effectiveness of homeopathic substances in treating diseases [10]. However, since the positive results have been reproduced numerous times, some scientists are suggesting a pointer towards the efficacy of homeopathic substances.

2.2. No better efficacy/ effectiveness than the placebo effect in clinical trials and safety questions

In some human observations, people who were taking homeopathic treatment produced similar results from those that were taking controls; thus, suggesting that homeopathy is primarily a result of the placebo effect [17-20].Over 150 clinical trials have failed to show that homeopathy works and the effect of the homeopathic medicine is no better than the placebo effect. For example, in an experiment that was done in the UAE, a meta-analysis study of about 3500 patients showed a positive homeopathic response in 60 patients and a positive placebo response in 55 patients, thus, discrediting homeopathic treatment [4].When all the evidence from many trials is pooled together, homeopathy is no better than a placebo. *Nevertheless,* between 1950 and 2009, 142 R.C.T there have been published studies that examined a total number of 74 infections . 63 R.C.T. reported a positive result 68 R.C.T. did not produce any convincing proof and 11 RCT reported a negative result [21]. The Homeopathy Faculty in London recognized 24 census takings having positive results in: allergy, diarrhea in children, influenza, post operational ileus, rheumatologic infections, seasonal allergic rhinitis , infection of the upper respiratory ducts comprising otitis media [19].Some researches claimed that small-scale studies have yielded positive results, but this is due to poor methodologies or random effects [22].

We have to underline that according to all manuals of biostatistics medicine studies of phase III and afterward imply millions of persons and multiple centers in order to prove the "effectiveness" (and not any longer the "efficacy" of a therapy).This is not certainly the case for the majority of clinical trials published . In many fields much smaller unpowered samples predominate and studies quality according to Jadad scale is low[21,22].So, it seems that there is a generalized need to improve the quality of clinical studies and the problem does not concern only homeopathic therapies.

In the case of innocuousness, even in large samples, there may be harmful side effects where there is a very scant probability of appearance. Conversely to the notion of the mean effectiveness, innocuousness is mostly an individual affair. So we can understand the danger emerging by these small trials to approve the wrong treatment in many cases. Also, this specific outcome (innocuousness), is one of the main reasons of their preference acceptable even by the critics. The alcohol that is usually used in homeopathic drugs is 96^0 that substantially evaporates and the information transmitted through water is only 4% so the probability to cause some reactions in patients is negligible. But even though the hazards from homeopathic products are modest in comparison with those of conventional medicines, the fast-growing popularity of homeopathy and its increasing use for self-medication signify the need for continued vigilance to ensure the quality and safety of these products .

Beyond the above arguments mentioned, there are some other problems concerning the degree which homeopathic therapies may be adapted to the conventional RCT's scheme . Some of the reasons are that homeopathic therapies treat symptoms and not diagnosis, the therapies are mostly individualized. Also, instruments for the quality of life measurement do not comprise any items that measure the potential benefits of homeopathy as claimed by homeopaths including stess and control management and life attitude. Additionally, especially in explanatory oriented clinical studies, where the class of patients suitable for the trial is redefined a posteriori, patients proving unsuitable for any reason to follow allopathic treatment are excluded. That can produce selection bias in favor of the allopathic treatment.

2.3. More costly than conventional medicine

According to many opposites homeopathy is not only less effective but implies also a higher cost that is, conventional therapies are dominant therapies under the point of view of health economics. We will examine the different cost parameters to see the differences between homeopathic and allopathic medicines in such parameters.

1. Consultation costs. Unlike contemporary medicine, homeopathic treatment is more personalized. Before prescribing medications, homeopathic consultants will need to review one's emotional state, his health, among other factors in addition to disease symptoms. The above arrangement means that homeopathic practitioners are required to spend more hours with their patients when compared with contemporary health practitioners. A direct result of such an arrangement is high consultation costs in homeopathic practice. However, there is often a low follow up consultation cost. The initial high consultation cost is usually fruitful as most patients report better health; thus, a low follow up cost. Since many homeopathic practitioners will extensively evaluate issues that are often ignored by contemporary health practitioners, their patients usually report better health within a short time [25]. Another implication that is worth mentionning here is the necessity of specialist practitioners for patients who are under contemporary medications. Specialists usually charge high fees as compared to ordinary practitioners. Researches by Rossi et al. showed that patients under homeopathic medication were in less need of specialists as opposed to patients who were under contemporary medication [26]
2. Medication costs. Usually, homeopathic drugs are prepared by a process that thoroughly mixes active ingredients with a solvent through a vigorous shaking process.

The process of diluting an active ingredient can be done for an infinite duration of time to obtain infinite quantities of medicine; thus resulting in homeopathic medications that have no molecule of an active ingredient per volume [2]. The economic implication of the above process is that homeopathic drugs can be prepared easily and at a low cost. Another factor that makes homeopathic drugs economical is the fact that homeopathic drugs are non-patented, generic, and can be easily reproduced. Consequently, costs that stem from copyright issues (among other costs that result from patented drugs) are eliminated. Also, as already mentioned homeopathy does not have the adverse events of conventional medicine implying additional costs. Also, a good part of homeopathic medicines according to homeopaths are preventive for some epidemic infections or contagious and they could assist to the better resistance against the prevention.

3. Diagnostic costs. Another factor that has helped to lower the cost of homeopathic medication as compared to ordinary medication is the lower requirement for laboratory procedures for patients that undergo homeopathic treatment as some studies indicated [25]. However, interpretation of these results are hampered due to the small sample size and the large variability between the practitioners.

3. Homeopathy in different countries: Overal evaluations of cost effectiveness

The high numbers of patients that are currently seeking homeopathic treatment in many countries suggest implications for health policy designers. More than a third of patients in the US that are suffering from allergy are seeking homeopathic treatment. [3].Among the countries that grant homeopathic therapies not of a lesser status we can site France, England, Germany, India, Bangladesh, the United States, Canada, Brazil, and many more. There has been a 60% growth in the homeopathic market in Europe over 10 years (1995-2005); from €590million to €930million. 90% of homeopathic products are consumed by France, Germany, Netherlands, Spain, Belgium, UK and Poland [26]. Relative to population, France and Germany have highest consumption - 59%-[27,28] More than half of the French declare that have already used homeopathic medicines, a number which constantly multiplies. (39 % in 2004, 53 % in 2010). [29].In India, alternative treatments, including homeopathy, are well established and integrated into the healthcare system, with 94 per cent of people saying that they have faith in alternative remedies, and 62 per cent trusting homeopathy[28]. 15% of the population in Britain trust the homeopathy as a form of treatment [32].In Germany in 2006, homeopathic remedies accounted for 3.16% of sold units (1.08% of business volume) in the pharmaceutical sector. 0.48% of prescriptions covered by public health insurance were for homeopathic remedies [33].

On the other hand, despite the extensive use of homeopathy few are the countries that reimburse homeopathic medicines. Some homeopathic treatment is covered by the national insurance of several European countries, including France, some parts of the United Kingdom, Denmark, and Luxembourg. In Austria, public insurance requires scientific proof of effectiveness in order to reimburse medical treatments, but exceptions are made for homeopathy[34]. In 2004, Germany which formerly offered homeopathy under its public health insurance scheme withdrew this privilege, with a few exceptions. In June 2005, the Swiss Government, after a 5-year trial, withdrew insurance coverage for homeopathy and four other complementary treatments, stating that they did not meet efficacy and cost-effectiveness criteria. However, following the result of a referendum in 2009 the five therapies were reinstated for a further 6-year trial period starting from 2012[35].

In this section, we will study the existing estimation of how homeopathy is more or less costly, less or more effective at the global level of an economy and the related consequences on their reimbursement.

Nevertheless, full-scale economic evaluation of homeopathy is very difficult to take place because of organizational, financial and ethical reasons. Systematic reviews to conclude not only whether homeopathy works or harms, but also whether its adoption will lead to a more efficient use of resources are also very difficult to be undertaken due principally to the small number of existing studies by indication.

Some observational and quasi-experimental studies recorded the outcomes and costs of treatment by General Practitioners (GPs) who integrated homeopathy in their practice, compared with those who did not: Also, national reports (governmental, federal and health authorities reports) conclude on the economic viability of using homeopathic therapies at a national level by studying the cost and/or the effectiveness of homeopathic therapies. These reports with the exception of the 1991 French Government Report that uses observational data have the form of narrative reviews .We will briefly examine these reports.

A. National reports and statements

A 1991 French Government Report making use of observational data revealed a significantly reduced cost from homeopathic care versus conventional medical care [34]. The totality of costs associated with homeopathic care per physicians was approximately one-half of the total amount of care provided by conventional primary care physicians. However, because homeopathy physicians, on average, saw significantly fewer patients, the overall cost per patient under homeopathic care was still a significant 15% less. It is also interesting to note that these savings appear to increase the longer a physician has been using homeopathy [36].

The most complete governmental report is that of Switzerland [37]. Drawing cost data of participating physicians from Swiss health insurers, this review included all expenditures covered from consultation costs (diagnostic and therapeutic procedures), costs for medication (directly dispensed or prescriptions), costs for external laboratory analyses, and costs for physiotherapy.

The Swiss report found that total practice costs for physicians who specialized in homeopathic medicine had an overall 15.4 percent reduction in overall health care costs associated with their practice, as compared with physicians who practiced conventional medicine as well as those physicians who practice other "complementary and alternative medicine" treatments (but not homeopathic medicine). The report comprises a highly-comprehensive narrative review of the wide body of preclinical and clinical and conclude that effectiveness of homeopathy can be supported by clinical evidence and professional and adequate application regarded as safe. Reliable statements of cost-effectiveness are not available at the moment, but the report states that cost- effectiveness studies on individual complementary medical treatments clearly indicate possible savings.

The Federal Centre of Expertise in Health Care (KCE)of Belgium has edited an analytical report, the second more completed national report based on narrative review[38] . This report concludes that the fees are higher than the other three non-conventional medical. This conclusion is based exclusively on cost data selected by secondary sources (patients) . Nevertheless, published economic evaluations are excluded from the review undertaken by this report .From a purely clinical perspective, by reviewing 26 systematic reviews , this report concludes that there is no evidence of the efficacy of homeopathy (evidence-based medicine) beyond the placebo effect. Nevertheless, it is not clear as to the exact exclusion criteria that concluded in 26 reviews having initially selected 80 studies retrieved for more detailed evaluation.

A national overview of homeopathy and other CAM therapies conclude for a significant improvement in health outcomes and after treatment an increase in days off work [39,37].

Beyond these reports no other reports use cost and effectiveness criteria to conclude about the economic viability of the homeopathic therapies. Recently, the House of Commons Science and Technology Committee advised that NHS funding should be stopped "since effectiveness of homeopathic medicines has not been proved superior than placebo effect"[40]. Despite this report, the Coalition stated homeopathy would continue to be funded, with PCTs responsible for making decisions locally.

The specific report followed a public statement by the National Health and Medical Research Council (NHMRC) attesting as a basic source the English report and is of the opinion that there is sufficient scientific evidence to conclude that homeopathy is no more efficacious than placebo [41]. We are not aware of any other national report or statement at this time.

Canada on the other hand (Canada Health, Ottawa) has established a research program with priority to the cost effectiveness evaluation for the natural products of health care such homeopathic medicines since it is stated that "the results of an important number of metaanalyses permits a cautious optimism [42].

B. Observational and quasi- experimental studies of the overall cost and effectiveness

A 1996 study of 130,000 prescriptions confirmed the results of the 1991 French government report (see above) and suggested significant benefits and savings as a result of homeopathic treatment. This survey also noted that the number of paid sick leave days by patients under the care of homeopathic physicians were 3.5 times less (598 days/year) than patients under the care of general practitioners (2,017 days/year). These figures suggest further benefit and savings to the homeopathic approach to care [43].

Smallwood's report included a study by Swayne et al. published in 1992 which examined the prescription costs of 22 doctors in the UK found that practices which included a GP using homeopathy prescribed 12% fewer items of medication per patient (including both conventional drugs and homeopathic medicines) compared with other local practices. Smallwood calculates that if this figure was extrapolated to a national level the number of items prescribed would be reduced by 41.5 million [44,45).

In Belgium, Wassenhoven and Yves studied 782 patients (most of who had serious conditions) who were undergoing homeopathic medication [25].

The findings of Wassenhoven and Yves suggest that ordinary doctors spend as much as three times on drugs as compared to their homeopathic counterparts. On the other hand, homeopathic doctors spend only a fifth of what is spent by contemporary doctors on antibiotics. Such a direction indicates massive savings (about 800 million Euros) that can be made if all doctors in Belgium were to prescribe medicines as homeopathic practitioners [25]

Further details for all these studies as well as for other cost studies are given in *Bornhöft* et al [37].Nevertheless, results of these studies have to be assessed with some caution because of some methodological limitations concerning especially their design and need of research to confirm the above mentioned results .

To conclude, in relatively few countries systematic efforts have been undertaken to estimate the cost and effectiveness of homeopathy at a national level despite its extensive use. Health Technology assessments are few and do not proceed to a systematic review of cost-effectiveness since the number of these studies by morbidity is too small. Observational and quasi experimental studies is well known that do not conveniently ensure the comparability of the groups. An attempt to understand the full economic impact of homeopathic practice at a macro scale level would have to consider an array of factors that are difficult to analyze (e.g consequences on the employment in the manufacturing sector). These are issues that are difficult to evaluate. The work of many researchers on the above issue can only be used to lay ground for a more detailed and exhaustive research. The evaluation of quality of life of the citizens by using adapted quality of life questionnaires and the avoidance at national level of adverse events by using homeopathy constitute central points for future research.

4. Cost and effectiveness of homeopathy by indication: A critical review of economic evaluation studies

Methods

For the assessment of the trial based economic evaluations we have used the International Society of Pharmacoeconomics and Outcomes Research (ISPOR) RCT CEA Task Force Report. For the other types of studies as well as for the global assessment and their comparison with studies of conventional medicine, we have used BMJ guidelines [47]. We have compared also these results with results from systematic reviews in conventional medicine [48,49].

More analytically, the results of a review [49] of conventional medicine have been used as well as the reviews for some studies of the Centre for Reviews and Dissemination of the University of York [51] that have been completed by the author in order to compare the criteria completion between homeopathic and conventional medicine in the case of Trial Based Economic Evaluations. As there are not yet specific guidelines for economic evaluations based on observational studies, items from the *BMJ* Checklist have been additionally used to make possible the assessment of all studies. The results of a review [49] of conventional medicine studies have been used and completed in order to compare statistically the criteria completion between homeopathic [53,66-70] and conventional medicine studies [71-79]. We have completed this review by Centre for Review and Dissemination Reviews for some studies [50] as well as by author review.

We have selected only full economic evaluations for our review focusing on special indications. Full economic evaluations compare at least 2 different strategies and measure both costs and health results (cost effectiveness/cost consequences, cost utility and cost benefit).Cost-benefit analysis attempt to value the consequences of programs in money terms [50]. The cost effectiveness analysis in its classical form, considers a single measure of output and the results are presented in the form of a cost effectiveness ratio. An other version of the cost effectiveness analysis, the cost consequences analysis presents an array of output measures alongside costs without aggregation. In the cost utility analysis the consequences are adjusted by health state preference scores [50].

Research strategy

We researched the following electronic databases from January 1999 to January 2012: DARE, NHS EED and HTA Medline, EMBASE, AMED, Alt-Health-Watch, and the Complementary and Alternative Medicine Citation Index via NCCAM and the National Library of Medicine (NLM). Researching has been restricted to English, French and Greek language journals and human studies with the keywords: homeopathy, and costs or cost analysis or cost-benefit, or cost-effective or cost utility economic analysis, or economic evaluation.

Data analysis

Because of too small sample size of studies selected, in the case of Trial Based Economic Evaluations no statistical test has been used to detect any differences between homeopathic and conventional medicine studies on the completion of the above mentioned criteria. *For the assessment of all economic evaluations based on BMJ* Checklist, *Fisher's exact mid-p test* has been used to test the homogeneity between the 2 groups for each quality criteria as well as for the total of the quality criteria. *Fisher's exact mid-p test is* the mid-*p* version of Fisher's exact conditional test, only half the probability of the observed outcome is included in the mid-*p*-value [80]. The resulting test is less conservative than Fisher's exact test, and its performance approximates that of an unconditional test. For the statistical analysis R software has been used [81].

Results

We have detected 186 records as well as 3 additional records identified by other sources (University of Lyon I). 80 duplicates have been detected and deleted. 25 full text articles have been detected and selected for eligibility (Figure 1) [82]. Eight of these publications met the criteria of full economic evaluations, whereas the others were partial economic evaluations and/ or did not focus on special indications. One of these publications comprises a randomized trial, an observational study and a review that we will study separately. So we will study 10 studies in the total comparing homeopathy with conventional medicine. Three of these studies were randomized clinical trials, 3 observational studies and one study was a review.

Trials based economic evaluations review

Details of the 3 studies [52-54] comparing homeopathy with conventional medicine [55-62] are given below (Table 1).

Authors , country and year of publication	Indication	Type of economic evaluation	Patients groups	Health Effects of Homeopathy compared to Conventional medicine	Cost of Homeopathy compared to Conventional medicine
Paterson et al, (2003),United Kingdom[52]	Dyspepsia	Cost effectiveness	a. acupuncture b. Homeopathy c. normal GP care	No significant differences (a=5%)	No significant differences (a=5%)
Kneis and Gandjour,2009, Germany[53]	Acute Maxillary Sinusitis	Cost utility	a. Homeopathy b. Placebo (no active treatment)	Significant differences in favor of homeopathy (a=5%)	Significant differences in favor of homeopathy (a=5%)
Thompson et al, 2011,United Kingdom[54]	Asthma	Cost effectiveness	a. Homeopathic treatment b. Usual care	No significant differences (a=5%)	No significant differences (a=5%)

Table 1. Trial Based Economic Evaluations comparing homeopathy with conventional medicine

Table 2 presents the results of the review. As can be seen, no important deviation has been observed between homeopathic and conventional medicine studies. All studies comparing homeopathy with conventional therapy (100%) are pragmatically oriented to measure the effectiveness versus efficacy with some stricter criteria for inclusion in the third study reasonable for this type of intervention (criterion1). Also, 5 out of 8 (63%) of conventional studies seem to follow a more pragmatic design oriented to measure effectiveness rather than efficacy despite the stricter inclusion criteria of 4 out of 8 studies of conventional medicine. Three of these studies are considered as more explanatory [63] since they do not use Intention to Treat Approach although this approach in recent years has almost universally dominated [64].

ISPOR's criteria[46]	Review of homeopathic medicines studies N (%)	Reviews of conventional studies N (%)
A. Clinical trial design		
1.Trial design should reflect effectiveness rather than efficacy when possible	3(100)	8(63)
2. Full follow-up of all patients is encouraged.	3(100)	8(75)*
3. Describe power and ability to test hypotheses, given the trial sample size.	3(0)	8(25)
4. Clinical end points used in economic evaluations should be disaggregated	3(100)	8(100)
5. Direct measures of outcome are preferred to use of intermediate end points.	3(100)	8(100)
B. Data elements		
6. Obtain information to derive health state utilities directly from the study population	2(50)	8(80)
7. Collect all resources that may substantially influence overall costs; these include those related and unrelated to the intervention	2(33)	8(38)
C. Database design and management		
8. Collection and management of the economic data should be fully integrated into the clinical data.	3(100)	8(63)
9. Consent forms should include wording permitting the collection of economic data, particularly when it will be gathered from third-party databases and may include pre- and/or post-trial records	3(0)	8(0)
D. Analysis		
10. The analysis of economic measures should be guided by a data analysis plan and hypotheses that are drafted prior to the onset of the study	3(0)	8(0)
11.1 Intention-to-treat analysis	3(100)	8(63)*
11.2 Common time horizon(s) for accumulating costs and outcomes	3(100)	8(75)
11.3 Within-trial assessment of costs and outcomes	3(100)	8(100)
11.4 Assessment of uncertainty is necessary for each measure	3(0)	8(13)

ISPOR's criteria[46]	**Review of homeopathic medicines studies N (%)**	**Reviews of conventional studies N (%)**
11.5 Common discount rate applied to future costs and outcomes	NA**	NA
11.6 An accounting for missing and/or censored data	3(75)	8(100)
12. Incremental costs and outcomes should be measured as differences in arithmetic means, with statistical testing accounting for issues specific to these data	3(33)	8(13)
13. One or more summary measures should be used to characterize the relative value of the intervention	3(33)	8(63)
14.1 Sampling uncertainty accounting	1(100)	8(63)*
14.2 Parameter uncertainty accounting	3(33)	8(38)
14.3 Protocol-driven resource use are addressed (in the design phase)	3(3)	8(13)
14.3 Unrepresentative recruiting centers are addressed	3(100)	8(100)
14.4 Inclusion of study sites from countries with varying access and availability of health-care services is addressed	3(0)	8(0)
14.5 Restrictive inclusion and exclusion criteria are addressed	3(100)	8(63)
14.6 Artificially enhanced compliance is addressed	3(100)	8(75)
15. Multinational trials require special consideration to address inter-country differences in population characteristics and treatment patterns	NA**	1(0)
16. When models are used to estimate costs and outcomes beyond the time horizon of the trial, good modeling practices should be followed..	NA	NA
17. Models should reflect the expected duration of the intervention on costs and outcomes.	NA	NA
18. Subgroup analyses (ex post) are encouraged	NA	NA
E. Reporting the results		
19. Patient demographics are reported	3(100)	8(63)
20. Trial setting is reported	3(100)	8(100)
21. Inclusion and exclusion criteria are reported	3(100)	8(100)

ISPOR's criteria[46]	Review of homeopathic medicines studies N (%)	Reviews of conventional studies N (%)
22. Protocol-driven procedures that influence external validity are reported	3(0)	8(13)
23. Intervention and control arms are reported	3(100)	8(100)
24. Time horizon for the intervention and follow-up are reported.	3(100)	8(100)
25. Key clinical findings are reported	3(100)	8(100)
26. Reporting should distinguish economic data collected as part of the trial vs. data not collected as part of the trial	3(100)	8(100)
27. Amount of missing and censored data	3(67)	8(63)*
28. If imputation methods are used, the method should be described.	1(100)	2(100)*
29. Methods used to construct and compare costs and outcomes, and to project costs and outcomes beyond the trial period should be described.	3(100)	8(75)
30. The results section should include summaries of resource use, costs, and outcome measures, including point estimates and measures of uncertainty	3(0)	8(0)
31. Results should be reported for the time horizon of the trial (and for projections)	3(100)	8(100)
32. Graphical displays are recommended for results not easily reported in tabular form	1(100)	6(33)

* Comparable estimates available from Polsky et al, 2006

** Not appropriate

Table 2. ISPOR's Good Research Practices

Power calculations, (criterion 3), were not performed in the planning phase of the study in none of the studies.(0%) treating homeopathy (however, power calculations were performed retrospectively in the first study [52].

One out of the three studies (33%) of homeopathy and 3 out of 8 (38%) of the studies of conventional medicine have measured some additional costs (criterion 7) beyond direct health costs.

None of the homeopathy (0/3) and conventional medicine studies (0/8) include in the consent form wording permitting for economic data collection (although in the study of Thompson et al [54] cost data are collected by children's parents.

None of the homeopathy (0%) or conventional medicine studies (0%) establish the hypotheses with a data analysis plan (criterion 10). No discount rate has been applied, (criterion 11.5), as the study period for each participant was 1 year in all studies.

Whereas all homeopathic medicine studies use p- values for hypotheses tests (100%), and respectively 6 out of 8 conventional medicine studies (75%), only one conventional medicine study reports confidence intervals for point estimates of all measures (criterion 11.4) and none homeopathic study.

Sensitivity analysis (criterion 14.2) has been used by the one of the three homeopathic studies (33%) whereas 3/8 conventional studies (38%) use sensitivity analysis for costs and outcomes. All homeopathic studies (100%) and 7 out of 8 of conventional studies (88%),, have been well addressed by the design the protocol induced procedures except one study of conventional medicine (criterion 14.3) . Nevertheless, in the report of results (criterion 23), there is no mention made in homeopathic studies (0%) concerning them as to whether there were observed and addressed or not except for one study of conventional medicine (13%) to which they have been spotted and measured).

Finally, the 2 categories of studies present proportional weakness and strengths with the biggest differences in favor of conventional medicine focused on aggregated outcomes (2/3 trials of homeopathy use cost consequences analyses). The trial based economic evaluations comparing homeopathy with conventional medicine do not seem to be of lower quality than studies of conventional medicine and complete the majority of the ISPOR's criteria. Also, homeopathy clinical trials are for some aspects more adapted to the traditional clinical trials guidelines offering better information on patient characteristics and flow [65].Additionally they avoid some aspects of explanatory design a more pragmatic design such as stricter eligibility criteria and no intention to treat approach. Nevertheless, no definitive conclusions can be extracted because of the too small sample sizes.

4.1. BMJ checklist including all full economic evaluations

Information for homeopathic studies included in this review is given on Table 3.The quality of homeopathic economic evaluation studies seems to constantly progress given that more recent studies are characterized by an improved design and more detailed reports, as is the case with conventional studies [4]. As can be seen,(Table 4), a significantly superior number of homeopathic studies defines clearly the aspect of the economic evaluation (criterion 3). Also, details of the subjects from which values were obtained are given more frequently by homeopathic studies (criterion 13). On the other hand, conventional studies use more frequently sensitivity analyses (criterion 27) as well as incremental analyses and aggregate clinical outcomes (criteria 31 and 32), as the majority of homeopathic studies included use cost consequences analyses (80%).Finally, both categories of studies present deficiencies concerning the justification of the form of economic evaluation chosen. The overall percentage of studies that complete BMJ criteria is 70.6 % for homeopathic studies and 78.6% for conventional studies. By the mid-*p* version of Fisher's exact conditional test we conclude that the differences observed between the 2 groups of studies aren't statistically significant. (mid p-value=0.20). Consequently, we accept the homogeneity between homeopathic and conventional medicine studies on the BMJ guidelines completion.

Authors year of publication and country	Morbidity studied	Type of economic evaluation	Patients groups	Cost of Homeopathy versus conventional medicine	Health Effects of Homeopathy versus conventional medicine
Stagnara et al, (2004), France [66]	Bronchiolitis (neonatal)	Cost effectiveness	a. Homeopathy b. usual care	Significant differences (a=5%) Less costly	significant differences (a=5%) More effective
Veinchtock et al, (2000) France [67]	Anxiety disorders	Cost consequences	a. Homeopathy b. Usual care	No significant differences (a=5%)	No significant differences (a=5%)
Trichard et al, 2005, France [68]	Acute Rhino-pharyngitis (Children)	Cost effectiveness	a. Homeopathy b. Usual care	Significant differences (a=5%) Less costly	Significant differences (a=5%) More effective
Witt et al, 2005, Germany [69]	Headache Low back pain Depression Insomnia	Cost effectiveness	a. Homeopathy b. usual care	No significant differences (a=5%)	Significant differences (a=5%) More effective
Witt et al, 2009, Germany [70]	atopic eczema (children)	Cost effectiveness	a. Homeopathy b. Usual care	Significant differences (a=5%) More costly	No significant differences (a=5%)
Kneis and Gandjour, 2009, Germany [53]	Acute Maxillary Sinusitis	Cost utility	a. Homeopathy b. Placebo	Significant differences (a=5%) Less costly	Significant differences (a=5%) More effective
Kneis and Gandjour, 2009 [53]	Acute Maxillary Sinusitis	Cost effectiveness	a. Homeopathy b. Antibacterials	Less costly	Significant differences in favor of homeopathy

Table 3. Non randomized studies for homeopathic treatment

Items from the BMJ Checklist [47]	Review of homeopathic medicines studies N(%)	Reviews of conventional studies N(%)	Mid p-value
Study design			
1.The research question is stated	10(100)	9(100)	0.5
2. The economic importance of the research question is stated	10(80)	9(78)	0.5
3. The perspective of the analysis is stated	10(100)	9(67)*	0.04
4. The rationale for choosing the alternatives is stated	10(90)	9(100)	0.5
5. The alternatives being compared are clearly described	10(90)	9(100)	0.5
6. The form of economic evaluation used is stated	10(50)	9(89)	0.07
7. The choice of form of economic evaluation is justified	10(0)	9(11)	0.09
Data collection			
8. The source(s) of effectiveness estimates are stated	10(100)	9(100)	0.5
9. Details of the effectiveness study are given	10(100)	9(100)	0.5
10. Primary outcome measures are clearly stated	10(90)	9(89)	0.5
11. Methods to value health states are stated	6(100)	9(89)*	0.5
12. Details of the method of synthesis or meta-analysis of estimates are given	1(100)	5(20)	-
13. Details of the subjects from which values were obtained are given	6(100)	9(56)	0.05
14. Productivity changes are reported separately	10(60)	9(44)	0.33
15. The relevance of productivity changes is discussed	10(20)	9(33)	0.31
16. Quantities of resources are reported separately from unit costs	10(70)	9(78)	0.5
17. Methods for the estimation of quantities and unit costs are described	10(100)	9(100	0.5

Items from the BMJ Checklist [47]	**Review of homeopathic medicines studies N(%)**	**Reviews of conventional studies N(%)**	**Mid p-value**
18. The currency and price date should be recorded	10(90)	9(89)	0.5
19. Details of any adjustment for inflation, or currency conversion are given	NA	3(75)	-
20. Details of any model used are given	NA**	6(100)	-
21. The choice of the model and its key parameters are justified	NA	6(33)	-
Analysis and interpretation of results			
22. Time horizon of costs and benefits is stated	10(100)	9(100)	0.5
23. The discount rate is stated	NA	6 (86)	-
24. The choice of discount rate is justified	NA	6(33)	-
25. An explanation is given if costs and benefits not discounted	10(30)	3(0)	0.5
26. Details of statistical tests and confidence intervals are given for stochastic data	9(56)	3(67)	0.5
27. The approach to sensitivity analysis is given	10(40)	9(89)*	0.03
28. The choice of variables for sensitivity analysis is justified	10(40)	9(67)	0.21
29. The ranges over which variables are varied are stated	10(40)	9(78)	0.08
30. Relevant alternatives are compared	10(100)	9(100)	0.5
31. Incremental analysis is reported	10(20)	9(89)	0.003
32. Major outcomes are presented disaggregated and aggregated	10(20)	9(89)	0.003
33. The answer to the study question is given	10(100)	9(100)	0.5
34. Conclusions follow from the data reported	10(100)	9(100)	0.5
35. Conclusions are accompanied by the appropriate caveats	10(80)	9(100)	0.23

* Comparable estimates available from Pirraglia et al, 2004

**Not Appropriate

Table 4. BMJ Checklist

5. Discussion

To conclude, few are the economic evaluation studies, but not of apparent or significantly lower quality than that of conventional medicine. And that despite the fact that the majority of the studies of the conventional medicines selected are published in journals with high impact factor [71-79]. The majority of homeopathic studies are observational whereas randomization is generally accepted as the most objective manner to have comparable groups. It is known that we should not generally use observational data to establish or attribute a difference between therapies, but they can be used to estimate the economic consequences of such a difference [83]

Nevertheless, some observational studies under evaluation particularly addressed this problem and prove that their groups are comparable in basic medico-demographic characteristics [66,67]. Also, many of the conventional studies comprised in the BMJ criteria evaluation use modeling approaches and one of them is based exclusively on expert opinion [78] that is classified in the lowest degree in the hierarchy of evidence. This probably is one of the reasons why the majority of these studies use sensitivity analysis in contradiction to homeopathic studies as is the dominating method of handling uncertainty in modeling studies (being nevertheless complementary and not substitute of the handle of uncertainty in stochastic approaches).

The limitations of these reviews are similar to those of other reviews. First, the only one reader was not blinded to journals and article authors, possibly having influenced results. To maximize accuracy, data extraction was performed many times -at least twice for each paper. Second, the measures of study quality depend on the information reported in an article, and no attempt was made to judge the merits of clinical or modeling assumptions and model choice made in the analyses. Also, no quality criteria exist for the amount of missing data that in some studies of conventional medicine not only surpass 15% of the data [85] in some RCT but reach even 79% in a specific study [59].Third, the number of reviewed studies was small. Nevertheless, to diminish the coservatiness of the statistical tests for type I error we have used Fisher's conditional mid-*p* test. Finally, while the strategy for identification, review, was rigorous, it is possible that some studies meeting finally the criteria of this review were not included [86].

6. Conclusions

Homeopathy is used almost worldwide by an important number of patients. Among the countries that grant homeopathic therapies not of a lesser status we can site France, England, Germany, India, Baglandesh, the United States, Canada, Brazil, and many more . France, England, Germany also are the countries that seem to dominate in the research on the efficiency of homeopathy. Some governmental reports support the financing of homeopathy based on reviews or on quasi experimental studies, some others are extremely negative. The financing or not of the homeopathic therapies by a third payer has clear consequences on the budgets of thousand of citizens who use homeopathy and on the accessibility of these therapies by the more vulnerable social categories. Because of their popularity, governments should be busy with homeopathy more seriously as well as with the framework of homeopathy and what it entails, that is:

Firstly, Good Manufacturing Practices such as cleanrooms must be applied on homeopathic products in order to ensure their quality.

Also, the need of assessing these therapies so as to find out which is the exact extension that truly is beneficial to the state and society making their funding necessary.

The debate with regard to efficacy/effectiveness and efficiency of homeopathy has dominated the scene the last decades. On the other hand, the quality of homeopathic economic evaluation studies seems to constantly progress given that more recent studies are characterized by an improved design and more detailed reports, as is the case with conventional studies. The trial based economic evaluations comparing homeopathy with conventional medicine do not seem to be of lower quality than studies of conventional medicine and complete the majority of the ISPOR criteria. Also, there are not statistically significant differences between studies of conventional and homeopathic medicine based on BMJ quality criteria. Certainly, the need for further improvement of both 2 categories of studies is obvious .And the greatest problem with homeopathic studies is their limited number.Nevertheless, despite objections there emerge serious indications of effectiveness and efficiency concerning homeopathic therapies. Yet the health effect ought to be proven through further well designed randomized trials.

Crossover design that allows robust estimates of intraindividual consistency of response using placeo-control groups and allows for preference assessments of benefit/tolerability ratios seem to be appropriate in case of moderate chronic diseases (e.g. allergy, rhumatology).Also, extended cross over designs or N of 1 trials seem to be more appropriate in diseases where treatments even of conventional medicine are highly individualized (e.g autism).

The trade off between conventional and homeopathic medicine concerning participant eligibility criteria is another crucial point of organized trials with homeopathic medicines. The development of multiple large and more pragmatically oriented clinical trials would make it possible to make viable effectiveness comparisons between specific patient groups. Additionally, it will permit to compare the resulting benefit to the avoidance of side effects in the case of homeopathic medicines.

Also, the enrichment of the quality of life questionnaires comprising such items in order to measure the potential benefits of homeopathy as claimed by homeopaths, including stess and control management and life attitude will be very useful in that they helped surface the effects of homeopathic treatments in the well being of citizens. Only by taking into consideration all the specific parameters we may a arrive at strong conclusions for the efficiency of homeopathy.

On a next stage the dimarginalization of homeopathy practitioners and the use of homeopathic treatments by all doctors in the fields where their efficiency would have been proven, would lead to optimization of medical practices for the benefit of society.

Author details

Vilelmine Carayanni
Technological Educational Institute of Athens, Greece

Acknowledgement

The author would like to thank Dr Spyros Diamantides and Dr Persa Kyvelou for her significant assistance in writing this paper.

7. References

[1] OECD , Health Data, OECD Editions ;2011
[2] Nahin, Richard et al. "Cost of Complementary and Alternative Medicine (CAM) and The Frequency of Visits to CAM practitioners: United States, 2007." National Health Statistics Report, 18:4 ;2009.
[3] CAMDOC Alliance. The regulatory status of Complementary and Alternative Medicine for medical doctors in Europe, http://www.camdoc.eu/Pdf/CAMDOCRegulatoryStatus8_10.pdf (accessed 8 June 2012).
[4] Herman P, Craig B., Caspi O., Is complementary and alternative medicine (CAM) cost-effective? a systematic review, Complementary and Alternative Medicine 2005;5-11.
[5] ECHAMP, The science of Homeopathy, http://www.alternative- training.com/docs/Blog/LUC_MONTAGNIER.pdf (accessed 8 February 2012)
[6] Benveniste, Jacques (2005) Ma vérité sur la 'mémoire de l'eau', Albin Michel; 2005.
[7] Official Homeopathy Resource, New Research From Aerospace Institute of the University of Stuttgart Scientifically Proves Water Memory and Homeopathy, http://homeopathyresource.wordpress.com/2011/12/28/new-research-from-aerospace-institute-of-the-university-of-stuttgart-scientifically-proves-water-memory-and-homeopathy/ (accessed 8 June 2012).
[8] Demangeat JL, Gries P, Poitevin B, Droesbeke JJ, Zahaf T, Maton F, Pierart C, Muller RN Low-field NMR water proton longitudinal relaxation in ultra-highly diluted aqueous solutions of silica-lactose prepared in glass material for pharmaceutical use. Appl Magn Reson 2004;26 465–481.
[9] Elia V, Niccoli M New physico-chemical properties of water induced by mechanical treatments. A calorimetric study at 25°C. J Thermal Analysis Calorimetry 2000; 61 527–537.

[10] Wolf U. et al. "Effectiveness, Safety and Cost Effectiveness of Homeopathy Practise" Forschende 2006;13.2:19-29.

[11] Linde K, Clausius N, Ramirez G, Melchart D, Eitel F, Hedges LV, Jonas WB Are the effects of homeopathy placebo effects? A meta-analysis of randomized, placebo controlled trials Lancet 1997 350 834–843.

[12] Righetti m., Baumgartne S., Ammon k. Homeopathy: Research and Research Problems (preclinical and clinical) In: Bornhöft, Gudrun; Matthiessen, Peter (Ed) Homeopathy in Healthcare Effectiveness, Appropriateness, Safety, Costs. Springer; 2012. p16-22.

[13] Bastide M, Doucet-Jaboeuf M, Daurat V (Action immunopharmacologique des preparations de thymus et d'hormone thymique utilisees a doses infinitesimales. Homeopathie Francaise1983;71v 185–189.

[14] Endler PC, Ludtke R, Heckmann C, Zausner C, Lassnig H, Scherer-Pongratz W, Haidvogl M, Frass M Pretreatment with thyroxine (10-(8) parts by weight) enhances a 'curative' effect of homeopathically prepared thyroxine (10-(13)) on lowland frogs. Forschende Komplementarmedizin und Klassische Naturheilkunde 2003; 137–142.

[15] Youbicier-Simo BJ, Boudard F, Mekaouche M, Bayle JD, Bastide M A role for bursa fabricii and bursin in the ontogeny of the pineal biosynthetic activity in the chicken. J Pineal Res 1996;21:35–43.

[16] Bellavite P, Ortolani R, Conforti ‧ Immunology and Homeopathy. 3. Experimental Studies on Animal Models, Evid Based Complement Alternat Med. 2006 ; 3(2) 171–186.

[17] Shang, A., Huwiler-Müntener K, Nartey L, Jüni P, Dörig S, Sterne JA, Pewsner D, Egger M. Are the clinical effects of homeopathy placebo effects? Comparative study of placebo-controlled trials of homeopathy and allopathy Lancet 2005; 366 726-732.

[18] Glaser, R Stress-associated immune dysregulation and its importance for human health: a personal history of psychoneuroimmunology' Brain, Behavior and Immunity 2005; 19 3-11.

[19] Lovallo, W.R. & W. Gerin 'Psychophysiological reactivity: mechanisms and pathways to cardiovascular disease' Psychosomatic Medicine, 2003;65 36-45.

[20] Kienle, G.S. & H. Kiene 'The powerful placebo effect: fact or fiction?' Journal of Clinical Epidemiology 1997; 50:1311-1318.

[21] European Network for Homeopathy Researchers (ENHRAn Overview of Positive Homeopathy Research and Surveys (http://hpathy.com/scientific-research/an-overview-of-positive (accessed 8 February 2012)

[22] Jonas W., Anderson R, Crawford C, Lyons J. A systematic review of the quality of homeopathic clinical trials BMC Complementary and Alternative Medicine 2001, 1-12.

[23] Tsang R, Colley L, Lynd LD J Clin Epidemiol. Inadequate statistical power to detect clinically significant differences in adverse event rates in randomized controlled trials.2009 ;62(6):609-616

[24] Hu JK, Chen ZX, Zhou ZG, Zhang B, Tian J, Chen JP, Wang L, Wang CH, Chen HY, Li YP Intravenous chemotherapy for resected gastric cancer: meta-analysis of randomized controlled trials. World J Gastroenterol 2002 ; 8(6) 1023-1028

[25] Wassenhoven Van M. and Ives Geoffrey "An Observational Study of Patients Receiving Homeopathic Treatment" Homeopathy 2004; 93 3-11.

[26] Rossi E, Crudeli L, Endrizzi C. and Garibaldi D."Cost-Benefit Evaluation of Homeopathy versus Conventional Therapy in Respiratory Diseases" Homeopathy 2009; 98 2-10.

[27] Ullman D. Homeopathic perspectives on infectious diseases, http://www.homeopathic.com/Articles/Using_homeopathy_for_ailments/A_Homeopathic_Perspective_on_Infectious_Dise.html (accessed12 May 2012)

[28] Global TGI Barometer, TGI; 2008.

[29] Complementary Medicines – UK Mintel;2007.

[30] ECHAMP's Facts & Figures, 2nd Ed ECHAMP; 2007

[31] Comparatif Mutuelle et Assurance Complémentaire Santé, L'homéopathie séduit de plus en plus de Français http://www.devismutuelle.com/article/267-l-homeopathie-seduit-la-france (accessed 8 June 2012)

[32] British Homeopathic Association, Popularity and the market place, http://www.britishhomeopathic.org/media_centre/facts_about_homeopathy/popularity_and_market_place.html (accessed 12 May 2012)

[33] Bundesverband der Pharmazeutischen Industrie e.V., Pharma-Daten 2007 http://whqlibdoc.who.int/hq/2001/WHO_EDM_TRM_2001.2.pdf. (accessed 12-6-2012)

[34] Legal Status of Traditional Medicine and Complementary/Alternative Medicine: A Worldwide Review" (PDF). World Health Organization. World Health Organization; 2001.

[35] Dacey J (14 January 2011). "Alternative therapies are put to the test". swissinfo.ch. (accessed 12 July 2012)

[36] French Government Report: Social Security Statistics, CNAM (National Inter-Regulations System) 61;1991

[37] Bornhöft G, Wolf U, Ammon K, Righetti M, Maxion-Bergemann S, Baumgartner S, Thurneysen AE, Matthiessen PF. Effectiveness, safety and cost-effectiveness of homeopathy in general practice – summarized health technology assessment. Forsch Komplementärmed 2006;13(suppl 2) 19-29

[38] Centre fédéral d'expertise des soins de santé Etat des lieux de lieux de l'homéopathie en Belgique KCE reports 154B https://kce.fgov.be/sites/default/files/page_documents/kce_154b_homeopathie_en_belgique.pdf (accessed 7 February 2012)

[39] Marstedt G, Moebus S Gesundheitsberichterstattung des Bundes Heft 9: Inanspruchnahme alternative Methoden in der Medizin. 2002; Verlag Robert Koch Institut, Berlin

[40] House of Commons Science and Technology Committee Evidence Check 2: Homeopathy Fourth Report of Session 2009–10 http://www.publications.parliament.uk/pa/cm200910/cmselect/cmsctech/45/45.pdf

[41] DRAFT NHMRC Public Statement on Homeopathy

http://images.theage.com.au/file/2012/03/14/3125800/Homeopathy%2520statement.pdf (access d 8 May 2012)
[42] SANTE CANADA Programme de recherche sur les produits de santé naturels Table ronde sur invitation dans le cadre d'une consultation sur l'établissement des priorités de recherche en médecine http://www.hc-sc.gc.ca/dhp-mps/pubs/natur/2008-nhprp_prpsn/index-fra.php (accessed 5 February 2012)
[43] Caisse Nationale de l'Assurance Maladie des Travailleurs Salaries, Rapport, 1996;CNAM
[44] Swayne, J. The cost and effectiveness of homeopathy. Br Homeopath J 1992; 81 148-150
[45] Smallhood C. The role of complementary and alternative medicine in the NHS http://www.getwelluk.com/uploadedFiles/Publications/SmallwoodReport.pdf (accesed 12 May 2012)
[46] Ramsey S, Willke R, Briggs A, Brown R, Buxton M, Chawla A,Cook J, Glick H, Liljas B, Petitti D, Reed S:Good research practicesfor cost-effectiveness analysis alongside clinical trials: theISPOR RCT-CEA Task Force report. Value Health 2005; 8 521–533
[47] Drummond MF, Jefferson TO, BMJ Economic Evaluation Working Party: Guidelines for authors and peer reviewers of economic submissions to the BMJ. BMJ 1996, 313:275-283.
[48] Polsky D, Doshi JA, Bauer MS, Glick HA. Clinical Trial-Based Cost-Effectiveness Analyses of Antipsychotic Use, Am J Psychiatry 2006;163:12.
[49] Paul A. Pirraglia, M.D., M.P.H.; Allison B. Rosen, M.D., M.P.H.; Richard C. Hermann, M.D., M.S.; Natalia V. Olchanski, M.S.; Peter Neumann, Sc.D. Cost-Utility Analysis Studies of Depression Management: A Systematic Review Am J Psychiatry 2004;161 2155-2162.
[50] Drummond MF, O'Brien B, Stoddart GL, Torrance GW: Methods for the economic evaluation of health care programmes .Second edition. Oxford, Oxford University Press; 1997:305.
[51] Center for Reviews and Dissemination http://www.york.ac.uk/inst/crd/index.htm (accessed 12 June 2012)
[52] Paterson C, Ewings P, Brazier J E, Britten N. Treating dyspepsia with acupuncture and homeopathy: reflections on a pilot study by researchers, practitioners and participants. Complementary Therapies in Medicine 2003; 11(2) 78-84 50.
[53] Kneis K C, Gandjour A Economic evaluation of Sinfrontal ® in the treatment of acute maxillary sinusitis in adults, Applied Health Econ Health Policy 2009; 7 (3): 181-191.
[54] Thompson EA, Shaw A, Nichol J, Hollinghurst S, Henderson AJ, Thompson T, Sharp D.The feasibility of a pragmatic randomised controlled trial to compare usual care with usual care plus individualised homeopathy, in children requiring secondary care for asthma. Homeopathy 2011; 100(3): 122-130.
[55] Chouinard G et al. A Canadian multicenter placebo-controlled study of fixed doses of risperidone and haloperidol in the treatment of chronic schizophrenic patients. Journal of Clinical Psychopharmacology 1993;13:25-40.

[56] Tunis S L, Johnstone B M, Gibson P J, Loosbrock D L, Dulisse B K. Changes in perceived health and functioning as a cost-effectiveness measure for olanzapine versus haloperidol treatment of schizophrenia. Journal of Clinical Psychiatry 1999; 60(Supplement 19): 38-45.

[57] Rosenheck R, Cramer J, Xu W, Grabowski J, Douyon R, Thomas J, Henderson W, Charney D. Multiple outcome assessment in a study of the cost-effectiveness of clozapine in the treatment of refractory schizophrenia. Health Services Research 1998; 33(5) 1237-1267.

[58] Rosenheck R, Cramer J, Allan E, Erdos J, Frisman L K, Xu W C, Thomas J, Henderson W, Charney D. Cost-effectiveness of clozapine in patients with high and low levels of hospital use. Archives of General Psychiatry 1999; 56(6) 565-572.

[59] Hamilton S H, Revicki D A, Edgell E T, Genduso L A, Tollefson G. Clinical and economic outcomes of olanzapine compared with haloperidol for schizophrenia: results from a randomised clinical trial. Pharmacoeconomics 1999; 15(5) 469-480.

[60] Essock S M, Frisman L K, Covell N H, Hargreaves W A. Cost-effectiveness of clozapine compared with conventional antipsychotic medication for patients in state hospitals. Archives of General Psychiatry 2000; 57(10) 987-994.

[61] Jerrell J M. Cost-effectiveness of risperidone, olanzapine, and conventional antipsychotic medications. Schizophrenia Bulletin 2002; 28(4) 589-605.

[62] Rosenheck R, Perlick D, Bingham S et al, Effectiveness and cost of olanzapine and haloperidol in the treatment of schizophrenia: a randomized controlled trial. JAMA 2003; 290(20) 2693-2670.

[63] Thorpe KE, Zwarenstein M, Oxman AD, et al. A pragmatic–explanatory continuum indicator summary (PRECIS): a tool to help trial designers. J Clin Epidemiol 2009; 62 464-75.

[64] Carayanni V, and Tsati E: Explanatory versus pragmatic trial-based economic evaluations: application to alternative therapies for burns Expert Rev. Pharmacoeconomics Outcomes Res. 2010; 10(1) 37–48

[65] CONSORT 2010 Statement: updated guidelines for reporting parallel group randomised trials BMJ 2010;340 available at: http://www.bmj.com/content/340/bmj.c332.full (accessed 23 Mars 2010).

[66] Stagnara J., Demonceaux A., Vainchtock A., Nicoloyannis N., Duru G. Etude sur la prise en charge de la bronchiolite du nourrisson en médecine ambulatoire. Etude observationnelle prospective à propos de 520 patients. Le Pédiatre 2004; (204),1-7

[67] Vainchtock A., Dansette G.Y., Nicoloyannis N., Duru G., Chaufferin G., Lamarsalla L. Medico economic evaluation of anxiety disorders management in outpatient care. Health and System Science 2000; 4 103-115.

[68] Trichard M, Chaufferin G, Nicoloyannis N. Pharmacoeconomic comparison between homeopathic and antibiotic treatment strategies in recurrent acute rhinopharyngitis in children. Homeopathy 2005 94(1):3-9.

[69] Witt C, Keil T, Selim D, Roll S, Vance W, Wegscheider K, Willich SN. Outcome and costs of homoeopathic and conventional treatment strategies: A comparative cohort study in patients with chronic disorders. Complementary Therapies in Medicine 2005; 13, 79-86

[70] Witt C M, Brinkhaus B, Pach D, Reinhold T, Wruck K, Roll S, Jäckel T, Staab D, Wegscheider K, Willich S N Homoeopathic versus conventional therapy for atopic eczema in children: medical and economic results, Dermatology 2009; 219 (4) 329-340.

[71] Revicki DA, Brown RE, Palmer W, Bakish D, Rosser WW, Anton SF, Feeny D: Modelling the cost effectiveness of antidepressant treatment in primary care. Pharmacoeconomics 1995; 8 524–540

[72] Lave J R, Frank R G, Schulberg H C, Kamlet M Cost-effectiveness of treatments for major depression in primary care practice. Archives of General Psychiatry 1998; 55(7) 645-651

[73] Schoenbaum M, Unutzer J, Sherbourne C, Duan N, Rubenstein L V, Miranda J, Meredith L S, Carney M F, Wells K. Cost-effectiveness of practice-initiated quality improvement for depression. JAMA 2001; 286(11) 1325-1330

[74] Valenstein M, Vijan S, Zeber J E, Boehm K, Buttar A. The cost-utility of screening for depression in primary care. Annals of Internal Medicine 2001; 134(5) 345-360

[75] Kamlet M S, Paul N, Greenhouse J, Kupfer D, Frank E, Wade M. Cost utility analysis of maintenance treatment for recurrent depression. Controlled Clinical Trials 1995; 16 17-40.

[76] Gournay K, Brooking J. The community psychiatric nurse in primary care: an economic analysis. Journal of Advanced Nursing 1995; 22 769-778.

[77] Revicki D A, Brown R E, Keller M B, Gonzales J, Culpepper L, Hales R E. Cost-effectiveness of newer antidepressants compared with tricyclic antidepressants in managed care settings. Journal of Clinical Psychiatry 1997; 58(2) 47-58.

[78] Hatziandreu E J, Brown R E, Revicki D A, Turner R, Martindale J, Levine S, Siegel J E. Cost utility of maintenance treatment of recurrent depression with sertraline versus episodic treatment with dothiepin. Pharmacoeconomics 1994; 5(3) 249-264.

[79] Nuijten MJ: Assessment of clinical guidelines for continuation treatment in major depression. Value Health 2001; 4 281–294.

[80] Agresti A. Categorical Data Analysis (2nd edn). Wiley: Hoboken, NJ;2002

[81] Moher D, Liberati A, Tetzlaff J, Altman DG, The PRISMA Group Preferred Reporting Items for Systematic Reviews and Meta-Analyses: The PRISMA Statement. PLoS Med 6(6): e1000097 2009; doi:10.1371/journal.pmed1000097

[82] MF Drummond. Experimental versus Observational Data in the Economic Evaluation of Pharmaceuticals. Med. Decis. Making 1998; 18 (S12 - S18)

[83] Shemilt I., Mugford M., Vale Luke, Kevin Marsh, Donaldson C., Evidence –Based Decisions and Economics. Health Care, Social Welfare, Education and Criminal Justice, Second Edition, BMJI Books, Wiley-Blackwell;2010.

[84] Piantadosi S. Clinical trials, a methodological perspective, 2nd Edition, Wiley Series in Probability and Statistics, Wiley; 2006.

[85] Fragkakis M. and Alexandris N. Outline of a trust and security model for multi-agent system platforms Advances in Computer Science and Engineering 2010; 6(1), 57 - 71

Section 2

Diagnostic Resources

Chapter 4

Review of Traditional Chinese Medicine Pulse Diagnosis Quantification

Anson Chui Yan Tang

Additional information is available at the end of the chapter

http://dx.doi.org/10.5772/50442

1. Introduction

Traditional Chinese medicine (tcm) pulse diagnosis is one of the four major assessments in tcm consultation. Through pulse palpation at three locations, i.e. cun, guan and chi, on both wrists, general health condition of a person and a particular organ can be fully recognized. Figure 1 illustrates the locations and their corresponding organs. tcm doctor is used to combine clinical data collected from pulse assessment and other clinical assessments to prescribe treatments to his patient and monitor his prognosis.

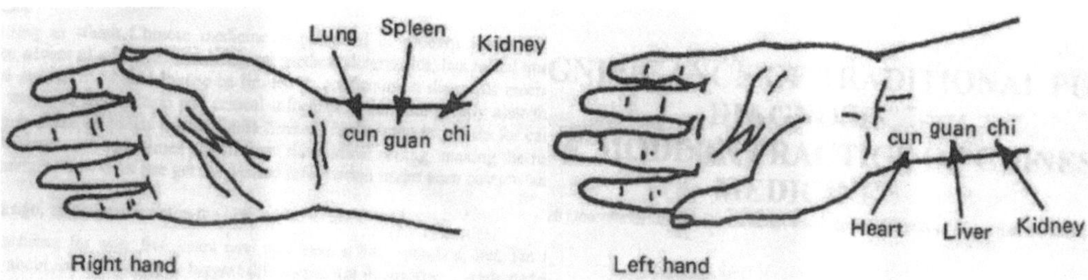

Figure 1. Distribution of organs at the six locations (Adapted from [1])

In view of the increasing popularity of tcm world wide, tcm pulse diagnosis has received much attention from the public concerning its scientific and clinical values. Much research work has been published since 1950s' to quantify tcm pulse diagnosis which aims at providing scientific base to tcm pulse diagnosis and so substantiating its clinical value. The aim of this review is to provide readers with a complete picture of current progression of tcm pulse quantification.

After reading this chapter, readers should be able to

1. acquire up-to-date scientific evidence on tcm pulse diagnosis quantification;

2. analyze strengths and weaknesses of current studies in terms of methodologies and statistical approaches; and
3. highlight future direction of tcm pulse diagnosis quantification.

The review is divided into five sections. The first three sections discuss and analyze qualification and quantification of tcm pulse diagnosis in ancient and recent literatures. Statistical approaches to quantify tcm pulse diagnosis are discussed. Section four presents a tcm pulse diagnostic framework proposed by the author in 2010 to illustrate the interrelationship of pulse conditions and arterial pulse. The last section highlights limitations of current studies and recommendations are suggested accordingly.

2. Qualification of tcm pulse diagnosis

Qualification of tcm pulse diagnosis means the elements that tcm pulse diagnosis should be included in order to have a complete and valid assessment on tcm pulse. Literatures show that there is much confusion about the assessment of pulse in tcm, mainly due to the ambiguous descriptions of pulse condition in Chinese medical texts [1].

Pulse itself is objective, but pulse condition is subjective. It is the quality of pulse as felt by a tcm doctor, and thus represents the subjective judgment of that doctor. More than 30 pulse conditions have been documented in Chinese medical texts. Some of them, e.g. floating, rapid, string-like are single pulse condition which describes one element of a pulse condition. Others describe more than one element of a pulse condition which is called compound pulse condition. For example, replete is the composite of forceful, long, large and stiff [2].

2.1. Description of pulse condition in ancient Chinese medical texts

Nei Jing [3] describes over 30 types, e.g. large, small, long, short, slippery, rough, sunken, slow, rapid, strong, tough, soft, moderate, hurried, vacuous, replete, scattered, intermittent, fine, and weak. Mai Jing [4] documents 24 types which are floating, sunken, hollow, large, small, skipping, tight, rapid, stirred, slippery, weak, string-like, faint, soft, dissipated, moderate, slow, bound, drumskin, replete, intermittent, vacuous, rough and hidden. The 28 pulse conditions most commonly used in clinical practice come from Bin Hu Mai Xue [5] and Zhen Jia Zhen Gyan [6]. They are floating, sunken, slow, rapid, surging, fine, vacuous, replete, long, short, slippery, rough, string-like, tight, soggy, moderate, faint, weak, dissipated, hollow, drumskin, firm, hidden, stirred, intermittent, bound, skipping, and racing.

Descriptions of pulse conditions in Chinese medical texts are mostly qualitative, and are often illustrated by similes and poems. For instance, the slippery is compared to "beads rolling" and the string-like is like pressing the string of a musical instrument [5]. A few of the descriptions, such as the rapid, the slow, the floating, and the sunken, are quantitative. The rapid and the slow describe the rate of a pulse, and can be quantified by the number of beats per breath. The floating and the sunken describe the depth of a pulse, and can be quantified by shu, the unit of weight used during the Warring States period (403-221BC) of ancient China, with floating corresponding to three shu and sunken nine shu [7].

Using analogies and poems to describe pulse condition is subject to the interpretation of the tcm doctor. For example, the string-like may be described as like pressing the string of a musical instrument and the tight as like pressing a rope, but the feeling of a string or a rope depends on the sensitivity of one's fingers. Qualifying words such as "a bit," "average," and "very" are used to describe the intensity of a pulse. For example, the difference between the fine and the faint is that the fine is a little bit stronger than the faint. "A little" is countable, but cannot precisely determine how much of this "little" differentiates the fine from the faint.

Descriptions of pulse conditions also overlap [8,9]. Some pulse conditions describe a single dimension of pulse. The floating, for example, describes the depth of a pulse, whereas the rapid describes the rate of a pulse. Others describe two or more dimensions. The firm means string-like, long, replete, surging, and sunken, whereas the drumskin is string-like, large, rapid, and hollow. The number of dimensions that a pulse assessment should encompass is controversial. Floating or sunken and slow or rapid are the two pairs of dimensions suggested in Bin Hu Mai Xue [5]. Nan Jing [7] and Mai Jing [4], in contrast, proposed three dimensions: floating or sunken, slippery or rough, and long or short. Nei Jing [3] described three dimensions: slippery or rough, slow or rapid, and surging or fine, whereas [2] suggested floating or sunken, slow or rapid, and vacuous or replete.

It is suggested that there are two reasons for the obscurity of descriptions of pulse condition. First, tcm doctors are accustomed to assessing pulse by their own perception, rather than on a rational basis [10]. Second, there are no concise and precise standards to guide tcm doctors in the diagnosis of pulse condition. It is likely that these two reasons are the causes of the low inter-rater and intra-rater reliability of pulse diagnosis by tcm doctors found by Craddock (1997) and Krass (1990) (as cited in [11]). As evidence-based practice emphasizes consistency of outcome [12], the low reliability of pulse diagnosis by tcm doctors reported in the literature demonstrates the need to standardize pulse diagnosis in tcm.

2.2. Eight elements: Milestone for standardizing tcm pulse diagnosis qualification

Zhou Xuehai's (1856-1906) early attempt to standardize pulse condition is a milestone in the quantification of tcm pulse diagnosis. He proposed that each pulse condition should have four elements. "Wei Shu Xing Shi Zhe, Zheng Mai Zhi Ti Wang. Qiu Ming Mai Li Zhe, Xu Xian Jiang Wei Shu Xing Shi Jiang De Zhen Qie, Ge Zhong Mai Xiang Liao Ran, Bu Bi Ju Ni Mai Ming" (as cited in [13], p. 31). He explicitly stated that position, frequency, shape, and trend are the four main elements of pulse condition, and that each pulse condition description should contain these four elements.

Various scholars have elaborated on this idea [2,14-18], and have extended the original four elements to eight: depth, rate, regularity, width, length, smoothness, stiffness, and strength.

Each pulse condition should contain these eight elements with different intensities [2,15,17,18].

Rate is the number of beats per breath. The definition of regularity is similar to that in modern medicine, it describes rhythm of a pulse condition. Rate and regularity gives information on the nature of a disease, whether heat or cold [19]. Depth is defined as the vertical position of a pulse, and indicates the location of a disease, whether interior or exterior [19]. Width and length describe the shape of a pulse, where width is defined as the intensity of a pulsation and length is defined as the range in which the pulsation can be sensed across the cun, guan, and chi [2]. Smoothness is defined as the slickness of a pulse, stiffness is defined as the sensation of arterial elasticity, and strength is defined as the change in forcefulness of a pulse in response to a change of applied pressure [19]. Width, length, smoothness, stiffness, and strength also describe the interaction of a pathogen and healthy qi in the body [2]. The eight elements thus provide a basis for qualifying pulse condition.

2.3. Recent works on qualifying tcm pulse diagnosis

King et al. (2002) [11] developed a measurement scale to standardize tcm pulse diagnosis. However, their scale does not reflect pulse condition adequately for several reasons. First, the six items included in the scale –depth, width, force, relative force, rhythm, and pulse occlusion –are not widely accepted as core items in tcm pulse diagnosis. Appropriate rating scales should include the six locations, as a complete tcm pulse diagnosis must include the eight elements at the six locations. Second, the definitions of the items are abstract. For example, force is defined as the overall intensity of a pulse and relative force is defined as a subtler version with overall force. Third, the scale is an ordinal scale that is anchored with descriptors to measure the items. For example, depth is measured at three levels: superficial, middle, and deep. However, an ordinal scale is not a sufficiently sensitive measure, as there are an insufficient number of available response categories to rate the items [20], and the words used to describe each ordinal level are not universal. Further, as the items have not been well quantified, using an ordinal scale would not reflect the actual sensation perceived by a tcm doctor.

To explore the uniqueness of each of the eight elements in tcm pulse diagnosis, Tang (2010) [21] used principal component analysis to explore the uniqueness of each of the eight elements in tcm pulse diagnosis. The result demonstrated that rate, regularity, width and smoothness represented four unique dimensions while it was not the case for depth, length, stiffness and strength.

The author believes that an appropriate content and rating scale must be chosen to measure pulse condition which should be relevant and should adhere to the fundamental concepts of pulse diagnosis in tcm. Since only a handful of studies have been conducted to qualify pulse condition, a rating scale which can genuinely reflect the sensation of pulse perceived by a tcm doctor should be used to minimize the influence of subjective judgment on a rating scale at a preliminary stage of qualification.

3. Quantification of tcm pulse diagnosis

In the qualification of pulse condition, the eight elements are measured unidimensionally. It is hypothesized that the eight elements are related to the arterial pressure waveform and that their intensity is a composite of the physical parameters of the arterial pressure waveform. Relating the eight elements to these physical parameters would thus make them quantitively measurable. Much research has been carried out on the quantification of pulse condition. Measurement of the arterial pressure waveform in the time domain and frequency domain are the two main approaches currently used, but due to the disparity of research aims, methodologies, and statistical approaches, the results of existing studies in this area are incomparable.

3.1. Time domain

The time domain is widely used in cardiovascular research [22] and is also popularly used in the quantification of pulse condition [23]. Time domain analysis looks at the arterial pressure waveform with respect to time, and a time domain graph shows how the arterial pressure waveform changes over time. Figure 2 shows a typical arterial pressure waveform.

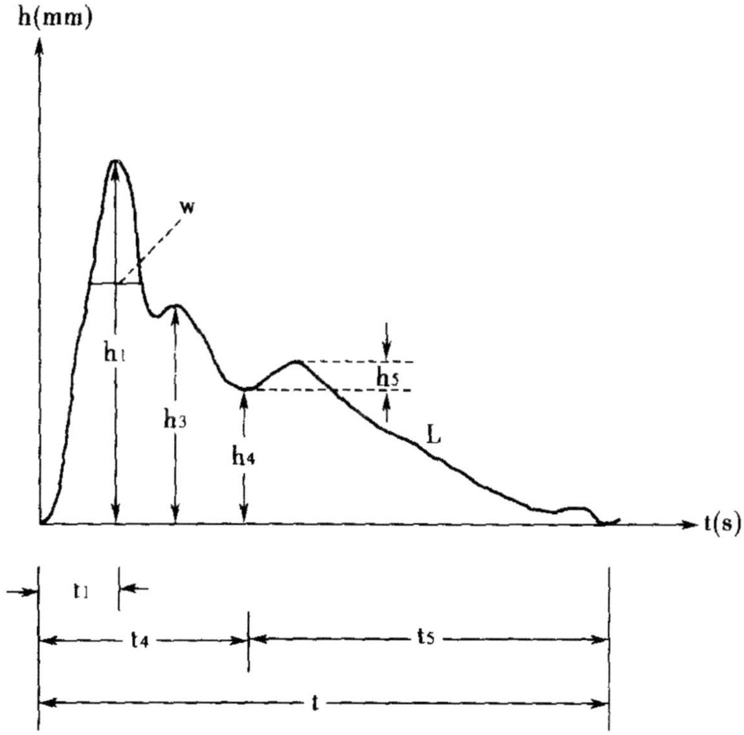

Figure 2. A typical arterial pressure waveform (Adapted from [2], p.163)

In time domain, researchers extracted physical parameters from the arterial pressure waveform, such as h_1, h_3, and generate new parameters from them. Yoon et al. (2000) [24]

proposed three parameters to measure depth, width, and strength. Depth was measured by the hold-down pressure with the relatively largest h_1 (Pamax). The maximum average h_1 (h_1) was used to quantify width, and strength was measured by the pressure difference at the 80% maximum average h_1 (Δ80%pamax). These three parameters have gained some acceptance as standard parameters for the measurement of depth, width, and strength [2,14].

The advantage of using the time domain for the quantification of pulse condition is that most of the physical parameters related to it have physiological meanings. Exploring their relationship with the eight elements should thus help to understand the elements from a modern medical perspective.

Many studies have demonstrated the association between the physical parameters of the arterial pressure waveform in time domain and the eight elements [2,13,24-31]. Depth has been associated with pamax, rate with t, and regularity with the interval between two individual arterial pressure waveforms and the consistency of the contour of the waveforms. Width has been associated with h_4/h_1, t_1, and h_1. The surging has been found to have a smaller h_4/h_1 and t_1 and a larger h_1. Length has been associated with h_1 at cun, guan, and chi. The short was observed to have small h_1, although association with the other physical parameters in the arterial pressure waveform was indiscernible. Smoothness has been related to W/t, h_4/h_1, t_1, h_5, and h_5/h_1. A smaller h_4/h_1 and a larger h_5 have been observed for the slippery, and h_3/h_1, h_4/h_1, and h_5/h_1 are associated with stiffness. A larger h_3/h_1 and h_4/h_1, and a smaller h_5/h_1 have been observed for the string-like. Four types of arterial pressure waveform have been identified for the string-like: lower h_1 than h_3, h_3 equal to h_1, h_3 higher than h_1, and h_3 merged with h_1. Strength is associated with a Δ80% pamax. Some of these observations have been explained in terms of hemodynamic, For example, the string-like was found to be caused by an increase in arterial stiffness and peripheral resistance, whereas width was determined by blood velocity, cardiac output, peripheral resistance, the diameter of the radial artery, and the spatial movement of the radial artery. Length has been related to the rate of arterial dilatation.

The incongruence of the results of these studies means that their postulations cannot be substantiated. Fei (2003) [2] reported that the superficial and deep levels of depth ranged from 25 to 175g and 100 to 250g, respectively. According to Xu et al. (2003) [27], the range of the superficial, middle, and deep levels was smaller than 100g, 100-200g, and greater than 200g, respectively. In these studies, depth is reported as a unit of force, whereas in other studies report as a unit of pressure [25,26]. Huang and Sun (1995) [26] reported that the superficial, middle, and deep levels ranged from 10 to 40 mmHg, from 50 to 80 mmHg, and 90-120 mmHg respectively, whereas Chen (2008) [25] reported ranges of 89.8 to 157.7 mmHg, 151.9 to 222.9 mmHg, and 279.3 mmHg for the superficial, middle, and deep levels, respectively. In terms of smoothness, Huang and Sun (1995) [26] characterized the slippery as having t_1 within the range of 0.07 to 0.09s, h_5 larger than 2 mm, obvious h_3, and h_4/h_1 smaller than 0.50, whereas Fei (2003) [2] found that the slippery was characterized as having W/t smaller than 0.20, an h_4/h_1 smaller than 0.40, and h_5/h_1larger than 0.10.

There appear to be four reasons for such inconsistency. First, none of the studies reports the surface area of the sensor used. As force varies with the surface area of a sensor with the same hold-down pressure, the lack of this information makes the results incomparable. Second, the characteristics of the subjects in the studies may have affected the results. Age, gender, and weight are all factors that affect pulse condition [2,26], yet these studies report no demographic data on the subjects. Hence, it is not possible to rule out that the incongruence is due to the diversity of the subjects. Third, there is no protocol that standardizes the pulse acquisition procedure, and few of the studies reported the procedure that they used to acquire the waveform. To mimic a tcm pulse assessment, the arterial pressure waveform is acquired with different hold-down pressure applied to the radial artery. Two procedures for pulse acquisition are known. Huang (2007) [13] developed a formula to calculate how much hold-down pressure should be used for the superficial, middle, deep, and hidden levels of depth in women and men. He also proposed that the ratio of actual body weight over ideal body weight is the determinant of the hold-down pressure (Table 1).

(Actual weight)/(Ideal weight)	**Hold-down Pressure at Different Levels of Depth**			
	Superficial	Middle	Deep	Hidden
< 0.8	50g	100g	200g	300g
0.8 – 1.0	70g	130g	250g	400g
1.0 – 1.2	100g	180g	300g	450g
> 1.2	150g	230g	350g	550g

Table 1. Weight ratio and corresponding hold-down pressure

Although several studies have adopted this protocol to acquire the waveform [28,32,33], the rationale for quantifying depth in this way is not explicated, and its credibility is thus suspect. The other procedure is that of Fei (2003) [2], who applied pressure from 0 g to 250 g at 50g intervals for each pulse acquisition. However, the interval of 50 g may be too wide, and does not allow for any change in the waveform within this interval.

Fourth, there is no standard measurement for the eight elements. The majority of the aforementioned studies focused on pulse condition rather than the eight elements. However, as each pulse condition embraces all eight elements with different intensities, even if the other seven elements have the same intensity, variation in one element will lead to a different waveform for the same pulse condition. Moreover, the sensation of a tcm doctor to the eight elements has not been standardized, and variation among the tcm doctors participating in the studies will inevitably have led to different results.

3.2. Frequency domain

The frequency domain can be used to analyze pulse condition based on the energy distribution of the arterial pressure waveform [34]. A frequency domain graph comprises two parts –amplitude versus frequency and phase versus frequency – and is converted from the time domain of the arterial pressure waveform using a transform, which is a pair of mathematical operators used to carry out a conversion. Fast Fourier transform is an example of a commonly used transform in signal processing. Usually, the amplitude versus frequency graph is examined in studies of pulse condition. A graph showing only the amplitude and frequency is called a power spectrum (Figure 3).

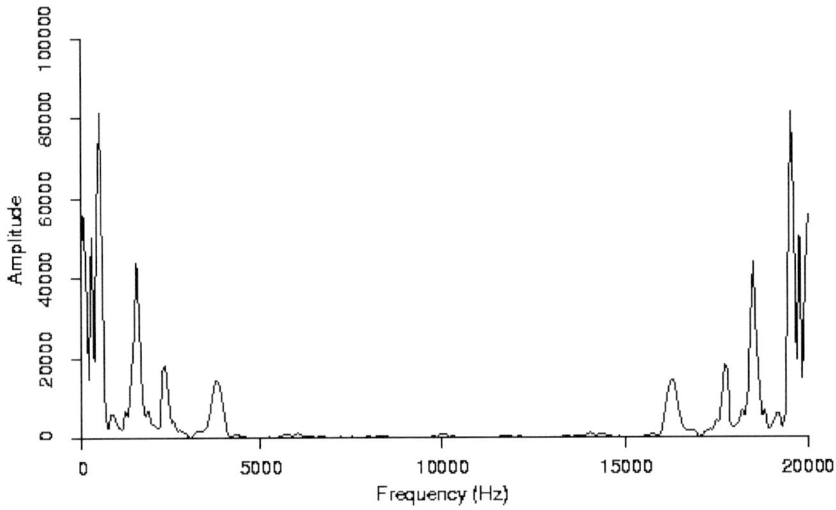

Figure 3. Example of a power spectrum (Adapted from [34])

The y-axis of a power spectrum graph, which is labelled "amplitude" represents the power of the frequency, whereas the x-axis shows the "frequency" in Hertz (Hz). A harmonic is the frequency component of an arterial pressure waveform.

The majority of the studies that use the frequency domain to analyze the arterial pulse have focused on differentiating diseases [35-37], examining the power spectrum in relation to the meridians [38,39], and investigating the relationship among disease, syndrome, and channels [23,40-43,45]. Only a few studies have explored the characteristics of the power spectrum for different pulse conditions [46,47].

Wang and Xiang (1998) [46] discovered that the power spectrum differed markedly for the normal, the slippery, the string-like, and the slow-intermittent. In general, the power spectrum of all pulse conditions decreased with increasing frequency and the frequency range was within 0 to 40Hz. However, the power spectrum of the normal was smoother than that of the other three pulse conditions. The slippery had more than ten harmonics, whereas the normal had eight harmonics. The string-like and the slow-intermittent had three to five harmonics. The frequency of the normal was distributed within the 25Hz range. The percentage of energy distributed below 10Hz was 99% for the normal and 97% for the string-like, and that distributed below 5Hz was 90.2% for the moderate, 83.7% for the slippery, and 60.9% for the string-like. Forty-five percent of the energy was distributed below 1 Hz for the moderate and 16% for the string-like. These findings suggest that the frequency of the normal falls within the 1 to 5Hz range, and those frequencies below 1 Hz and over 10 Hz may indicate illness. Xu et al. (2002) [47] suggested that counting the number of harmonics in the power spectrum could be used to differentiate pulse conditions. Their study reported that the slippery possessed three main harmonics that were much higher than those of the normal, and the drumskin had two main harmonics. The amplitude of the harmonics in the normal decreased with increasing frequency. The reasons for the different results for the slippery are the same as those proposed for the time domain quantification.

Both the time domain and frequency domain are based on the arterial pressure waveform, but differ in the way in which they interpret it. Although the available evidence supporting the applicability of the frequency domain to quantify pulse condition is weaker than that supporting the use of the time domain, this may simply due be to the lack of studies on the frequency domain. However, the time domain is to a certain extent more advantageous than the frequency domain for quantifying pulse condition because the physical parameters in the time domain have physiological meanings, which means that the physiological implications of the eight elements could be revealed if their relationship with these physical parameters were traced. It is thus more prudent and beneficial to adopt the time domain in the quantification of pulse condition.

4. Statistical approaches

Though regression analysis is commonly used in medical research for function approximation and classification [48,49], failure of modelling the relationship of the eight elements and the physical parameters [21] suggested that the relationship is not linear. It has been suggested that more advanced statistical techniques, such as fuzzy inference and artificial neural network (ANN) may be more appropriate for modelling the relationship of the eight elements at the six locations and the physical parameters [50-52].

Fuzzy inference is a modelling technique that is based on fuzzy set theory. Fuzzy set theory deals with the degree of truth in a vaguely defined set, where truth is represented as a value that ranges from 0 to 1. Lee et al. (1993) [53] used fuzzy inference to assess the health state of a subject with renal problems before and after taking herbal medicine. The arterial pressure waveform was acquired at the right chi, and the physical parameters in the time domain were used to construct the fuzzy model. The results showed that the model could successfully predict the prognosis for a patient. The authors thus proposed applying fuzzy inference to assess health status using pulse condition.

ANN is a nonlinear statistical modelling technique commonly used in the modelling of complex nonlinear relationships among independent variables and dependent variables [49,54]. It resembles regression analysis, but has much more flexibility because it is not restricted by any statistical assumptions or prespecified algorithms. In other words, ANN is a self-adaptive and data-driven modelling technique [54,55]. The presence of hidden layers in the network greatly increases its capacity to deal with various complicated relationship. Figure 4 shows the basic architecture of an ANN.

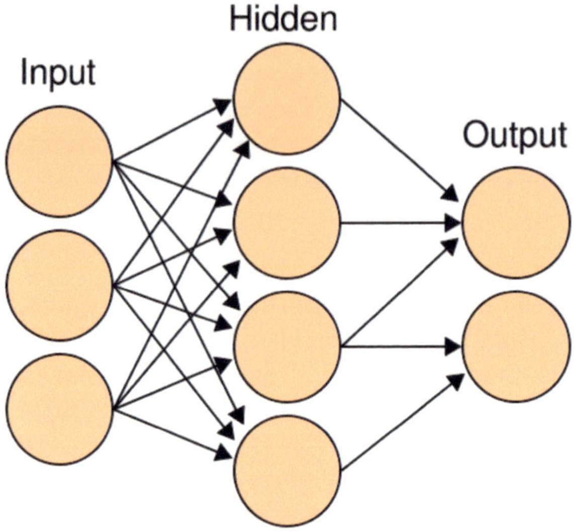

Figure 4. Basic architecture of an ANN (Adapted from [56])

The architecture shown in Figure 4 is commonly used in the type of ANN known as a multilayer perceptron. This consists of an input layer, a hidden layer, and an output layer. The input layer and output layer also appear in the architecture of linear regression, but the distinguishing characteristic of an ANN is the hidden layer in between the input and output layers. The number of hidden layers can be manipulated by the researcher until a satisfactory result is obtained. The input layer contains input neurons, which represent the number of independent variables in the study. The output neurons in the output layer are the dependent variables. The number of hidden neurons in the hidden layer(s) and the number of hidden layers in the model are determined by trial and error using the sum-squared error in function approximation and the cross entropy function in classification. The cross entropy function can be regarded as analogous to the likelihood function in logistic regression [54]. They are the cost functions that determine when to stop training the model.

Backpropagation is the most popular training algorithm for ANNs. This utilizes the steepest gradient descent in a multilayer perceptron to minimize the sum-squared error. The steepest gradient descent is a mathematical algorithm that locates the local minimum of a function by taking steps proportional to the negative of the gradient of the function at the current point. In backpropagation, the weights of the hidden and input neurons are modified according to the sum-squared error fed back from the output neurons until the mean squared error is minimized.

Wang and Xiang (2001) [57] compared the accuracy of fuzzy inference and ANN in predicting pulse condition. They reported the successful application of ANN in identifying the normal, the string-like, the slippery, and the fine, and showed that ANN had a 87% predictive accuracy, which was 12% higher than that of fuzzy inference. Xu et al. (2007) [58] compared the predictive accuracy of traditional ANN and fuzzy neural network in predicting eight pulse conditions. Three traditional ANNs using backpropagation were developed, each of which had 3 layers: an input layer, a hidden layer, and an output layer. The input neurons were seventeen physical parameters of the arterial pressure waveform in the time domain and the output neurons were the eight pulse conditions, which were, however, not specified. The numbers of hidden neurons used in the three traditional ANNs were 10, 15, and 20. The fuzzy neural network was a composite of four sub-fuzzy neural networks, and was used to model seventeen physical parameters and the four elements (position, frequency, shape and trend) proposed by Zhou Xuehai (1856-1906) (as cited in [13]) separately. The four sub-fuzzy neural networks were then combined to predict the eight pulse conditions. The three traditional ANNs obtained 86-88% accuracy, but the fuzzy neural network outperformed these networks by 4%. They concluded that it was beneficial to combine fuzzy inference and ANN to quantify pulse conditions.

The successful application of these advanced statistical techniques for quantifying pulse conditions is encouraging, and at least indicates that the various pulse conditions have a physiological basis. However, medical research emphasizes the explanatory power of a model, and values statistical techniques with a high explanatory power [59-61]. According to these criteria, ANN can be condemned as black box [49], which means that the internal knowledge of the system cannot be readily known by researchers [59].

5. tcm pulse diagnostic framework: Integration of the East and the West

A dice model has been formulated by Tang (2010) [21] to explain the interconnection and interrelation between the arterial pulse and the eight elements of pulse condition at the six locations, and between the eight elements at the six locations and health status in tcm. This framework serves as the backbone to quantify tcm pulse diagnosis.

The dice model comprises two levels. Level one includes the arterial pulse and the eight elements at the six locations, and level two covers the eight elements at the six locations and health status in tcm. More specifically, level one deals with the sensation of the arterial pulse as perceived by a tcm doctor, and level two gives an interpretation of the eight elements at the six locations to determine health status. These two concepts are interconnected. The symbolic meaning of a dice and a dice roll with respect to the arterial pulse and the health status in tcm are explicated below.

5.1. Arterial pulse and the eight elements at the six locations

It is postulated that the eight elements are influenced by the arterial pulse at the six locations (left and right cun, guan, and chi). Depth, rate, regularity, width, length, smoothness, stiffness, and strength are the eight elements of pulse condition at the six locations. The intensity of each element is determined by the sensation of the arterial pulse perceived by a tcm doctor. Thus, the eight elements at the six locations are operationalized as a rating along a continuum with Yin and Yang at the extremes.

Specifically, depth is operationalized as the vertical position of the arterial pulse, and is rated along a continuum with the deepest being Yin and the most floating being Yang.

Rate is the number of beats in a minute, with the slowest being Yin and the most rapid being Yang. Regularity is the rhythm of the arterial pulse, which is categorized as either regular or irregular. Width is the intensity of the arterial pulse, with the smallest being Yin and the largest being Yang. Length is the range of the arterial pulse that can be sensed across cun, guan, and chi, with the shortest being Yin and the longest being Yang. Smoothness is the slickness of the arterial pulse, where the roughest is Yin and the smoothest is Yang. Stiffness is the elasticity of the radial artery, with the least stiff being Yin and the stiffest being Yang. Finally, strength is the forcefulness of the arterial pulse relative to the change in pressure applied by a tcm doctor, with the least forceful being Yin and the most forceful being Yang.

5.2. The eight elements at the six locations and health status

In tcm pulse diagnosis, health status is determined by the pulse condition at the six locations, with each location reflecting the health status of a specific organ. Left cun, guan, and chi reflect the health status of the heart, the liver, and the kidneys, whereas right cun, guan, and chi reflect the health status of the lungs, the spleen, and the kidneys (lifegate). The eight elements are the assessment criteria for the health status of the organs. Health status is the outcome measure of tcm pulse diagnosis, and is a composite measure of the health status of the organs.

5.3. The dice model

In the model, a dice is used to embody the intertwining and cascading relationship among the arterial pulse, the eight elements at the six locations, and health status (Figure 5). Figure 5 shows a diagrammatic presentation of the dice model.

5.3.1. Assumptions

The dice model is formulated under three assumptions. The first is that the eight elements carry the same weight in the assessment of overall pulse condition. Second, the mid-point along a continuum indicates the balance of Yin and Yang. Third, the six locations have the same weight in determining health status.

5.3.2. Symbolic meaning

The dice is analogous to the concept of health in tcm. Health is perceived as the balance of Yin and Yang, which in turn relies on the individual functioning and interaction of the organs. The six pyramids that make up a dice are thus analogous to the organs at the six locations.

The inside of the dice represents the blood flow within the organs, the combination of which constitutes the arterial pulse. Hence, any change in the blood flow from any of the organs is reflected in the arterial pulse. By assessing the six pyramids, the health status of the organs and thus overall health status can be revealed.

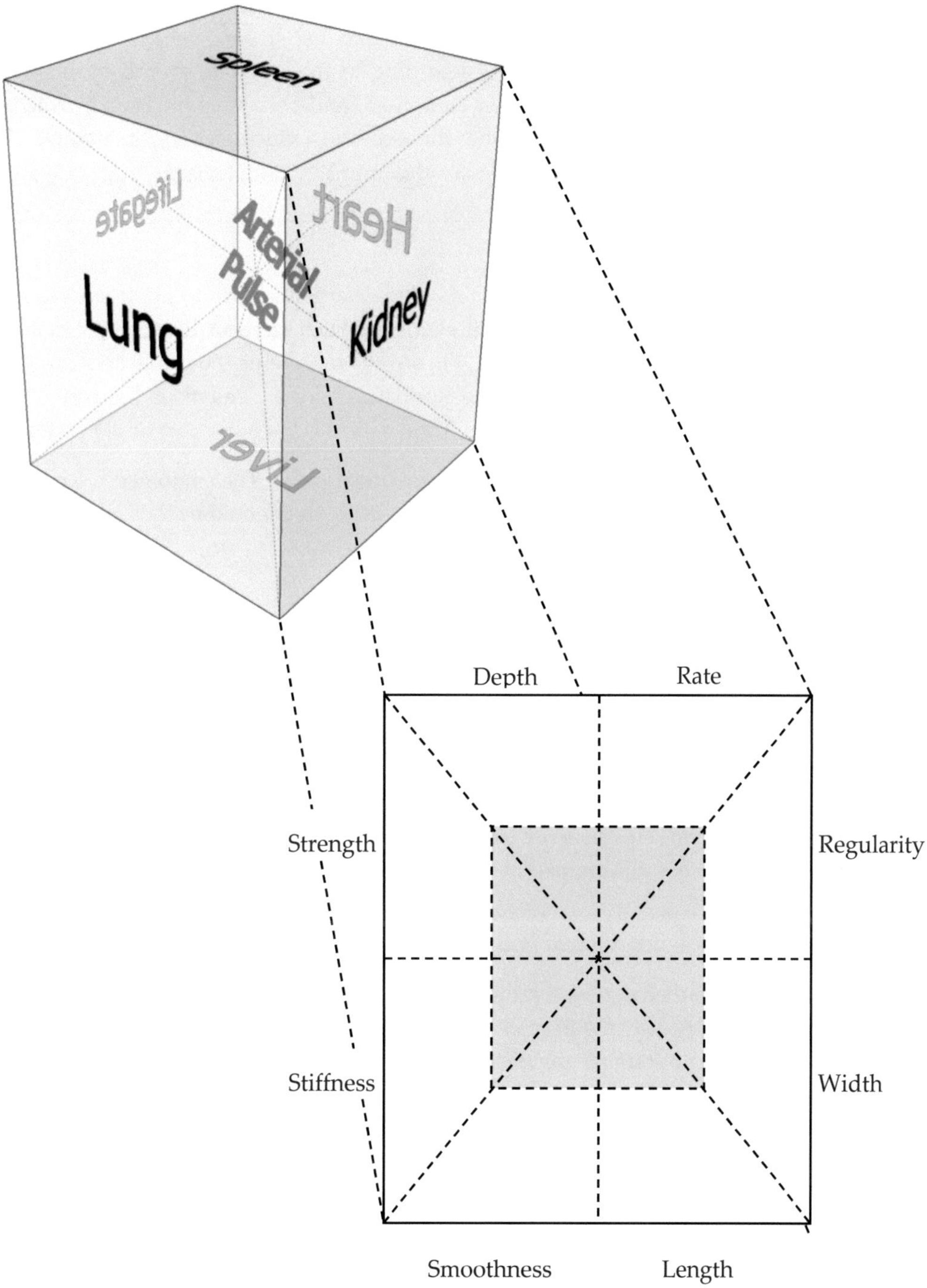

Figure 5. The dice model

5.3.3. Position of the six organs

As has been stated, the six pyramids represent the six locations where the pulse is assessed by a tcm doctor. The lungs and the heart, the liver and the spleen, the kidneys and the lifegate are arranged in opposite pyramids according to their role in overall health. This arrangement is based on the notion that left cun, guan, and chi assess the blood, which is Yin in nature, whereas right cun, guan, and chi assess qi, which is Yang in nature. The position of the organs arranged in the dice thus adheres to Yin Yang theory.

5.3.4. The eight elements

Each pyramid is made up of the eight elements. The enlarged square to the lower right of Figure 5 shows the interrelation of the eight elements. Each element is a complementary Yin-Yang pair. According to Yin Yang theory, Yin always represents the inside and Yang the outside. Thus, the black square indicating the Yin nature of the elements is the core of the pyramid, and the white square indicating their Yang nature is the outer part of the pyramid.

The intensity of the eight elements depends on the arterial pulse. The combined intensity of the eight elements thus indicates the health status of the organ denoted by that pyramid.

5.3.5. Interconnection in the dice model

The dice model of tcm pulse diagnosis is inspired by the Taiji symbol. The dotted line that links the six pyramids together symbolizes the interchanging and dynamic relationship among the organs. In the model, the Yin and Yang of each element, the eight elements in each pyramids, and the six pyramids of the dice are connected with dotted lines, which means that they are Yin and Yang composites and are always interchanging and balancing one another. The solid outline of the dice represents the absolute of health, just as the Taiji circle represents the world. Health is not expandable or reducible: it is only the health status that can be altered, which is determined by the interaction of Yin and Yang in the body.

5.3.6. Analogy between a dice roll and health status

To further elaborate the dice model, a roll of the dice is taken as analogous to health status. With a balanced or "fair" dice, the probability of rolling each pyramid is equal, because the areas and weights of the pyramids are identical. A "fair" dice is thus analogous to a healthy status, in which the blood flow within the organs is normal, the wave reflection and wave resonance occur in the proper way, the intensity of the eight elements is around the mid-point of the continuum and forms a regular shape in the middle of the pyramid, and the six pyramids are equal and balanced. Yin and Yang are balanced and harmony is attained.

However, if any one of the pyramids is intentionally altered in terms of its area or weight, then the dice is no longer "fair" and can be called a loaded dice. With a loaded dice, the probability of rolling each pyramid is unequal, and varies with the area and weight of the pyramids. A loaded dice is analogous to an unhealthy status, in which the abnormal functioning of any of the organs affects the wave reflection and wave resonance within the circulatory system, blood flow is altered, and thus the weight of the pyramid representing that organ is altered. The arterial pulse changes in accordance with the health status of the organ, and thus the intensity of the eight elements also changes. The pyramid formed by the eight elements is no longer regular, but is smaller or larger and skewed. An imbalance thus occurs in the six pyramids, Yin and Yang are imbalanced, and health is compromised.

5.4. Recent works on validating the framework

Several works have been done to verify the hypotheses of the framework. Tang et al. (2012) [62] conducted a study to validate the content and diagnostic ability of the framework. Content validation index was 0.73 which was acceptable. And the criterion validation was conducted by comparing the accuracy, sensitivity and specificity of the models generated by artificial neural networks. About 80% accuracy was attained among all ANN models. Their specificity and sensitivity carried, ranging from 70% to nearly 90%. It suggested that the tcm pulse diagnostic framework was valid in terms of its content and diagnostic ability.

Tang et al. (2012) [63] reported that the nonlinear relationship of the eight elements at the six locations and the physical parameters in time domain were successfully established by Levenberg-Marquardt algorithm with an r-squared ranged from 0.60-0.86.

6. Conclusion: What's next?

The tcm pulse diagnostic framework is a novel direction suggested by Tang (2010) [21] to guide tcm pulse diagnostic quantification. Despite studies [62,63] have been conducted to verify the hypotheses in the framework, the results were preliminary and yet verified the framework fully. Much more effort has to be made in the future. This session highlights limitations of the studies and corresponding recommendations are given.

6.1. Limitations

6.1.1. Methodology

tcm doctors usually assess pulse at the six locations both individually and simultaneously. However, pulse acquisition device used was usually a single-probe type, as no validated three-sensor pulse acquisition device is available, and the arterial pressure waveforms could only be acquired one at a time. Thus, the simultaneous manipulation of pulse at the six locations carried out in a typical tcm pulse diagnosis could not be examined.

The pulse acquisition process was fairly long at about one hour as reported by [62], [63], which may have provoked motion artifacts in the subjects that affected the quality of the arterial pressure waveforms acquired. Also, the baseline of the arterial pressure waveform fluctuated due to the movement and breathing pattern of the subjects, and the feature extraction program was insufficiently developed to remove this noise from the waveforms. The rescaling of the fluctuating baseline into a horizon would have distorted the arterial pressure waveform and introduced errors into the features extracted. One of the physical parameters, peak-to-peak interval, could not be extracted by the program and thus could not be used in the modelling. Further, the pulse acquisition device limited the hold-down pressure to a maximum of 400 mmHg, but the amplitude of the arterial pressure waveform did not decrease in some of the subjects, and thus Δ80%pamax could not be calculated.

Another limitation is about characteristics of the subject recruited. Those subjects recruitment in [62], [63] were rather stable, the intensity of the eight elements was therefore confined to a narrow range, and such homogeneity in the samples may have lowered the r-squared.

6.1.2. Statistical approaches

ANN was suggested to verify the relationships in the framework because of their nonlinear nature. There are several limitations with this approach needed to be overcome. First, the sample size required by the ANN was too large to be recruited in a clinical study, and the smaller sample size used may have lowered the effect size of the models. Second, as mentioned before, the low explanatory power of ANN does not allow researchers to fully analyzing the models generated.

6.2. Recommendations

In view of the limitations of the studies, five recommendations are made for further studies in this area.

6.2.1. Methodology

It is suggested that a validated three-sensor pulse acquisition device be developed so that the effect of simultaneous hold-down pressure on the arterial pressure waveforms at cun, guan, and chi can be examined. Also, the feature extraction program requires further enhancement to extract all of the necessary features from the arterial pressure waveform. The development of the feature extraction program is a major part of the study because the physical parameters are calculated based on the features extracted by the program.

6.2.2. Statistical approaches

A program should be generated that can extract the underlying relationships among the physical parameters and the eight elements at the six locations and the relationships among the eight elements at the six locations and health status. Increasing the explanatory power of the models in this way would provide modern scientific theoretical backing for tcm pulse diagnosis and more evidence to support tcm theories.

Another suggestion is on subject recruitment. More diverse subjects should be recruited to verify the models. The models established are preliminary models that demonstrate the nonlinearity of the physical parameters and the eight elements, but a larger sample is required to validate them fully. As those studies recruited subjects with stable hypertension, the models cannot be extrapolated to patients with severe hypertension or hypotension. It is thus recommended to recruit subjects with severe hypertension or hypotension in future studies to increase the generalizability of the models. In addition, patients with other diseases should also be recruited to examine the models' ability to differentiate hypertension from other diseases.

Author details

Anson Chui Yan Tang
School of Nursing, Caritas Medical Centre, Hong Kong

7. References

[1] Dharmananda S. The Significance of Traditional Pulse Diagnosis in The Modern Practice of Chinese Medicine. http://www.itmonline.org/arts/pulse.htm (accessed 26 January 2004)
[2] Fei Z. Zhongguo Mai Zhen Yan Jiu. Shanghai: Shanghai Zhong Yi Xue Yuan Chu Ban She; 2003.
[3] Li Z, Liu X. Yellow Emperor's Canon of Medicine Plain Conservation II. Xi'an: World Publishing Corporation ; 2005.
[4] Wang SW. Mai Jing (1st ed.). Beijing: China Economic Publishing House; 2002.
[5] Li SZ. The Lakeside Master's Study (1st ed.). (B. Flaws, Trans.) ; 1998. http://www.netlibrary.com/Reader/ (accessed 20 October 2008).
[6] Li ZZ. Zhen Jia Zheng Yan. Beijing: Huaxia chu ban she ; 1997.
[7] Li SZ. The Classic of Difficulties: A Translation of Nan Jing. (B. Flaws, Trans.) ; 1999. http://www.netlibrary.com/Details.aspx (accessed 19 November 2007).
[8] Ma J, Yan H. Bin Hu Mai Xue Tong Jie. Xi'an Shi: San Qin Chu Ban She; 2001.
[9] Yang Z, Chen Y. Zhong Yi Mai Zhen Ru Men. Shantou Shi: Xhantou Da Xue Chu Ban She; 1999.
[10] Guan X. Mai zhen: Ge Shi Hua, Shen Mi Hua, Ke Guan Hua - Mai Zhen Yan Jin Zhong Ruo Gan Zhong Da Wen Ti. Medicine and Philosophy 2001; 22(5) 58-60.
[11] King E, Cobbin D, Walsh S, Ryan D. The Reliable Measurement of Radial Pulse Characteristics. *Acupuncture in Medicine 2002* Vol.20, No.4, pp. 150-159.
[12] Water P. Evidence-based Practice (Three Series)-Part 1 What Is Evidence-Based Practice. http://www.scattc.org/pdf_upload/Beacon001.pdf (accessed 1 July 2009).
[13] Huang JB. Zhong Yi Mai Zhen Tu Pu Zhen Duan. Taibei Shi: Zhi Yin Chu Ban She; 2007.
[14] Li J. The Objective Detection and Description of The Types of Pulse Based on The Chinese Traditional Medical Science. Medical Instrumentation 2005;18(5) 7-11.
[15] Liu W, Wang Y, He H. Ba Wei Mai Xiang Dang Yi. Journal of Beijing University of Traditional Chinese Medicine 1997; 20(6) 18-20.
[16] Luo Z. Sheng Wu Li Xue Zai Zhong Yi Mai Xiang Fen Lei Zhong De Ying Yong. Journal of Basic Information 1983; 1 21.

[17] Wei R. Duo Yin Su Mai Tu Ren Mai Fa – Mai Zhen Ke Guan Hua De Yi Zhong Chang Shi. Medical Instrumentation 1981; 6(4), 291.
[18] Xu YJ, Niu X. Exploration of Detecting Character of Digital Phase in TCM Pulse Diagnosis. Chinese Journal of Integrated Traditional and Western Medicine 2003; 23(6), 467-470.
[19] Deng T, Guo Z. Zhong Yi Zhen Duan Xue. Shanghai: Shanghai Ke Xue Ji Shu Chu Ban She; 1983.
[20] Chung WY. The Construction and Evaluation of A Tool for The Assessment of Cancer Pain in A Chinese Context. PhD thesis. The University of Hong Kong; 1998.
[21] Tang CY. Developing An Objective Traditional Chinese Medicine Pulse Diagnostic Model in Essential Hypertension. PhD thesis. The Hong Kong Polytechnic University; 2010.
[22] Vlachopoulos C, O'Rourke MF. Genesis of The Normal and Abnormal Arterial Pulse. Current Problems in Cardiology 2000; 25(5), 298-367.
[23] Su YC, Huang KF, Chang YH, Li TC, Huang WS, Lin JG. The Effect of Fasting on The Pulse Spectrum. American Journal of Chinese Medicine 2000; 28(3-4) 409-417.
[24] Yoon YZ, Lee MH, Sah KS. Pulse Type Classification by Varying Contact Pressure. The Institute of Electrical and Electronics Engineers Engineering in Medicine and Biology Magazine 2000;19(6), 106-110.
[25] Chen J J. Application of The Chinese Medicine Pulse Diagnoses to Clinical Diseases. Yearbook of Chinese Medicine and Pharmacy 2008; 26(5), 189-220.
[26] Huang S, Sun M. Zhong Yi Mai Xiang Yan Jiu. Taibei Shi: Zhi Yin Chu Ban She ; 1995.
[27] Xu L, Wang K, Zhang D, Li Y, Wan Z, Wang J. Objectifying Researches on Traditional Chinese Pulse Diagnosis. Informatica Medica Slovenica 2003; 8(1), 56-62.
[28] Yang J, Niu X. Ultrasound-Videotex Detection on Three Dimensional Movement of Radial Artery on Cunkou. China Journal of Traditional Chinese Medicine and Pharmacy 2006;21(5), 264-266.
[29] Zhang ZG, Niu X, Yang XZ, Si YC. A New Opinion on Detection Methods for Pulse Shape and Pulse Force. Journal of Chinese Integrative Medicine 2008; 6(3), 243-248.
[30] Zheng J, Wang J, Wang Z. Preliminary Study on 45 Pulses from Healthy Young People. Journal of Yunnan College of Traditional Chinese Medicine 1994;17(3), 25-27.
[31] Zhu X, Niu X, Gao W, Niu S, Guo Z, Zhang Z, et al. Ultrasound Pulse-Based Technology Research Ideas to Explore Potential Properties. Chinese Journal of Management in Chinese Medicine 2007;15(4), 252-254.
[32] Chang HH. The Association between Left Ventricular Function and Sphygmogram of Heart Failure Patients. Yearbook of Chinese Medicine and Pharmacy 2005; 23(2), 375-424.
[33] Tyan CC, Chang HH, Chen JC, Hsu YT. A Study of Radial Sphygmogram on Yin Vacuity Syndrome in Patients with Systemic Lupus Erythematosus. Journal of Chinese Medicine 2001; 12(3), 145-154.
[34] Cassidy S. Speech Recognition. http://www.ics.mq.edu.au/~cassidy/comp449/html/index.html (accessed 19 April 2009).

[35] Fu SE, Lai SP. A System for pulse measurement and analysis of Chinese medicine. Proceedings of The Annual International Conference of the Institute of Electrical and Electronics Engineers of Engineering in Medicine and Biology Society 1989; 5, 1695-1696.

[36] Wang BH, Luo J, Xiang JL, Yang Y. Power Spectral Analysis of Human Pulse and Study of Traditional Chinese Medicine Pulse Diagnosis Mechanism. Journal of Northwest University (Natural Science Edition)2001;31(1), 21-25.

[37] Zhang A, Yang F. Study on Recognition of Sub-Health from Pulse Signal. Proceedings of International Conference on Neural Networks and Brain 2005; 3, 1516-1518.

[38] Wang W. *Qi De Yue Zhang*. Taibei Shi: Da KuaiWen Hua Chu Ban Gu Fen You Xian Gong Si; 2002.

[39] Wang WK, Bau JG, Hsu TL, Lin Wang YY. Influence of Spleen Meridian Herbs on The Harmonic Spectrum of The Arterial Pulse. American Journal of Chinese Medicine 2000; 28(2), 279-289.

[40] Kuo YC, Lo SH, Wang WK. Harmonic Variations of Arterial Pulse during Dying Process of Rats. Proceeding of The Twenty-third Annual International Conference of The Institute of Electrical and Electronics Engineers of Engineering in Medicine and Biology Society 2001;1, 519-521.

[41] Kuo YC, Chiu TY, Jan MY, Bau JG, Li SP, Wang WK, et al. Losing Harmonic Stability of Arterial Pulse in Terminally Ill Patients. Blood Pressure Monitoring 2004; 9(5), 255-258.

[42] Lu WA. Pulse Spectrum Analysis in 205 Patients with Abnormal Liver Function Test. Taipei City Medical Journal 2006;3(3), 240-247.

[43] Lu WA, Cheng CH, Lin Wang YY, Wang WK. Pulse Spectrum Analysis of Hospital Patients with Possible Liver Problems. American Journal of Chinese Medicine 1996; 24(3-4), 315-320.

[44] Lu WA, Lin Wang YY, Wang WK. Pulse Analysis of Patients with Severe Liver Problems. The Institute of Electrical and Electronics Engineers Engineering in Medicine and Biology Magazine 1999; 18(1), 73-75.

[45] Wang WK, Hsu TL, Chiang Y, Lin Wang YY. The Prandial Effect on The Pulse Spectrum. American Journal of Chinese Medicine 1996; 24(1), 93-98.

[46] Wang B, Xiang J. Detecting System and Power-Spectral Analysis of Pulse Signals of Human Body. Proceedings of The Fourth International Conference on Signal Processing 1998; 2,1646-1649.

[47] Xu L, Wang K, Zhang D. Modern researches on pulse waveform of TCPD. Proceedings of The International Conference of The Institute of Electrical and Electronics Engineers on Communications, Circuits and Systems and West Sino Expositions 2002; 2,1073-1077.

[48] Kleinbaum DG, Kupper LL, Chembless LE. Logistic Regression Analysis of Epidemiologic Data: Theory and Practice. Communications in Statistics Theory and Methods 1998; 11(5), 485-547.

[49] Sargent DJ. Comparison of Artificial Neural Networks with Other Statistical Approaches: Results from Medical Data Sets. Cancer 2001; 91(8 suppl), 1636-1642.

[50] Hu JN. Ren Gong Te Zheng Ren Gong Wang Luo Fen Lei Qi. Journal of China Medical University 1996 ; 25(6), 571.

[51] Lu X, Shi Q, Xing S, Cao H. Several Approaches on Criteria Investigation of TCM Pulse Diagnosis. Journal of Tianjin University of Traditional Chinese Medicine 2007; 26(3), 113-115.
[52] Yu L. The Objectivity and Digital of Diagnosis by Pulse Based on Traditional Chinese Medical Science. Liaoning Journal of Traditional Chinese Medicine 2006; 33(2), 129-131.
[53] Lee HL, Suzuki S, Adachi Y, Umeno M. Fuzzy Theory in Traditional Chinese Pulse Diagnosis. Proceedings of The International Joint Conference on Neural Networks 1993; 1, 774-777.
[54] Zhang GP. Neural Networks for Classification: A Survey. The Institute of Electrical and Electronics Engineers Transactions on Systems, Man, and Cybernetics – Part C: Applications and Reviews 2000; 30(4), 451-462.
[55] Wu Y, Giger ML, Doi K, Vyborny CJ, Schmidt RA, Metz CE. Artificial Neural Networks in Mammography: Application to Decision Making in The Diagnosis of Breast Cancer. Radiology 1993; 187, 81-87.
[56] Wikimedia. Basic Architecture of ANN. http://commons.wikimedia.org/wiki/Image:Gray1237.png (accessed 11 March 2009).
[57] Wang B, Xiang J. Fuzzy Clustering of Human Body Pulse Signals Based on AR Model. Applied Acoustics 2001; 20(5), 21.
[58] Xu LS, Meng MQH, Wang WQ. Pulse Image Recognition Using Fuzzy Neural Network. Proceedings of The Twenty-ninth Annual International Conference of the Electrical and Electronics Engineers of Engineering in Medicine and Biology Society 2007; 3148-3157.
[59] Hart A, Wyatt J. Evaluating Black-Boxes As Medical Decision Aids: Issues Arising from A Study of Neural Networks. Informatics for Health & Social Care 1990; 15(3), 229-236.
[60] Lisboa PJG. A Review of Evidence of Health Benefit from Artificial Neural Networks in Medical Intervention. Neural Networks 2002; 15,11-39.
[61] Silver D, Hurwitz G. The Predictive and Explanatory Power of Inductive Decision Trees: A Comparison with Artificial Neural Network Learning As Applied to The Non-Invasive Diagnosis of Coronary Artery Disease. Journal of Investigative Medicine 1996; 45(2), 99-108.
[62] Tang ACY, Chung JWY, Wong TKS. Validation of A Novel Traditional Chinese Pulse Diagnostic Model Using An Artificial Neural Network. Evidence-based Complementary and Alternative Medicine 2012; doi:10.1155/2012/685094.
[63] Tang ACY, Chung JWY, Wong TKS. Digitalizing Traditional Chinese Medicine Pulse Diagnosis with Artificial Neural Network. Telemedicine and e-Health 2012. (accepted and will be published on 18/6/2012)

Chapter 5

Does the Cognitive Top-Down Systems Biology Approach, Embodied in Virtual Scanning, Provide Us with a Theoretical Framework to Explain the Function of Most Complementary and Alternative and Most Orthodox Biomedical Techniques?

Graham Wilfred Ewing

Additional information is available at the end of the chapter

http://dx.doi.org/10.5772/50441

1. Introduction

Perhaps the greatest challenge faced by advocates of complementary or alternative therapies is the lack of a theoretical concept to explain why such techniques can have a therapeutic or diagnostic effect. If there is not a theoretical concept or explanation it follows that the use of such techniques often cannot be adapted in a methodical or scientific manner. If there is not an objective and/or accurate means of identifying the emergence of the health problem then there cannot be an objective means of treating the problem. It may also mean that the outcomes of such techniques are experiential and unreliable, different practitioners get variable results, different techniques or combination of techniques could have adverse side-effects, etc. The lack of a robust theoretical concept to explain the body's dysfunction and the role of drugs, which are only circa 50% effective in 90% of the population [1], is also a fundamental limitation of orthodox biomedicine. No-one has yet been able to explain how the body regulates its function.

Many clinical studies have illustrated that some CAM techniques are able to provide a diagnostic or therapeutic effect. Moreover many drugs and medical techniques have their origins in what we know as CAM. The therapeutic application of plant extracts, the development of penicillin, the use of X-rays, etc; are all derived from naturally occurring phenomenae.

Any explanation for CAM techniques must fit into established concepts and theories which prevail in science. Anything which cannot be thus explained should be discarded in favour of more robust explanations. If a technique has a proven diagnostic or therapeutic effect it will be adapted for use by the medical profession although perhaps in recent years it has become more difficult to introduce new technologies into the major regulated markets i.e. due to the increased cost of developing and validating such techniques, lack of basic research in non-pharma techniques, and perhaps also opposition from those with established market share and hence of vested interests who seek to maintain the status quo. Nevertheless if the technology has a commercial significance entrepreneurs will evaluate the opportunity, invest and develop the opportunity e.g. light-based techniques are used in different forms of optometry.

Orthodox biomedicine has selectively assimilated CAM research into its realm e.g. the pharmaceutical company GSK has been researching polyclonal antibodies which are more typically associated with the antibody response in homeopathy, yet despite the proliferation/dominance of pharmacological research there is not an accepted understanding of the processes which lead to morbidity and mortality. There is no accepted understanding of how the body regulates its function [2]. Moreover, the requirement for medical care has increased by a factor of ten or more in the last 30 years. No-one has yet been able to offer a significant explanation for this explosion of morbidity. Despite the emphasis upon vaccines and drugs the occurrence of cognitive and physiological dysfunction in society continues to increase. Morbidity and mortality are associated with genetic and non-genetic changes. This leads us to consider the various factors (i) which lead to genetic change and (ii) which suppress the processes which the body requires to maintain its regulated function and which we recognise as our health and wellbeing i.e. the effect which viruses and hence of vaccines, bacterial infections, psychological or environmental stresses, genetically modified foods, and drugs have upon the body's function.

In general, drugs are designed to treat the symptoms of disease. As most disease is caused by the aforementioned factors it becomes evident that drugs do not and cannot treat the cause of disease but instead act upon the biological processes of dysfunction which arise from the dysregulation or destabilisation of the body's function. Drugs modulate, suppress or alter the production of metabolites from pathological processes and/or otherwise adapt the use of pharmacological entities to modify the body's function and reduce the symptoms of disease and associated causes of discomfort and morbidity. It is perceived that such effects may allow the natural process of regulation or homeostasis to be re-established. This overlooks that the brain is continually seeking, assessing and computing the means to better maintain or re-establish the body's physiological stability i.e. it will in many cases compensate for the effect which drugs have on the body's function. For example (i) psychological traumas influence heart function e.g. bereavement, divorce [3], social isolation [4], illnesses. In such cases drugs treat the symptoms of dysfunction caused by the trauma. (ii) Diabetes may be the first step in a cascade of pathologies leading to heart dysfunction, Alzheimer's disease, circulatory problems, etc. It is ultimately caused by the cognitive dysfunction and altered behaviour [5] which governs calorific intake and the expenditure of energy.

The idea that autonomic regulation takes the body back to a base or homeostatic state lacks validity. Every change to genotype and phenotype makes changes which are to some degree reversible or irreversible. Some genetic changes can be reversed, some relatively quickly, others more slowly over a longer period, and others may be irreversible e.g. changes to our DNA due to viral or vaccinal RNA, may be relatively short-lasting (months), or may last for the duration of our lifetime.

The historical evolutionary pathways of medicine have resulted in what we know as physiology and psychology i.e. the function of the body and the brain are studied separately. This historical legacy continues to influence the prevailing psychological/physiological paradigm and regards the brain's function to be almost completely separate from the body's function. In recent years there has been greater research in the biological processes taking place in the brain however this neuroscientific approach often overlooks the significance of visceral pathologies upon brain development, brain plasticity and hence upon neural function. In principle, this means that psychology is the mirror of physiology i.e. that what we see/experience from our external environment influences our internal environment and what we experience in our internal environment influences our cognition and behaviour i.e. the development of pathologies influences our behaviour (mood, emotional response, the way in which we behave, etc). In other words one person's output or behaviour (or that of external influences) can influence another person's sensory input and their expectations. This can be illustrated if we consider how the medical profession benefits from the power of association i.e. when a patient's ailment has reached the stage that they decide to consult their doctor (i) they make an appointment to see the doctor who (they perceive and better than anyone else) can improve their health; (ii) they travel to their local health clinic confident that this is the place where better health is prescribed; (iii) they meet the doctor who receives them in a positive yet sympathetic manner, who examines them and advises how their ailment can be cured; (iv) they are prescribed a pill or potion which the doctor assures them will alleviate their symptoms; (v) they are prescribed time away from the stresses of life. Irrespective of the healing power of the pharmaceutical product this is a hugely powerful psychological therapy or placebo effect.

By contrast the psychological environment in a hospital is a more complex and potentially more brutal environment. The patient attends the hospital in varying degrees of trepidation. The experience is largely negative i.e. they are in varying degrees of ill-health; feel vulnerable, lonely and perhaps scared; do not know anyone, and hence mistrust those involved in their treatment. The wards in which they reside during their hospital treatment often have abnormal levels of natural lighting or ventilation. The beds are often standard issue hospital beds which may leave them in some degree of discomfort. They will be advised of both positive outcomes and the risk of increased morbidity and the potential of mortality although they can expect to receive reassurance from staff. They will see others who have been treated leave the hospital in better health but also can expect to see the problems faced by other patients. It is a stressful environment lowering the level of the immune response which is not conducive to the healing process - hence the current emphasis upon getting patients to recuperate in their home environment at the earliest opportunity.

2. The sensory interface

We experience our external and internal environments through the sensory [6] and visceral interfaces i.e.

i. Sensory input: light/sight, odour/smell, sound/hearing, taste, touch and voice.
   The sensory perception i.e. of vision, hearing, smell, taste, touch and the vocal spectrum; is influenced by the extent of prevailing pathologies.

ii. Frequency
   - Flashing lights can cause photosensitive epilepsy and migraine but can be also adapted to treat photosensitive migraine and dyslexia. They are indications of systemic function and dysfunction.
   - The EEG frequency(s) are indicators of the physiological significance of an event e.g.

Frequency Range	Effect
Gamma (30-60hz):	taking a picture of our environment; experiencing a smell, hearing a sound
Beta (15-30hz):	coordinated sensory/physical activity
Alpha (8-15hz):	conscious thought; linking activity to physiological activities or objectives such as hunger, thirst, warmth, sleep, procreation; recognising danger.
Theta (4-8hz):	pain is an indicator of an inflammatory response, a precursor of damage; the link between conscious thought and systemic function/dysfunction.
Delta (1-4hz):	systemic function and regulation; damage; processes of repair; critical illness/coma and sleep.

Table 1.

Gamma, Beta and Alpha frequencies function during the wakened hours and hence are associated with sensory perception and processing whilst Theta and Delta frequencies are evident throughout the 24 hour cycle and hence are associated with the body's physiology.

Changes to cell morphology are associated with the EEG or resonant frequencies e.g. theta frequencies are associated with pain management, altered cell morphology, the subconscious thought processes and fixation of memories whilst delta frequencies are linked to physical damage (e.g. in the comatose state) and the processes of repair (e.g. which require sleep to facilitate or enhance the production of essential hormones). They are the evidence for the body's multi-level function.

- Accordingly knowledge of the resonant or frequency-related properties of organs and organ systems may be adapted with therapeutic effect e.g. to stimulate healing processes, to re-establish homeostasis, to improve sensory perception and coordination, to improve the fixation of memories, etc.

  This is an area of research in which eminent Russian researchers have excelled [7,8] for many years.

iii. Visceral input: breathing/air, temperature/warmth, acidity/pH, moisture/dry, food/diet, and drink.

These environmental influences are our phenotype: each altering the rate at which physiological reactions and extractions proceed. It is through these mechanisms that we interact with our environment and deal with adverse influences.

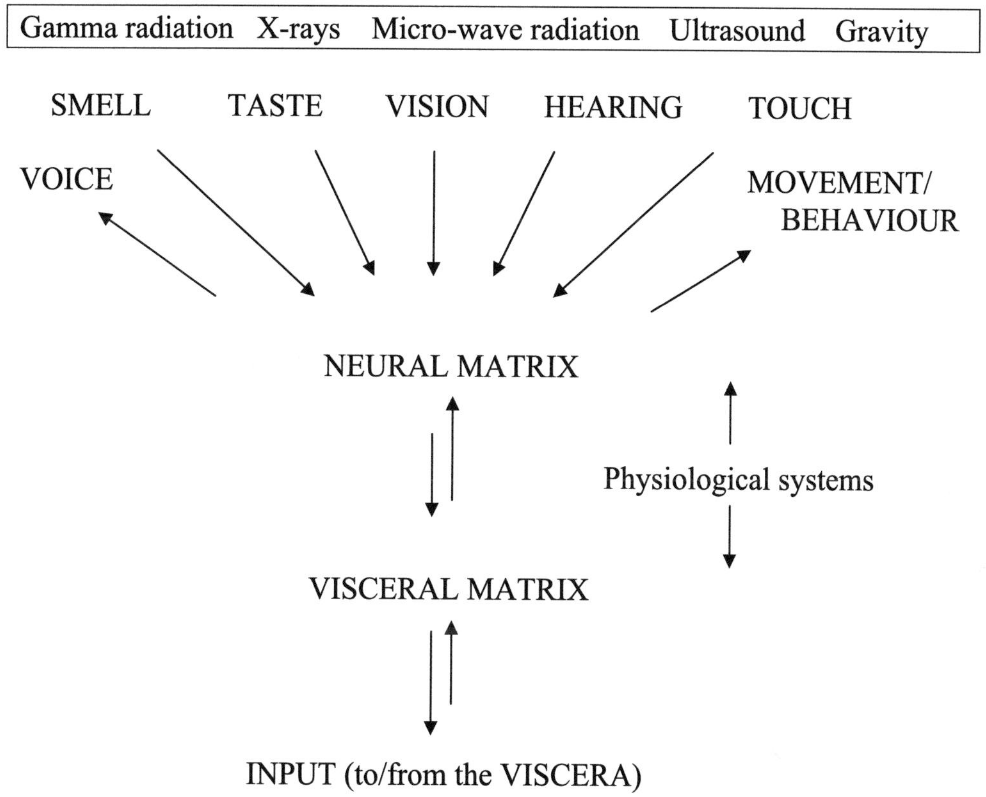

Figure 1. Sensory Input from the External Environment

The nature, structure and conformation of our genes influences the nature and level of the proteins which are expressed however it is our phenotype (influences such as pH and temperature) which influence protein conformation, the levels of minerals and cofactors, and the rate at which expressed proteins react.

An adequate level of exposure to light is essential to maintain the levels of calcitriol (vitamin D3), bilirubin, nitric oxide and many other neural and visceral processes. Light of specific wavelengths activates many of the physiologically significant proteins [9]. The action of light stimulating the production of Vitamin D3 influences the function of up to 3,000 of the estimated 10-25,000 genes which encode for proteins and the production of an estimated 200 antimicrobial peptides.

Light comprises an estimated 85% of sensory input and hence is the predominant way in which we experience and perceive our environment. It is therefore the dominant way in which we experience the positive and negative (stress) influences. For instance if we see a car crash but cannot hear, smell or touch the event it becomes somewhat surreal. It takes the combined effect of vision and hearing to transmit the significance of the event and of the urgency to act e.g. to extract car passengers from further danger and injury. For instance a person who does not have hearing may be oblivious of impending danger even if they see the danger unfolding e.g. someone running towards them – with what purpose?

Light or vision requires other sensory inputs (hearing, smell, taste or touch) in order to give significance [10] (see Figure 1). Multi-sensory input is an essential component of the body's complex multi-level function [11] i.e. mono-sensory input on its own cannot convey the significance of an event. The spectrum of light absorbed and emitted by proteins influences cognition, in particular colour perception and visual contrast (b/w) i.e. of the magno- and parvo-cellular pathways. This is often seen in developmental dyslexia in which the speed and coordination of sensory processing is altered by prevailing biological deficits [12].

The frequency of sensory input (at EEG frequencies) influences system function i.e. networks of organs and cells [13]. Visceral input influences the reaction conditions (temperature, pH, levels of minerals and vitamins), protein conformation, cell morphology and the rate at which proteins react. Altered protein conformation, pH, levels of minerals and cofactors influences the spatial distribution of proteins in the cell and ultimately alters cell morphology and the function of different physiological systems. The orthodox or prevailing understanding of physiological systems [13].

3. Physiological systems

Brain function to manage unregulated physiological activity. It does so through a mechanism involving the autonomic nervous system which includes an understanding of the significance, nature and structure of the physiological systems.

Historical definition: Cardiovascular, Respiratory, Nervous, Skin, Musculoskeletal, Blood, Digestive, Endocrine, Urinary, Male & Female Reproductive

Amended Definition: Breathing, Blood pressure, Blood Glucose, Blood Volume, Blood Cell Content, Digestion, Elimination, Sexual, **pH**, **Temperature**, Osmotic pressure, Posture, **Sleeping, Communication**

This revised understanding of the significance of the physiological systems incorporating acid/base regulation, temperature, and sleep allows a greater understanding of how many

CAM techniques can be of value i.e. treating the causes of dysfunction; and allows us to look critically at the role of pharmaceuticals i.e. which treat the biochemical consequences of systemic dysfunction.

4. Therapeutic sub-types

Pharmaceuticals are essential components of modern medicine. They block the developing pathological processes which are ultimately manifest as symptoms. They block the production and/or absorption of key metabolites which influence brain function but they do not prevent the onward manifestation of the stress-related processes. There is a distinct difference between cause and symptom. If not, how can nutrients (antioxidants, vitamins, minerals, cofactors, etc) obtained from diet [18] protect against disease or vice versa i.e. the lack of nutrients contribute to the onset of disease(s) [19]?

In addition most pharmaceuticals are mono-biological yet the processes of dysfunction may have many causes and have a multi-systemic nature [14,15,16]. This is recognised in combination drug products e.g. involving a heart drug and diuretic. This revised understanding or definition of the physiological systems and sensory input leads us to an improved understanding of the role played by many CAM techniques [17].

i. Systems-based Biofeedback
Breathing Buteyko, Meditation ™, Exercise (swimming, walking, running), Ayurvedha
Digestion: Nutrition/Diet, Ayurvedha
Elimination: Colonic Irrigation
Posture: Alexander Technique, Chiropathy, Osteopathy, Kinesiology, Massage techniques, Pilates, Yoga.
Temperature: Sauna, Turkish baths
and **Sleep**

ii. Frequency-based Biofeedback
Biofeedback, Hemi-Sync, Neurofeedback; Psychological interventions, Cognitive Behavioural Therapy (CBT); Hypnosis.

iii. Sensory-based Biofeedback
Light[20,21]**:** Colour/Light Therapy, Syntonic Optometry, Coloured lenses, Light-based biofeedback systems, Ayurvedha
Sound: Sound-based Biofeedback systems, Sound-based relaxation techniques, Music
Touch: Massage techniques
Smell: Aromatherapy
Taste:
Vocal: Biosonics

iv. CAM Techniques which Lack an Apparent Scientific Rationale

4.1. Acupuncture

As acupuncture can replace the use of anaesthetics e.g. in open-heart surgery, there can be little doubt that it adapts a most significant medical concept. It appears likely to be a pseudo-pharmacological intervention which links the EEG theta frequencies and the production of pain masking mu-opioids/cannabinoids [22]. The idea that Acupuncture can be explained by a network of energy channels or Qi which run beneath the skin's surface appears to contradict orthodox biomedical research findings. If someone undergoes surgery would this interrupt the flow of Qi? Nevertheless this flow of energy, or Qi, is influenced by hereditary factors, stress, trauma, grief, infection and nutrition. This indicates a link with the autonomic nervous system. Furthermore, that acupuncture points are distributed around the body, and also that stimulating these biologically active points (singly or in combination) can relieve pain, links the function of acupuncture to that of the physiological systems (e.g. breathing, blood pressure and digestion), autonomic nervous system, and to cellular and molecular biology. In addition, the acupuncture points can be stimulated by different modalities e.g. light, sound (Sonopuncture) and micro-currents (Voll electroacupuncture [23], Rydoraku)

Changes to cell morphology are linked to the EEG or resonant frequencies e.g. delta frequencies are linked to physical damage and the processes of repair whilst theta frequencies are, arguably, associated with pain management and advanced thought processes. They are the clear evidence of the body's multi-level function. In essence, the lower the frequency the greater the indication of physical damage and the need for neuropeptides or mu-opioids. For example it takes up to 30 seconds for pain to develop following a significant trauma (e.g. car accident, bullet wound, etc). This is indicative of the speed of transmission by the central nervous system but also of the rapid response by pain-modulating cannabinoids. Changes of cellular morphology have biochemical, structural, resonant and electrochemical properties, each in a dynamic relationship with the others. Changes to one parameter will influence the stability of the others. In addition the acupuncture points have lower electrical resistance than the surrounding skin. This may be evidence of altered local structures e.g. accumulation of neuropeptides at acupuncture points [24].

4.2. Homeopathy

Arguably this is a pharmacological intervention [25]. We cite the example of Materia Medica Holding, a major research-based Russian pharmaceutical company which, for more than 10 years, has developed and manufactured a new class of medicines based upon a homeopathic technology i.e. which are based upon the use of ultra low doses of (polyclonal) antibodies. Such is the significance of their work, that major and minor pharmaceutical companies have established research groups to investigate this potentially fruitful area of research.

5. Proof of concept

It is completely disingenuous to dispute the efficacy of CAM techniques especially so when such modalities are used throughout the world with clear therapeutic effect. Moreover that such techniques have inherent side-effects indicates that such techniques can have a positive or negative effect e.g. side-effects, contraindications or risks are associated with flashing-light therapies, acupuncture, homeopathy, colonic irrigation, osteopathy etc. There is a significant scientific principle involved e.g.

- **Flashing lights** can cause photosensitivity but can also be used with therapeutic effect e.g. flashing lights can invoke photosensitive migraine and epilepsy but can also be adapted with therapeutic effect (Biofeedback) to treat migraine.
- Reported side-effects with **acupuncture** include accidental injury to visceral organs and nerves, bleeding, muscle spasms, bruising, fainting [26].
- There are several published reports of patients experiencing extremely dangerous side effects as a result of **colon hydrotherapy**. These side effects include potentially fatal electrolyte imbalances and perforations of the colon during the insertion of the colonic tube.
- The potential of side-effects when combining different CAM techniques which have differing modes of action.

That many get relief from using CAM techniques indicates the value of such techniques [27] and of the limitations of orthodox biomedicine (which largely ignores the influence of phenotype).. Often patients use CAM techniques when orthodox biomedicine fails to provide relief or the expected level of medical recovery. CAM techniques are based upon re-establishing balance and of lowering the overstimulation of the autonomic (or visceral) sympathetic nervous system and/or perhaps of raising the understimulation of the parasympathetic nervous system. This is increasingly linked to the function of the medulla and vagus nerve - polyvagal theory [28,29]. This is a different physiological context by comparison with pharmaceuticals. It addresses the fundamental cause whereas drugs treat only the symptoms of dysfunction.

6. Virtual scanning

Light is fundamental to the body's physiological stability [6,9]. It is the medium which delivers circa 85% of our sensory input. The benefit of a summer vacation in the sun to recharge our metaphorical batteries has long been accepted. Different light frequencies can stimulate different physiological processes e.g. the production of calcitriol (Vitamin D), bilirubin, nitric oxide [30], etc.

Virtual Scanning is a cognitive technique which has diagnostic and therapeutic significance. It is based upon the light absorbing and emitting properties of proteins. Accordingly (i) by measuring the spectrum of light emitted it is possible to determine the levels of proteins expressed and the rate at which such expressed proteins react in each pathological process (see Appendix 1, example report; and Appendix 3, case studies), (ii) to identify the location and state of development of developing pathologies and changes to cell morphology (see Appendix 2), and (iii) provide a mono-chromatic light-based biofeedback therapy [31,13] which can activate inactivated processes and proteins and hence contribute to improved homeostasis and lessened morbidity (see Appendix 4). Such technique holds the prospect of being a better and more cost-effective option than genetic screening.

Virtual Scanning arose out of research into the medical application of industrial lasers. From these origins a research team led by I.G.Grakov established a biological response to a waveform i.e. that the body responded to monochromatic light. This led to the development of a mathematical model which linked cognitive input, in particular the visual perception of colours, to the autonomic nervous system. Ultimately this model (and associated algorithms) was developed to include an understanding of the nature and significance of the physiological systems - an area of great significance to medicine - because a doctors' consultation is based upon a rudimentary assessment of physiological stability i.e. of systemic stability. This has been overlooked by researchers as they seek to adapt a systems-biology approach (i.e. of bottom-up systems biology) to better understand the vagaries of molecular biology.

It is widely recognised that the visceral organs are organized in systems however the prevailing or orthodox explanation (see section 3) has inhibited further research in this area. How is it possible to research such phenomena? What tools are available to conduct the validating research? Moreover, if the visceral organs are organized in systems/structures, as is widely accepted, how are these structures regulated? Systems may not be able to be biochemically regulated. This is a major dilemma for orthodox biomedicine which, in recent years, has focussed upon genetic research to the apparent exclusion of almost every other aspect of biomedical research. For example in their efforts to cultivate cells using artificial animal embryos and uterus, leading embryologist Dr Hung-Ching Liu and coworkers found that cells began to divide and went to full term but all produced significantly deformed embryos. What is not yet known is the process which the brain/body uses to regulate cell growth.

The evidence that twins (identical and otherwise) can have completely different health outcomes illustrates that phenotype is far more significant than genotype i.e. that our sensory experiences and nutritional habits can be manifest as stress and ultimately as greater levels of morbidity and premature mortality. The stresses to which we are exposed can overcome our genetic characteristics.

Each and every medical condition must have a genetic component and an environmental component (phenotype) i.e. (i) of proteins expressed, (ii) of the rate at which expressed proteins subsequently react with their reactive substrates, and (iii) include the reaction conditions (pH, temperature, levels of substrates, etc) which influence the rate at which expressed proteins react with their reactive substrates. These reaction conditions (physiological systems) influence the rate of every physiologically significant reaction and extraction. They are part of the neuro-regulatory system which manages all aspects of the body's function.

7. Discussion

This understanding of how CAM techniques function forms the basis for a mathematical model of the consequences of cognition, in particular of visual perception, which has been linked to the function of the physiological systems [32-34] and the autonomic nervous system [5,6].

It includes a first mathematical model of the physiological systems. This has been incorporated into a medical technique 'Virtual Scanning' [35-37] which has diagnostic and therapeutic significance, and which uses cognitive input as the data sets for this particular mathematical model. As outlined it may provide a theoretical framework or explanation for most CAM techniques. Furthermore this leads us to consider the biological manifestation of the laws of physics in which the flow of current i.e. of biophotons, through the body's electromagnetic field(s) has a physiological effect.

- Different metallic acupuncture needles have a different effect/polarity [38]. This is especially significant in bimetallic acupuncture needles.
- The insertion of acupuncture needle stimulates nerve fibres which send a stimulus to nerve fibres in the spinal cord and mid brain. This releases endophins which have the effect of modulating what we perceive to be pain.
- In addition the acupuncture effect stimulates the release of beta-endorphin and ACTH from the pituitary gland. ACTH stimulates the release of cortisol from the adrenal glands i.e. the acupuncture effect is an anti-inflammatory effect acting upon inflammatory processes at the cellular level.
- Altered flow of biophotons i.e. of electrical current.
    i. Greater levels of natural sunlight act to re-establish homeostasis whilst lowered levels of natural sunlight act to restabilise homeostasis.
    ii. Different colours influence the energetic characteristics of the electrical current.
    iii. The light emitted by proteins as they react provides a flow of biophotons with different energetic characteristics
    iv. Different pulsed/EEG frequency of the electrical current will influence the physiological effect
    v. The characteristics of biophotons/light emitted will alter depending upon the characteristics of the medium in which the light is being transmitted
- Altered physiology causes variation to the prevailing electromagnetic field [39] and can have a local or systemic effect.

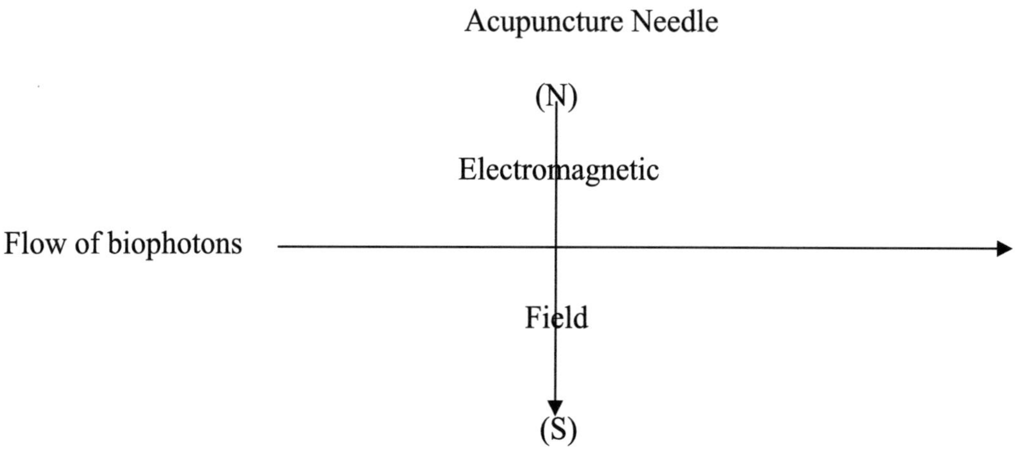

Figure 2. Diagram

There is a biodynamic relationship between an electric current (the flow of energy/biophotons through the meridians), the local electromagnetic field (a factor of the local physiology/ pathology), and the polarity of the needle. In an electric motor an electric current in a magnetic field will experience a force however in the body this dynamic cannot be similarly expressed. In the body changes to the electric current or flow of biophotons, and the polarity of the needle (by selecting needles of different metals or thickness), will influence the local electromagnetic field and hence must influence local physiology, in particular that of the autonomic nervous system and physiological systems i.e. it can influence coordination and function but not the basic structures. The meridians are components in a sophisticated electrical transmission system which has outlets along this sophisticated electrical circuitry i.e. the acupoints are electromagnetic focal points or plugs which have a strong electromagnetic effect. This effect changes when pathologies develop within organs and organ systems.

7.1. Physiological principles

As outlined, most CAM techniques function at different levels of physiological significance. They are applied independently of other CAM modalities – a criticism which is usually leveled at orthodox biomedicine! Nevertheless at which level of physiological significance can the CAM modality be expected to function? The use of acupuncture e.g. in open-heart surgery, clearly illustrates the significance of such technique. Despite this there is not yet an accepted understanding of how acupuncture works. In India Ayurvedha is widely used. The complexity of such approaches are such that it can only be applied by the most experienced, well trained and intelligent practitioners.

7.2. Clinical applications

A good diagnosis is essential for any trained practitioner irrespective of their specialism. Orthodox medicine lacks an inexpensive screening modality therefore they only find what they are looking for. Doctors are fallible. Genetic screening is now being introduced yet such technique identifies the genes associated with a medical condition yet this makes the erroneous assumption that specific genes or gene groups of gene associations can be markers for specific diseases. It is known that in type 2 diabetes the genetic associations differ between racial sub-types. It is also known that altered lifestyle e.g. of improved diet, exercise and better lifestyles, alters the genetic profile i.e. that phenotype is a more significant factor than genotype. The theoretical basis upon which pharmaceutical medications is based is gene-based and hence is limited. Every person is different and will respond differently to any form of medication. Areas of potential clinical application and benefit for phenotype-based approaches include:

- The use of an appropriate CAM therapy to complement the use of a drug, as in neuro-oncology.
- to stimulate the lymphatic system in order to better eliminate neurotoxins produced by chemotherapy or radiotherapy

- to re-establish the balance of the digestive and eliminatory systems i.e. without drugs
- to suppress overstimulation of the autonomic nervous system e.g. in asthma, hay fever, etc.
- to work alongside nutritional deficits in cases of mineral supplementation.
- to prevent the onset or progression of stress-related conditions
- to re-establish synchronized neural activity e.g. in Parkinsonism/as an option to deep brain stimulation [40].
- to re-establish the stability of the nervous structures [41,42].

7.3. Summary

It is inconceivable that the human body is not a neurally regulated system. Moreover the nature of this regulated system can only be explained by what has hitherto been researched in the name of the medical sciences and this must include feedforward by the brain to the organs and feedback by the organs to the brain. There must also be a recognition of the link between sensory input and its ultimate expression as changes to cellular and molecular biology. For there to be a regulated system there has to be an understanding of what exactly is the role of the brain i.e. 'to regulate the body's function and unregulated physical activity, process cognitive input, fix and access memories, and the process which we recognise as thought/compute/plan/calculate'.

Secondly, it is not possible to have a comprehensive approach to the management of health unless you address both the fundamental stress-related origins AND the symptoms of disease.

Thirdly, the extent or level of the ailment leads to changes to cell morphology and ultimately to the onset of pathologies. Throughout all forms of medicine the same theme arises i.e. of balance, of the sympathetic and parasympathetic nervous system, of 'hyper'function and 'hypo'function, fight or flight, nature and nurture, the brain and the body, of yin and yang. What we recognise as pathologies is due to 'autonomic dysfunction' and ultimately to autonomic failure i.e. 'degeneration'.

Such a wholistic concept illustrates the theoretical superiority of an integrative approach to medicine. The question is no longer whether CAM techniques work but instead (i) to what extent do they work and (ii) how viable are such techniques in the hands of trained practitioners? Practitioners cannot just apply a frequency or flashing light without an appreciation that such techniques have the potential, not just to treat autonomic dysfunction, but also to induce dysfunction and side-effects. All forms of medicine must be applied by the most experienced, well trained and intelligent practitioners.

Computer-based techniques have been introduced in all walks of life to improve the quality of products and services offered. They are used in manufacturing and in surgical procedures to eliminate the variability due to human involvement i.e. 'doctors are human and humans make mistakes'. Virtual Scanning may be such a technology.

Appendix

Example report

Last Name	
Name	
Sex	Woman
Age	59 years.
Weight	77,000 kg.
Additional information	Migraine
Diagnostics date	31August 2004 (15:03:45)

BRAIN

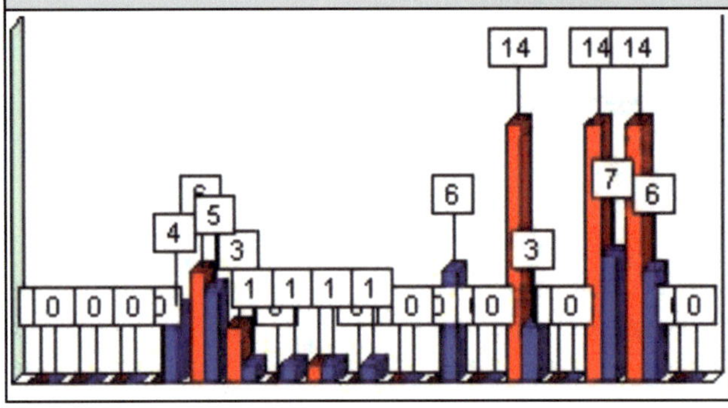

Functional Changes:
Epilepsy:
Migraine:
Verterbral Artery Syndrome:
Consequences of Brain Traumas:

SPINAL CORD

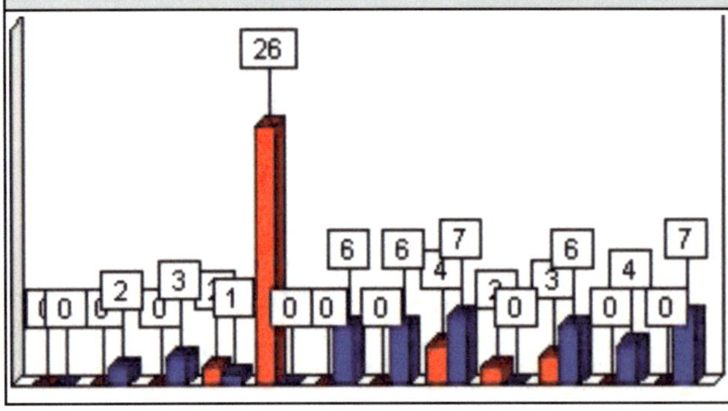

Impairment of Spinal Circulation:
Spinal Arachnoiditis:
Post-Stress Effects:

PERIPHERAL NERVOUS SYSTEM	
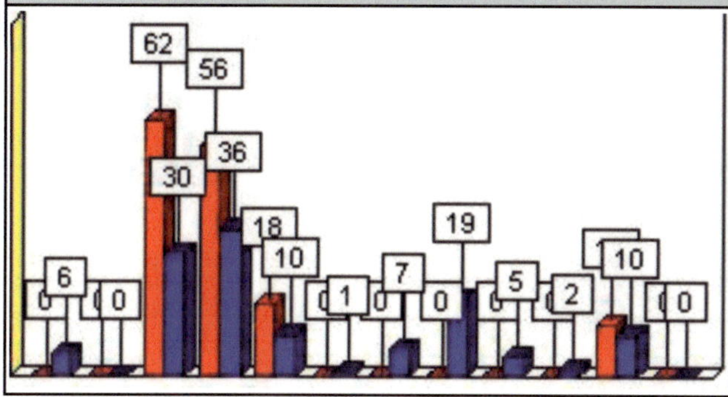	**Chronic Fatigue:** **Spinal Osteochondrosis with Neurological Effects:** **Allergic Process:** **Hereditary-Degenerative Process:** **Intoxication Effects:** **Polyneuropathy:**

EAR	
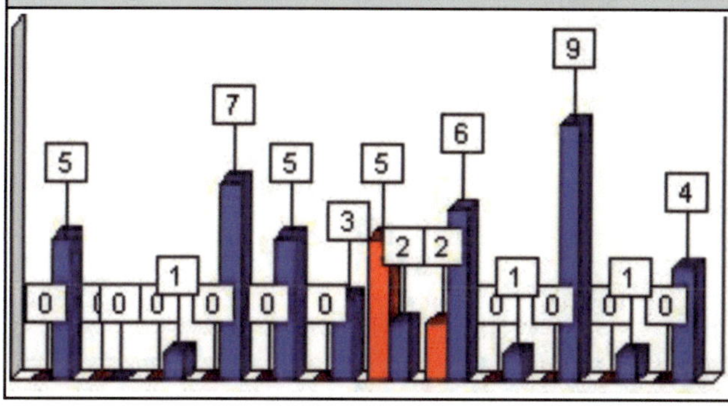	**Degenerative Process:** **Chronic Fatigue:**

NOSE	
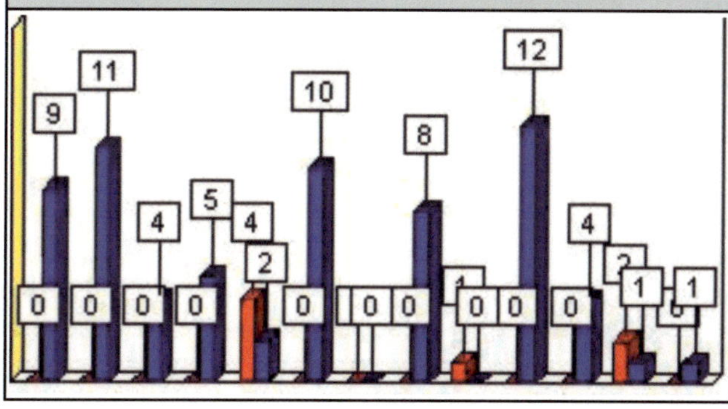	**Tension of compensatory abilities.**

PITUITARY GLAND	
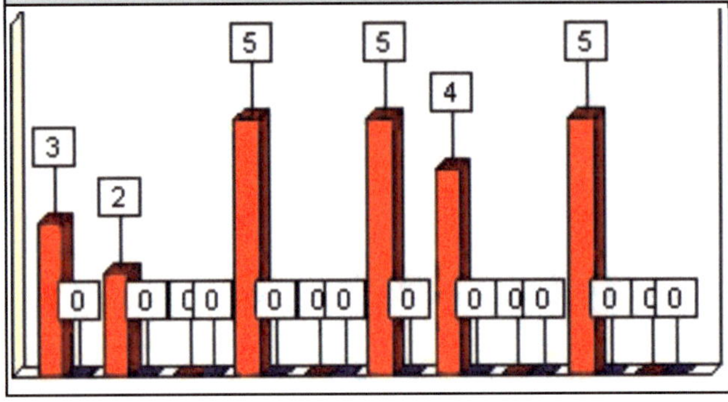	**No changes detected.**

THYROID GLAND	
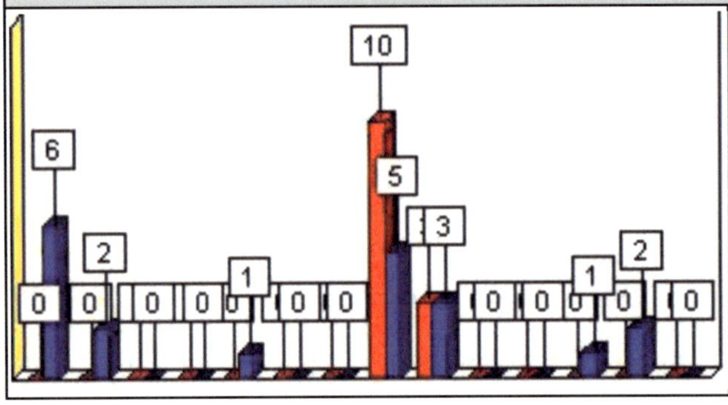	**Allergic Process:** **Abnormalities of Development:**

ADRENAL GLANDS	
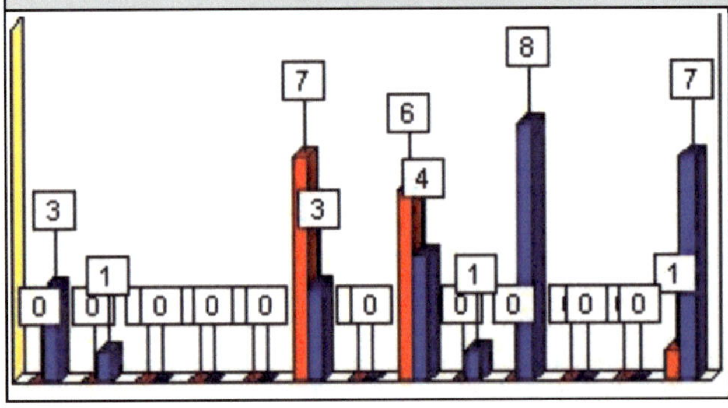	**Allergic Process:** **Cushing Syndrome:** **Functional Changes:**

OVARIES

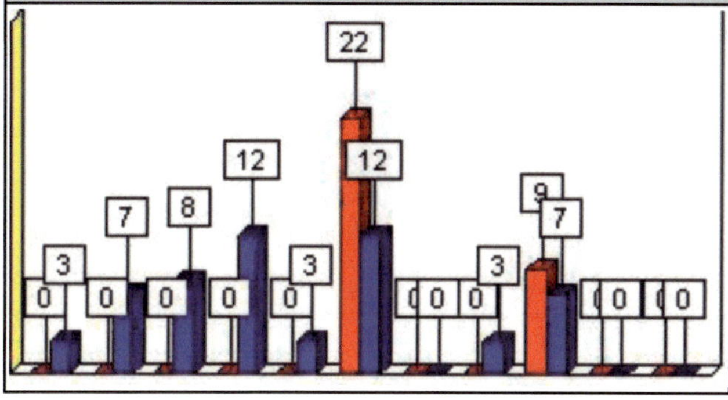

Degenerative Process:
Allergic Process:
Post-Stress Effects:
Ovarian Cyst:

MAMMARY GLAND

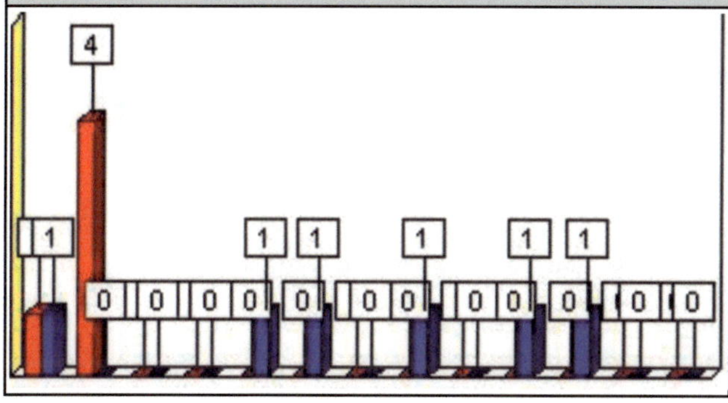

No changes detected.

LIVER

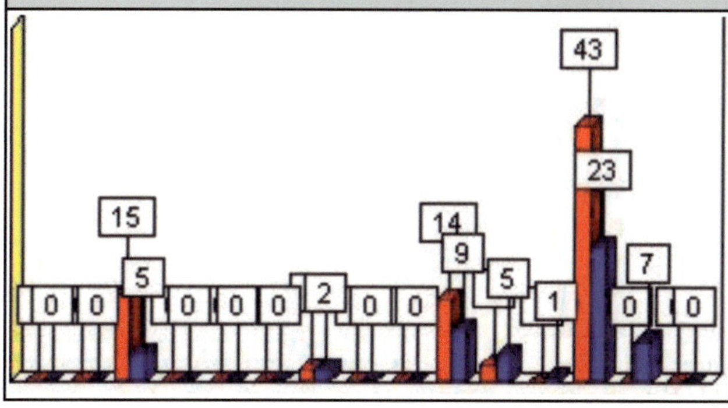

Allergic Process:
Disruption of Bilirubin Metabolism:
Liver Insufficiency:
Growth of New Cells:

GALL BLADDER

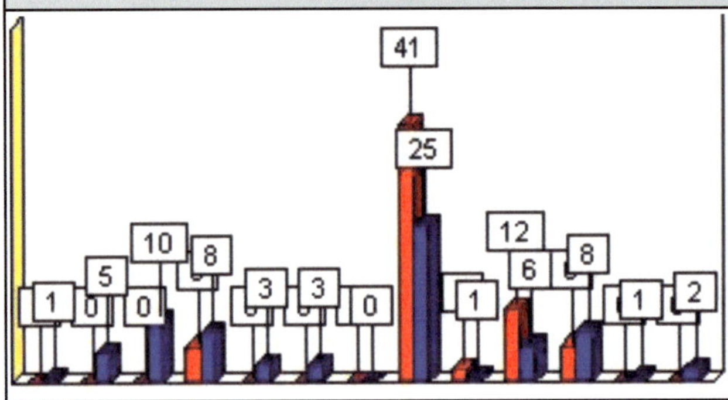

Dyskinesia of Biliary Ducts and Gall Bladder:
Chronic Fatigue:
Post-Stress Effects:
Tissue Growth:
Cholangitis:

PANCREAS

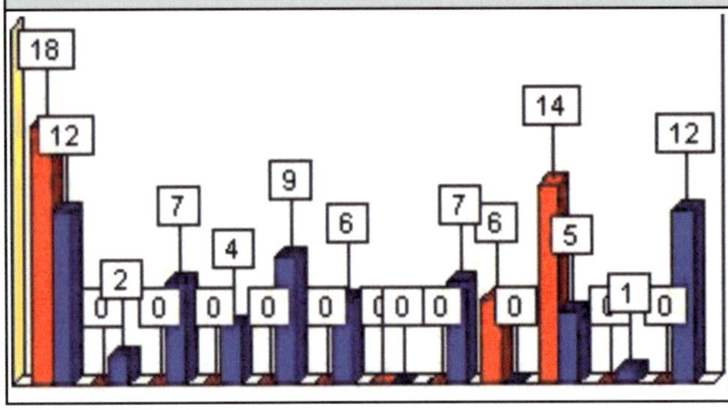

Chronic Fatigue:
Pathology of Islands of Langerhans:
Post-Stress Effects:
Age-Related Changes:
Functional Changes:
Abnormalities of Development:

HEART

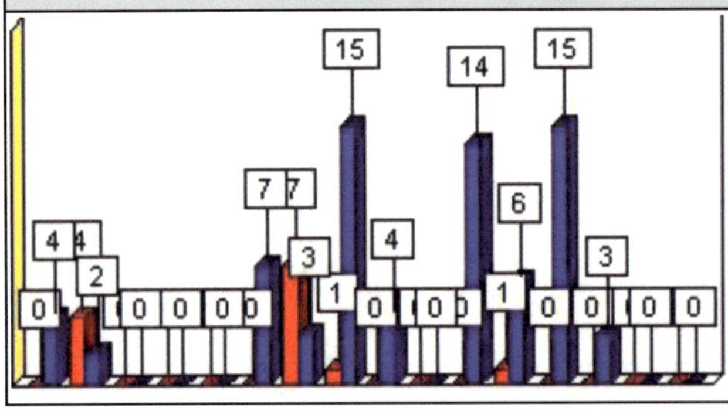

Chronic Fatigue:
Cardiosclerosis:
Myocardial Dystrophy:
Intoxication Effects:
Cardiac Insufficiency:
Cardiac Myopathy:

BLOOD AND PERIPHERAL BLOOD VESSELS

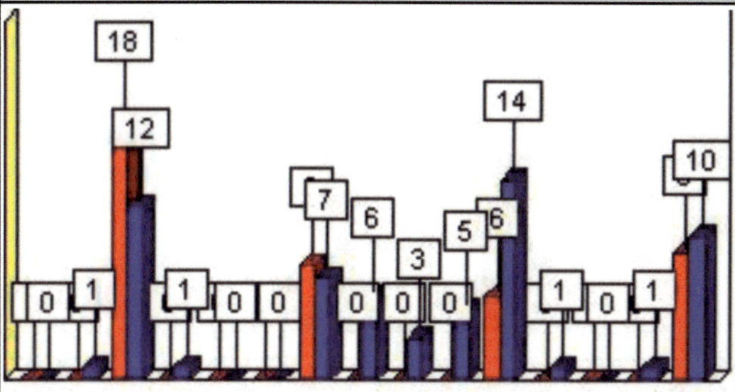

Leukopenia:
Hemorrhagic Vasculitis:
Idiopathic Hypotension:
Post-Stress Effects:
Growth of New Cells:

SPLEEN

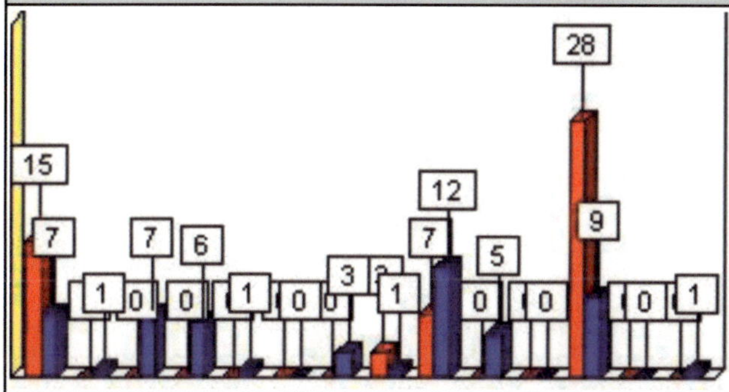

Chronic Fatigue:
Hyposplenism:
Chronic Staying Splenomegaly:
Splenomegaly:
Functional Changes:

LUNGS AND BRONCHI

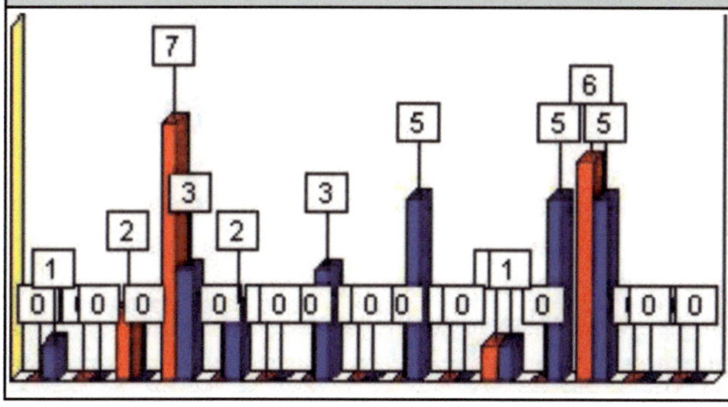

Bronchiectatic disease:
Post-Stress Effects:

SKIN

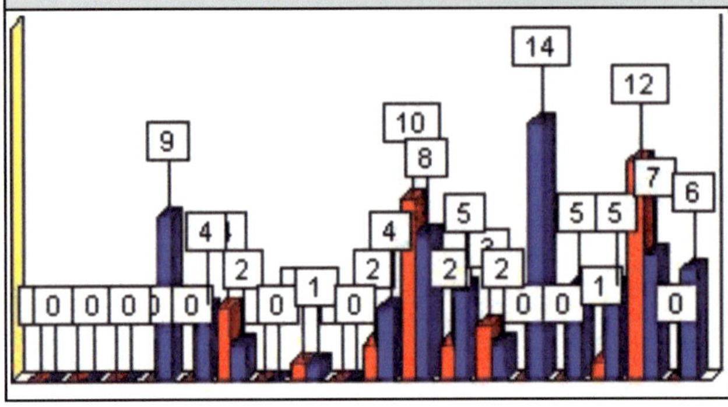

Eczema:
Herpes:
Growth of New Cells:
Age-Related Changes:
Degenerative Process:
Erythema:
Post-Stress Effects:
Intoxication Effects:

OESOPHAGUS

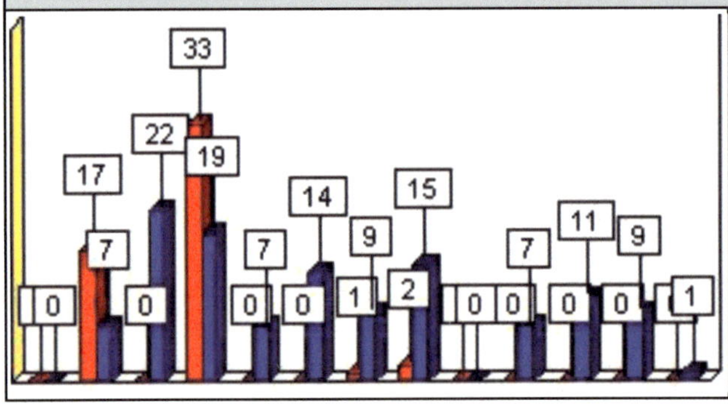

Degenerative Process:
Chronic Fatigue:
Tension of compensatory abilities.

STOMACH

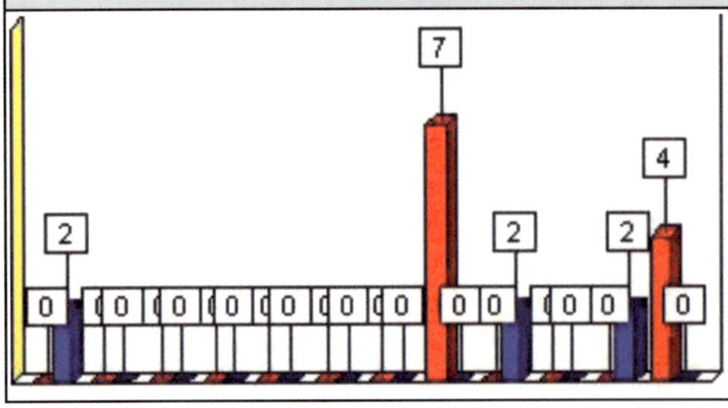

Ulcerative Disease:

DUODENUM

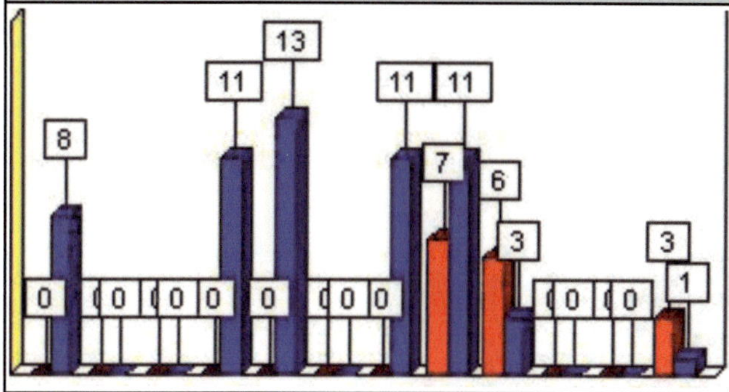

Allergic Process:
Growth of New Cells:
Duodenitis:
Intoxication Effects:
Ulcerative Disease:

SMALL INTESTINE

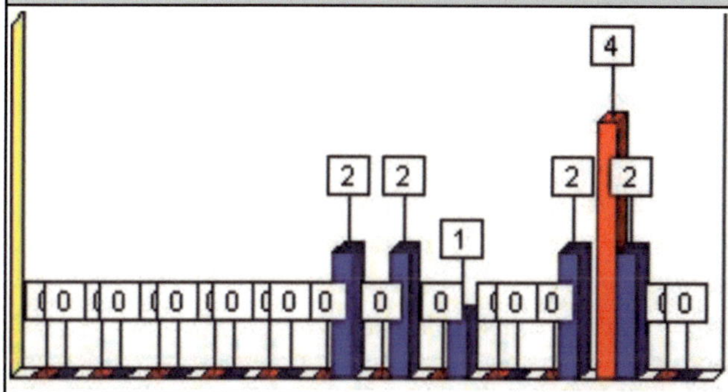

No changes detected.

LARGE INTESTINE

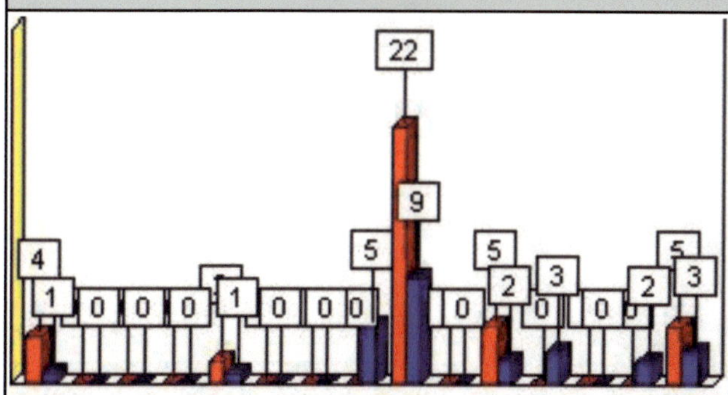

Degenerative Process:

KIDNEYS

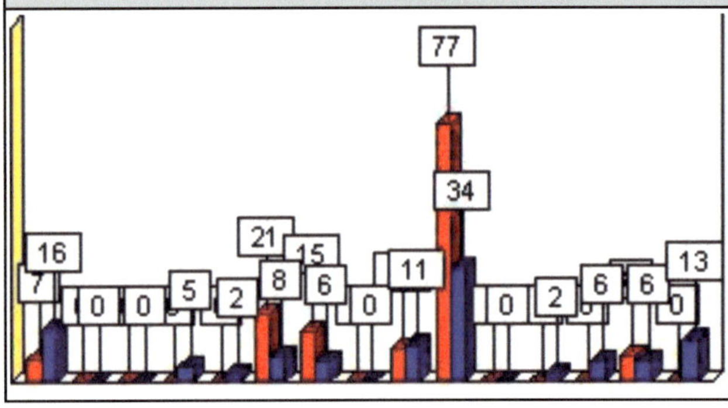

Glomerulonephritis:
Tissue Growth:
Urolithiasis:
Functional Changes:

URINARY BLADDER

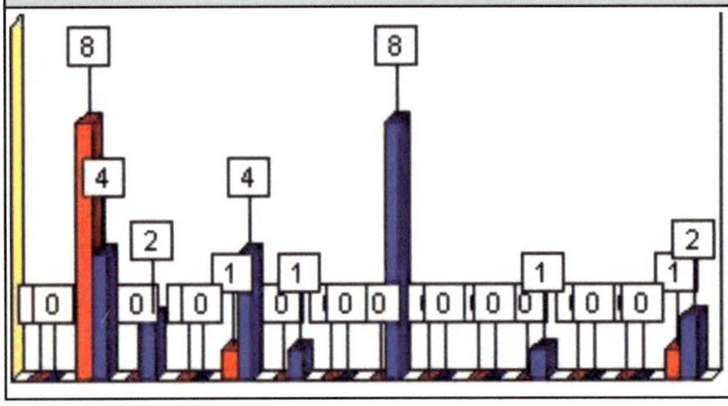

Chronic Fatigue:
Age-Related Changes:

WOMB AND APPENDAGES

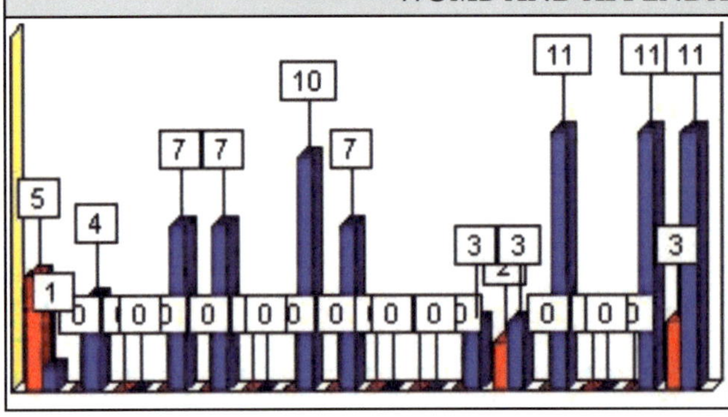

Allergic Process:

SKELETAL AND MUSCULAR SYSTEM	
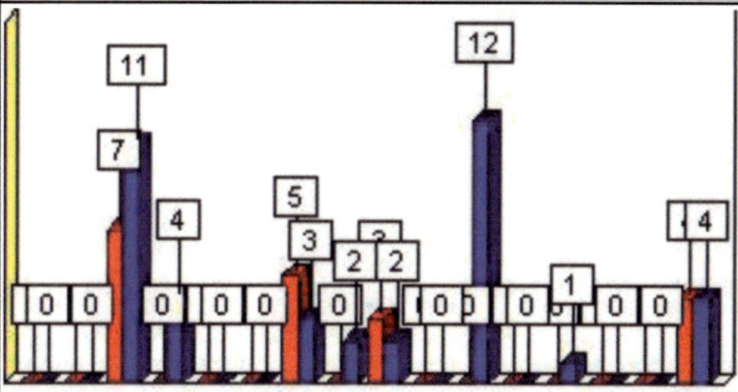	**Age-Related Changes:** **Chronic Fatigue:** **Functional Changes:**

Images of cell morphology

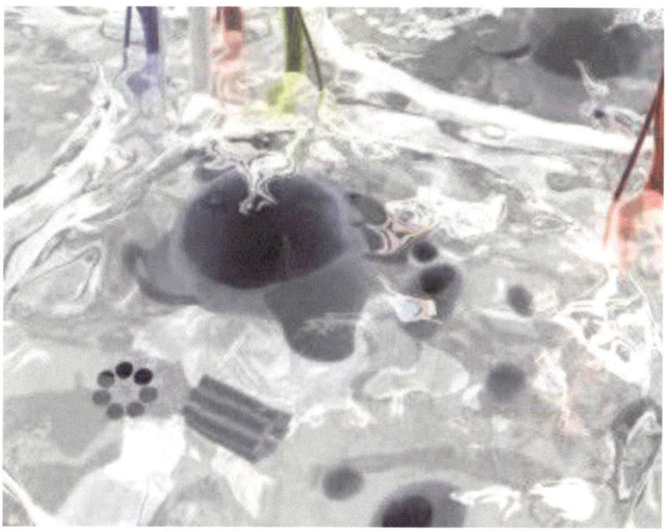

Normal cellular processes

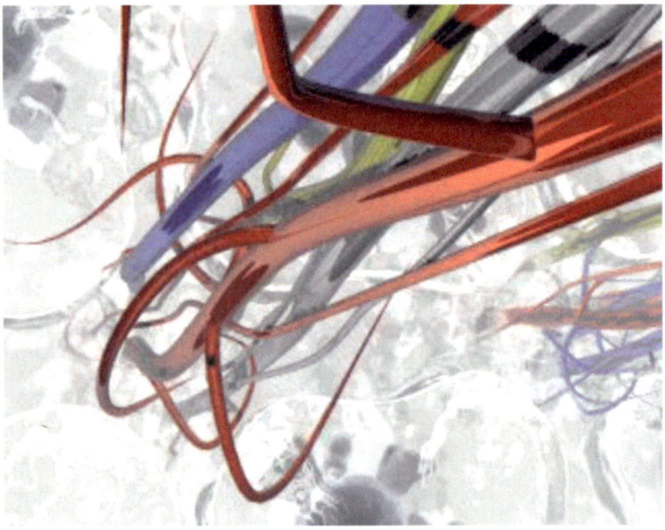

Inc blood flow/ Inflammation

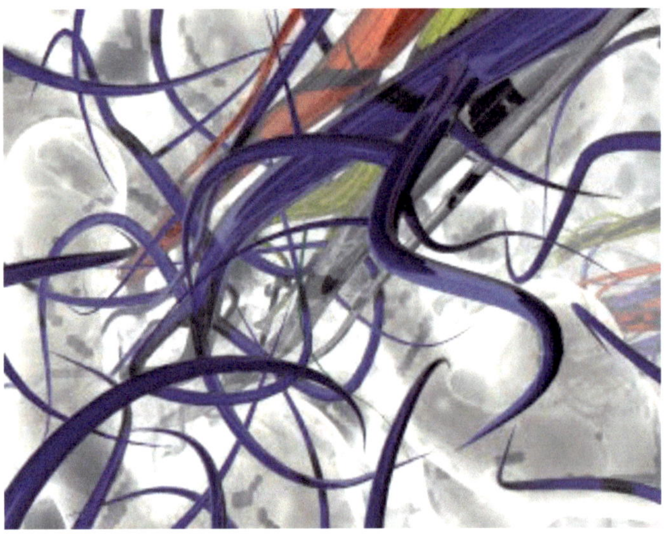

Ischaemia

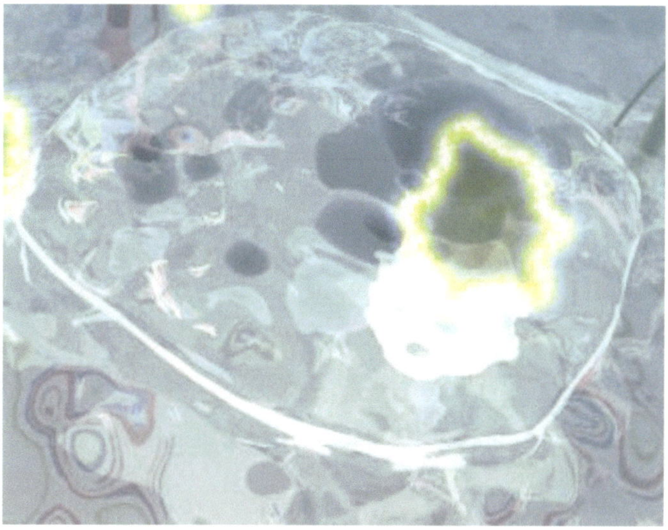

Cell hypofunction

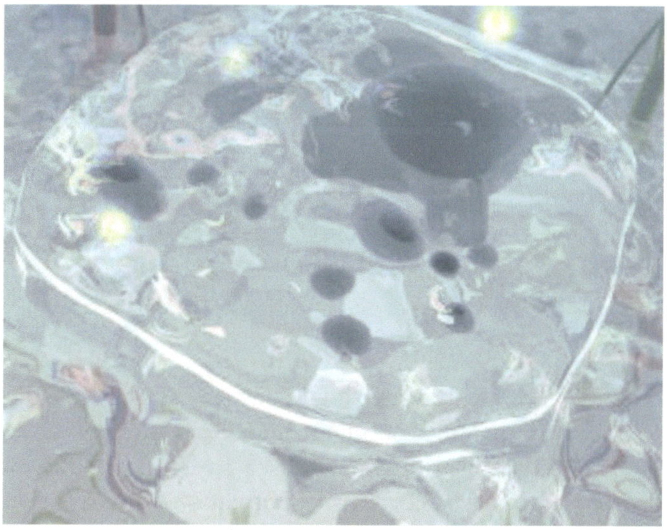

Cell hyperfunction

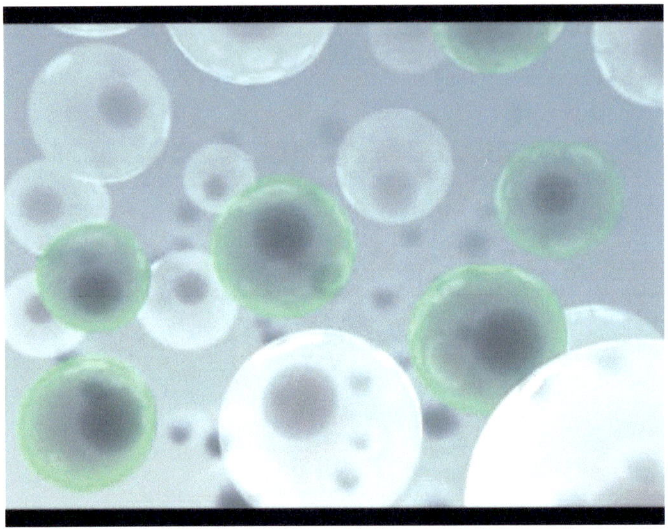

Abnormality of a limit of cell division

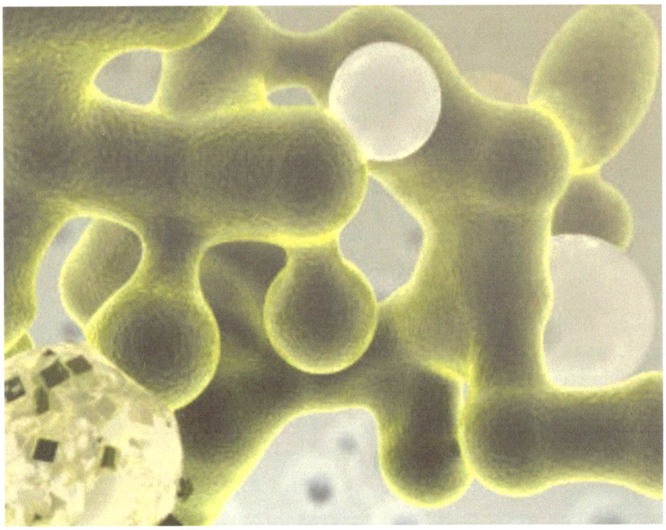

Old cells

Examples of diagnostic effect

1. female, 50 yrs. A VS practitioner with history of **lymphoblastic leukaemia**. VS identified the reoccurrence of the condition although medical tests had shown a steady level of leukocytes. As she had previously been treated for leukaemia and her most recent test had shown a steady level of leukocytes she discounted the possibility of reoccurrence of her lymphoblastic leukaemia. A subsequent medical check identified the reoccurrence of leukaemia.

2. female, c45 yrs. A lady with fatigue had been receiving acupuncture for several years. Medical testing was not able to identify the problems. VS indicated a number of issues including the early onset of pancreatic cancer. The lady died of **pancreatic cancer** several years later.
3. female, 50 yrs with **duodenal problem.** GP advised that she did not have a problem. Virtual Scanning detected process of duodenal ulcer. GP under duress carried out a further consultation and again gave a negative report. She was admitted to hospital with blood discharges just one week later and spent over one week in hospital being treated for a perforated duodenal ulcer. The lady gained a compensatory settlement as a result of the misdiagnosis by the GP.
4. the Medical Director of a reputable hospital in England asked Montague Healthcare to illustrate the scope of Virtual Scanning to diagnose the health of a patient. Within 15 minutes of completing the test Montague Healthcare had advised a list of five medical conditions. The results were confirmed by the Medical Director. He commented that his hospital did not have the ability to provide such diagnosis.

Examples of therapeutic effect

1. female, 59 years, who experienced **migraines** from the age of 11 until 59 years. Increasingly severe migraine attacks - the most recent resulted in her being Admitted to hospital in a semi-conscious state.
   The VS health assessment showed indications of migraine, epilepsy, impaired cerebral circulation, impaired spinal circulation as a result of vertebral artery syndrome, osteochondrosis and idiopathic hypotension. Since starting VS therapy she has not had any further migraine symptoms and is now completely free of migraines. In addition, several years previously she had a single mastectomy to remove cancer. This involved removal of the lymph nodes which resulted in poor drainage and hence swelling of her arm. After 4 months Virtual Scanning therapy there was little, if any, remaining swelling in her arm.
2. male, 78 years was dissatisfied with his GP's diagnosis when he consulted him with **type 2 diabetes, circulatory problems and a swollen foot**. He became disillusioned with the diagnosis when prescribed antibiotics. After a 6 month course of VS colour therapy he has improved stability of blood sugar levels, improved mobility, improved circulation, improved energy, and dramatically improved quality of life.
3. male, c65yrs suffering from **dysarthria** who could only mumble gutturally for almost 5 years. His hospital could not identify the problem despite using MRI, checking for Parkinsonism and Alzheimers, and finally was unable to assist him. Virtual Scanner detected encephalopathy, impairment of cerebral circulation, etc. VS colour therapy enabled him to recover the ability to speak clearly within **6 days**.
4. dyslexic female, 11yrs. The first indications of improved writing (distinct) and reading were indicated by the third VS consultation. Her end of term report commented that her reading ability had been re-assessed as that of a 14yo. Following a change of school this child completed her first examinations. Of the 11 examinations 9 were passed at

grades 1 & 2 (greater than 70%) whilst the remaining two examinations were grade 3 (60-70%).

5. male, 76 years with **prostate and asbestos-induced lung cancer.** Poor prognosis, required assistance to walk. Following chemotherapy and radiotherapy he had severely restricted breathing due to fluid on the lungs which required surgical intervention to drain fluid from his lungs but which failed to cure the problem of accumulating fluid. After a course of VS colour therapy, medical scanning techniques (x-rays) showed the complete absence of fluid on his lungs. As a result he no longer had chronic breathing insufficiency, he could walk unaided and his overall health was much improved. He lived for 1-2 years more than medical expectations.

Author details

Graham Wilfred Ewing
Montague Healthcare, Nottingham, United Kingdom

8. References

[1] Spear BB, Heath-Chiozzi M, Huff J. Clinical Applications of Pharmacogenetics. *Trends in Molecular Medicine* 2001; 7(5):201-204

[2] Ewing GW, Grakov IG. Fashion or Science? How can orthodox biomedicine explain the body's function and regulation? *N.Am.J.Med.Sci.* 2012;4(2):57-61.

[3] Malarkey WB, Kiecolt-Glaser JK, Pearl D, Glaser R. Hostile behaviour during marital stress alters pituitary and adrenal hormones. *Psychosomatic medicine* 1994;56(1):41-51.

[4] Grippo AJ, Lamb DG, Carter CS, Porges SW. Social isolation disrupts autonomic regulation of the heart and influences negative affective behaviors. *Biological Psychiatry* 2007;62:1162-1170.

[5] Ewing GW, Ewing EN. NeuroRegulation of the Physiological Systems by the Autonomic Nervous System – their relationship to Insulin Resistance and Metabolic Syndrome. *J. Biogenic Amines* 2008;22(4-5):208-239.

[6] Ewing GW, Ewing EN. Cognition, the Autonomic Nervous System and the Physiological Systems. *J. Biogenic Amines* 2008;22(3):140-163.

[7] Sudakov KV. The basic principles of the general theory of functional systems. *Medicine* 1987;S.26-49.

[8] Kryzhanovskii GN, Adrianov OS, Bekhtereva NP, Negovskii VA, Sudakov KV, Khananashvili MM. Integrative activity of the nervous system in health and in disease. *Vestnik Rossiĭskoĭ akademii meditsinskikh nauk* 02/1995.

[9] Ewing GW, Parvez SH, Grakov IG. Further Observations on Visual Perception: the influence of pathologies upon the absorption of light and emission of bioluminescence. *The Open Systems Biology Journal* 2011;4:1-7.

[10] Chifferstein HNJ, Talke KSS, Oudshoorn D-J. Can Ambient Scent Enhance the Nightlife Experience? *Chemosensory Perception* 2011;4(1-2):55-64.

[11] De Araujo IE, Simon SA. The gustatory cortex and multisensory integration. *International Journal of Obesity* 2009;33(Suppl. 2): S34-43.

[12] Ewing GW, Parvez SH. The influence of Pathologies and EEG frequencies upon sense perception and coordination in Developmental Dyslexia. A Unified Theory of Developmental Dyslexia. *N.Am.J.Med.Sci.* 2012;4(3):109-116.

[13] Ewing GW. A Theoretical Framework for Photosensitivity: Evidence of Systemic Regulation. *Journal of Computer Science and System Biology* 2009;2(6):287-297.

[14] Ewing GW, Parvez SH. The Dynamic Relationship between Cognition, the Physiological Systems, and Cellular and Molecular Biochemistry: a Systems-based Perspective on the Processes of Pathology. *Act. Nerv. Super. Rediviva* 2010; 52(1):29-36.

[15] Ewing GW. There is a need for an Alternative or Modified Medical Paradigm involving an understanding of the nature and significance of the Physiological Systems. *N.Am.J.Med.Sci.* 2010;2(6):1-6.

[16] Ewing GW, Parvez SH. The Multi-systemic Nature of Diabetes Mellitus: genotype or phenotype? *N.Am.J.Med.Sci* 2010;2(10):444-456.

[17] Ewing GW. Does an improved understanding of the nature and structure of the Physiological Systems lead to a better understanding of the therapeutic scope of Complementary & Conventional Medicine? *Journal of Computer Science and Systems Biology* 2009;2(3):174-179.

[18] Bowman GL, Silbert LS, Howieson D, Dodge HH, Traber MG, Frei B, Kaye JA, Shannon J, Quinn JF. Nutrient Biomarker Patterns, Cognitive Function and MRI Measures of Brain Aging. *Neurology* 2012;78:1-1.

[19] Ewing GW. The Regulation of pH is a Physiological System. Increased Acidity alters Protein Conformation and Cell Morphology and is a Significant Factor in the onset of Diabetes and other common pathologies. *The Open Systems Biology* 2012;5:1-12.

[20] Ewing GW, Parvez SH, Grakov IG. Further Observations on Visual Perception: the influence of pathologies upon the absorption of light and emission of bioluminescence. *The Open Systems Biology Journal* 2011;4:1-7.

[21] Horwitz LR, Burke TJ, Carnegie DH. Augmentation of Wound Healing Using Monochromatic Infrared Energy. *Advances in Wound Care* 1999;12:35-40.

[22] Melzack R, Wall PD. Pain mechanisms: a new theory. *Science* 1965;150(3699): 971-9.

[23] Voll R. Twenty years of electroacupuncture in Germany: a progress report. *Am.J. Acupunct* 1975;3:7-17.

[24] Ji-Sheng Han. Acupuncture: neuropeptide release produced by electrical stimulation of different frequencies. *Trends in Neurosciences* 2003;26(1):17-22.

[25] http://www.materiamedica.ru/en/

[26] Ernst E. Deaths after acupuncture: A systematic review. *The International Journal of Risk and Safety in Medicine* 2010;22(3):131-6.

[27] Vasquez A. "Allopathic Usurpation of Natural Medicine: The Blind Leading the Sighted." [Editorial] *Naturopathy Digest* 2006, February.

[28] Porges SW. The Polyvagal Perspective. *Biological Psychology* 2007;74:116-143.

[29] Porges SW. The Polyvagal Theory: phylogenetic contributions to social behavior. *Physiology and Behavior* 2003;79:503-513.

[30] Belvisi MG, Stretton CD, Yacoub M, Barnes PJ. Nitric oxide is the endogenous neurotransmitter of bronchodilator nerves in humans. *European Journal of Pharmacology* 1992;210(2):221-2.

[31] Vysochin Yu et al, 2001. Methodology and Technology of Invigoration of Different Population Orders. In: Consolidated 5 year Research Plan of Physical Training, Sports and Tourism State Committee of the Russian Federation. 2000. English translation available at: http://www.montaguehealthcare.co.uk/files/Vysochin/Vysochin.pdf

[32] Ewing GW, Parvez SH. The Multi-systemic Nature of Diabetes Mellitus: genotype or phenotype? *N.Am.J.Med.Sci* 2010;2(10):444-456.

[33] Ewing GW. Mathematical Modeling the Neuroregulation of Blood Pressure using a Cognitive Top-down Approach. *N.Am.J.Med.Sci.*2010;2(8):341-352.

[34] Ewing GW, Parvez SH. Mathematical Modeling the Systemic Regulation of Blood Glucose: 'a top-down' Systems Biology Approach. *NeuroEndocrine Letters* 2011;32(4):371-9.

[35] Grakov IG. Strannik Diagnostic and Treatment System: a Virtual Scanner for the Health Service. *Minutes of Meeting No. 11 of the Praesidium of the Siberian of the Academy of Medical Sciences of the USSR* (AMN) held in Novosibirsk 4 December 1985.

[36] Hankey A, Ewing EN. New Light on Chromotherapy: Grakov's 'Virtual Scanning' System of Medical Assessment and Treatment. *eCAM* 2007;4(2):139-144.

[37] Ewing GW, Ewing EN, Hankey A. Virtual Scanning - Medical Assessment and Treatment. *Journal of Alternative and Complementary Medicine* 2007;13(2):271-286.

[38] Gaponiuk Pia, Perov IuF. Electrode potentials of acupuncture needles made of different metals [Article in Russian]. *Vopr. Kurortol. Fizioter. Lech. Fiz. Kult.* 1981 Jan-Feb;(1):46-9.

[39] Eachou Chen. De-chi and propagated sensation along meridian. *Journal of Accord Integrative Medicine* 2011;7(3):116-118.

[40] Kringelbach ML, Jenkinson N, Owen SLF, Aziz TA. Translational principles of deep brain stimulation. *Nature Reviews Neuroscience* 2007;8:623-635.

[41] Salansky N, Fedotchev A, Bondar A. Responses of the Nervous System to Low Frequency Stimulation and EEG Rhythms: Clinical Implications. *Neuroscience and Biobehavioural Reviews* 1998;22(3):395-409.

[42] Bell G, Marino A, Chesson A, Struve F. Electrical states in the rabbit brain can be altered by light and electromagnetic fields. *Brain Research* 1992;570(1-2):307-315.

Chapter 6

Musical Auditory Stimulation and Cardiac Autonomic Regulation

Vitor Engrácia Valenti, Luiz Carlos de Abreu, Heraldo L. Guida, Luiz Carlos M. Vanderlei, Lucas Lima Ferreira and Celso Ferreira

Additional information is available at the end of the chapter

http://dx.doi.org/10.5772/52186

1. Introduction

Humans discovered the effects of the musical auditory stimulation on their own wellness at the dawn of the pre-historical age, i.e., during the Cro-Magnon and the Neanderthalian cave cultures. Charles Darwin hypothesized that musical auditory stimulation may have been a protolanguage in ancient times. Under a cultural perspective, the definition of musical auditory stimulation is subtle and not well established, since it has varied through history, in different regions, and within societies. The fifteenth edition of the Encyclopædia Britannica describes that "while there are no sounds that can be described as inherently unmusical auditory stimulational, musical auditory stimulationians in each culture have tended to restrict the range of sounds they will admit". In his 1983 book, Musical auditory stimulation as Heard: A Study in Applied Phenomenology, Thomas Clifton affirms that "musical auditory stimulation is the actualization of the possibility of any sound whatever to present to some human being a meaning which he experiences with his body—that is to say, with his mind, his feelings, his senses, his will, and his metabolism" (Clifton, 1983). On the other hand, the French musical auditory stimulationologist Jean-Jaques Nattiez has affirmed that "the border between musical auditory stimulation and noise is always culturally defined — which implies that, even within a single society, this border does not always pass through the same place; in short, there is rarely a consensus. By all accounts there is no single and intercultural universal concept defining what musical auditory stimulation might be (Clifton, 1983).

Some authors believe that the first ancient musical auditory stimulational rituals, such as wooden-drums beating, vocalizing (either as animal voice imitation, or as an extension of spoken language) and body swaying and shaking, may represent the oldest form of religion and perhaps of medicine, searching and often obtaining a sense of depersonalization and well-being (Révész, 1953). The power of the musical auditory stimulation in eliciting physical reactions has been known probably since the ancient Assyrian and Greek cultures, although the relationship between musical auditory stimulation and body responses was at that times believed to belong to the field of magic. During the Olympic Games in ancient Greece, musical auditory stimulationians were paid for playing flute and kithara (a harp-like string instrument) with the aim of improving athlete's performance (Révész, 1953). In that era, Pythagoreans were the first to disclaim the mathematical relationships of musical auditory stimulational notes, and Plato, in "The Republic", wrote that "Musical auditory stimulation is most sovereign because rhythm and harmony find their way to the inmost soul and take strongest hold upon it, imparting grace, in one is rightly trained". Musical auditory stimulation was mostly based on three distinct "modes" (dorian, lydian, and phrygian) in ancient Greece, each further subdivided in two or three sub-modes, representative of different musical auditory stimulational scales. This organization was strongly related to the feeling, each "mode" being characterized by specific properties (e.g., to arouse pity, or fear, or enThereforeiasm – this last word having itself a mystic connotation: εν τηεοσ (én Theos), meaning, according to the majority of authors, "having a God inside", or "being in a God-like state") and sometimes allowing to "heal and purify the soul" (Aristotle) (Révész, 1953). In ancient Rome, Plinius reported that Cato recalled a melody specific for the treatment of muscular distractions, and Varro another one for the treatment of gout (Révész, 1953). In the Middle Ages there was an "epidemic of dances": choreic patients were used to dance continuously for several hours, in the belief that this might heal them. The southern-Italy dance "tarantella" was also thought to cure some tarantula-spider (Lycosa tarantula, Latrodectes tredecimguttatus and other species) bites (Sacks, 2007).

Robert Burton wrote in his "Melancholy's Anatomy" in 1632: "musical auditory stimulation is the more grateful and effective remedy for sadness, fear and mood disorders". Peter Lichtenthal, an Austro-Hungarian scientist and musical auditory stimulationian, wrote in his "Dissertation About the Influence of Musical auditory stimulation on the Human Body" (1811): "Worthy of the experiment of a physician is, in my opinion, research into the impact of musical auditory stimulation on man and, led by philosophical reasoning, use it in the treatment of illnesses". The great German surgeon C.A.T. Billroth (also a good violin and cello player), in his "Wer ist musikalish?" published in 1894, attempted first to correlate musical auditory stimulational abilities with the anatomy and physiology of the brain [6]. It was only in 1899, however, that "The Lancet" published an article by J.T.R. Davison, entitled "Musical auditory stimulation in Medicine", leading to the now growing field of scientific investigation in musical auditory stimulation and health (Davison, 1899). In 1914 E. O'Neil Kane published in JAMA the first experiment describing the effects of musical auditory stimulation in medical procedures, demonstrating that the use of a phonograph within operating and recovery room was able to decrease the need for pharmacological analgesia and decrease anxiety of patients undergoing "horrors of surgery" (Davison, 1899). In 1918 Hyde and Scalapino reported, in the first technology-based experiment in this field (e.g., EKG recording), that minor tones enhanced pulse rate and lowered blood pressure, whereas stirring musical auditory stimulation enhanced both blood pressure and heart rate (Hyde and Scalapino, 19289). In recent years, musical auditory stimulation has been increasingly used as a therapeutic tool in the treatment of different diseases, although the physiological basis in healthy and ill subjects is still poorly understood.

There has been considerable recent interest in the cardiovascular, respiratory, and neurophysiological effects of listening to musical auditory stimulation, including the brain areas involved, which appear to be similar to those involved in arousal. Responses to musical auditory stimulation appear to be personal, particularly when skin tingling or "chills" occur, which suggests individual reactions to musical auditory stimulation that are dependent on individual preferences, mood, or emotion (Koelsch et al, 2005). However, a previous study showed consistent cardiovascular and respiratory responses to musical auditory stimulation with different styles (raga/techno/classical) in most subjects, in whom arousal was related to tempo and was associated with faster breathing (Bernardi et al, 2006). The responses were qualitatively similar in musical auditory stimulationians and nonmusical auditory stimulationians and apparently were not influenced by musical auditory stimulation preferences, although musical auditory stimulationians responded more. That original study concerned average responses to musical auditory stimulation rather than to dynamic changes during a track, because we used artificial tracks with 2 or 4 minutes of consistent style and tempo. Changes in tempo and emphasis were less evident, which is important for originating "chills."

As mentioned, musical auditory stimulation is known to elicit various psychological responses, but the effects of musical auditory stimulation on physiological phenomena have not been as well studied. Auditory stimulation with musical auditory stimulation lowers the heart rate and blood pressure (BP) in human beings (Lee et al, 2005) or spontaneously hypertensive rats (Sutoo and Akiyama, 2004), suggesting that musical auditory stimulation can affect autonomic and cardiovascular function.

Overall, comprehending the process which musical auditory stimulational auditory stimulation modulates cardiac autonomic regulation will provide further procedures as therapies for cardiovascular disorders. In this chapter we summarize concepts regarding musical auditory stimulational auditory stimulation and cardiac autonomic regulation.

2. Musical auditory stimulational auditory stimulation and cardiovascular system

The analysis of texts selected for this review indicated that harmonic musical auditory stimulation is able to improve the cardiac autonomic regulation. The literature on the effect of musical auditory stimulation on autonomic nervous system (ANS) activity in healthy subjects is quite large. On the other hand, the literature on how musical auditory stimulation affects individuals with cardiovascular dysfunction is less developed.

A previous study (Alvarsson et al, 2010) tested whether physiological stress recovery is faster during exposure to pleasant nature sounds than to noise. As a main finding, they suggested that nature sounds facilitate recovery from sympathetic activation after a psychological stressor. The mechanisms behind the faster recovery could be related to positive emotions (pleasantness), evoked by the nature sound as suggested by previous research using non audio film stimuli13. Other perceptual attributes may also influence recovery. In the study of Alvarsson et al (2010), the ambient noise was perceived as less familiar than the other sounds, presumably because it contained no identifiable sources. One may speculate that this lack of information might have caused an enhanced mental activity and thereby an enhanced skin conductance level compared with the nature sound reported by them. An effect of sound pressure level may be seen in the difference between high and low noise, this difference is in line with previous psychoacoustic research14 and is not a surprising considering the large difference (30 dBA) in sound pressure level.

Another study investigated the effects of musical auditory stimulation therapy on drugs-induced cardiac autonomic regulation injury (Chuang et al, 2011). Considering that anthracycline is a compound known to induce cardiovascular disorders (Chuang et al, 2011), Chuang and coworkers indicated that long-term musical auditory stimulation therapy improved heart rate variability in anthracycline-treated breast cancer patients. The findings of a previous study also suggest that the parasympathetic nervous system is activated by musical auditory stimulation therapy and appears to protect against congestive heart failure events in elderly patients with cerebrovascular disease and dementia by reducing the levels of both epinephrine and norepinephrine (Okada et al, 2009). Therefore, musical auditory stimulation therapy intervention may also help breast cancer patients control the progression and relieve symptoms of cardiac damage, which is a result of treatment with anthracycline-containing chemotherapy. As a main conclusion, Chuang et al. (2011) suggested that regular musical auditory stimulation therapy appears to be useful for promoting autonomic function, although further research is necessary to determine whether more (or more frequent) sessions of musical auditory stimulation therapy intervention can promote and maintain autonomic function after musical auditory stimulation therapy is stopped.

A very elegant study performed by Nakamura et al. (2007) indicated that in rats musical auditory stimulation decreases renal sympathetic nerve activity and blood pressure through the auditory pathway, the hypothalamic suprachiasmatic nucleus, and histaminergic neurons. Moreover, the authors suggested that only certain types of musical auditory stimulation affect renal sympathetic activity and blood pressure in rats. Animals with bilateral lesions in the auditory cortex may discriminate a simple sound, suggesting that there is another auditory sensing pathway that is not mediated by the auditory cortex (Butler et al, 1957) but lesions of the cochleae or the auditory cortex eliminated musical auditory stimulation-induced changes in the renal sympathetic activity and blood pressure (Salimpoor et al, 2011), indicating that the changes to renal sympathetic activity and blood pressure did depend on signaling through the auditory system.

In the same context, a recent investigation presented the first direct evidence that the intense pleasure experienced when listening to musical auditory stimulation is associated with dopamine activity in the mesolimbic reward system, including both dorsal and ventral striatum (Salimpoor et al, 2011). One explanation for this phenomenon is that it is related to enhancement of emotions (Salimpoor et al, 2009). The emotions induced by musical auditory stimulation are evoked, among other things, by temporal phenomena, such as expectations, delay, tension, resolution, prediction, surprise and anticipation (Huron and Hellmuth Margulis, 2009).

Another study (Bernardi et al, 2009) reported that the cardiovascular (particularly skin vasomotion) and respiratory fluctuations were associated to the musical auditory stimulation profile, especially if it contained a crescendo. They also showed that specific musical auditory stimulation phrases (frequently at a rhythm of 6 cycles/min in famous arias by Verdi) may synchronize inherent cardiovascular rhythms, Therefore, modulating cardiovascular control. This occurs regardless of respiratory modulation, which suggests the possibility of direct entrainment of such rhythms and allows us to speculate that some of the psychological and somatic effects of musical auditory stimulation could also be mediated by modulation or entrainment of these rhythms. Furthermore, musical auditory stimulationians and nonmusical auditory stimulationians showed similar qualitative responses, however, musical auditory stimulationians presented closer and faster cardiovascular and particularly respiratory modulation induced by the musical auditory stimulation. The same authors suggested that musical auditory stimulation induces predictable physiological cardiovascular changes even in the absence of conscious reactions, which suggests that these changes may "precede" the psychological appreciation. Their finding may explain the apparent discrepancy between individual appreciation (subjective) and physiological reactions (common to all subjects despite different musical auditory stimulation culture and practice) and provide a rational basis for the use of musical auditory stimulation in cardiovascular medicine.

The studies cited in this chapter present considerable implications for the use of musical auditory stimulation as a therapeutic tool, because all subjects, whether musical auditory stimulationally trained or not, responded in a similar manner. Musical auditory stimulation is used more and more frequently as a therapeutic tool in different diseases (Okada et al, 2009; Chuang et al, 2011). It is also hypothesized that a distracting effect of musical auditory stimulation can prolong exercise by increasing the threshold for pain or dyspnea (von Leupoldt et al, 2007). An externally driven autonomic modulation could be of practical use to induce body sensation (eg, enhance in heart rate or by skin vasoconstriction), which might finally reach the level of consciousness or at least create a continuous stimulus to the upper brain centers. This may better explain the efficacy of musical auditory stimulation in pathological conditions such as stroke (Särkämo et al, 2008), and it opens new areas for musical auditory stimulation therapy in rehabilitative medicine.

3. Musical auditory stimulation and autonomic nervous system

The literature on the effect of musical auditory stimulation on autonomic nervous system (ANS) activity in healthy subjects is quite large; the literature on how musical auditory stimulation affects individuals with ANS dysfunction (especially within the context of musical auditory stimulational interventions) is less developed. In both literatures, however, changes in physiological activity (e.g., heart rate, blood pressure, electrodermal activity) are often investigated and discussed from one of two distinct (and tacit) perspectives: as either (1) the byproducts of arousal, mood, anxiety, and other psychological states that are the primary target of study; or (2) definitive barometers of those psychological states. The second perspective assumes that statistically significant changes in ANS activity reflect meaningful changes in the state of the organism (when in fact they may not). Conversely, the first perspective assumes that, since physiological changes are the downstream consequences of changes in "central" states, they have only limited diagnostic utility. Neither perspective addresses a fundamental issue: that the autonomic nervous system (and activity in its targets) is exquisitely linked, bidirectionally, with the central nervous system, endocrine system, and immune system. Given that the ANS is both associated with physiological health and responsive to musical auditory stimulation, the ANS may serve as one path by which musical auditory stimulation exerts its therapeutic effect. The implications of such an association have yet to be fully explored.

The influence of the ANS on the heart is dependent on informations from baroreceptors, chemoreceptors, atrial receptors, ventricular receptors, changes on the respiratory system, vasomotor system, the renin-angiotensinaldosterone system and the thermoregulatory system, among others (Valenti et al, 2007; Valenti et al, 2009a; Valenti et al, 2009b; Valenti et al, 2011a; Valenti et al, 2011b; Valenti et al, 2011c).

This neural control is closely linked to heart rate (HR) and baroreceptor reflex activity (Valenti et al, 2007). From the afferent informations, by means of a complex interaction between stimulation and inhibition, the responses from sympathetic and parasympathetic pathways are formulated and modify the HR, by adapting to the needs of each moment. The heart is not a metronome and its beats do not have the regularity of a clock, so changes in HR, defined as heart rate variability (HRV), are normal and expected and indicate the heart's ability to respond to multiple physiological and environment stimuli, among them, breathing, physical exercise, mental stress, hemodynamic and metabolic changes, sleep and orthostatism, as well as to compensate disorders induced by diseases (Colombari et al, 2001).

In general, HRV describes the oscillation of the intervals between consecutive heart beats (RR intervals), which are related to the influences of the ANS on the sinus node, being a noninvasive measurement that can be used to identify phenomena related to the ANS in healthy individuals, athletes and patients with diseases (Task Force, 1996). Figure 1 shows rate tachogram obtained from the RR intervals of a normal young adult and a normal newborn. It is observed that the HRV is much smaller in the newborn.

Currently, the HRV indexes have been used to understand various conditions, such as coronary artery disease (Carney et al, 2007), cardiomyopathy, arterial hypertension, myocardial infarction, sudden death, chronic obstructive pulmonary disease, renal failure, heart failure, diabetes, stroke, Alzheimer's disease, leukemia, obstructive sleep apnea, epilepsy, headache, among others (Vanderlei et al, 2009).

A decreased HRV has been identified as a strong indicator of risk related to adverse events in healthy individuals and patients with a large number of diseases, reflecting the vital role that ANS plays in maintaining health (Task Force, 1996).

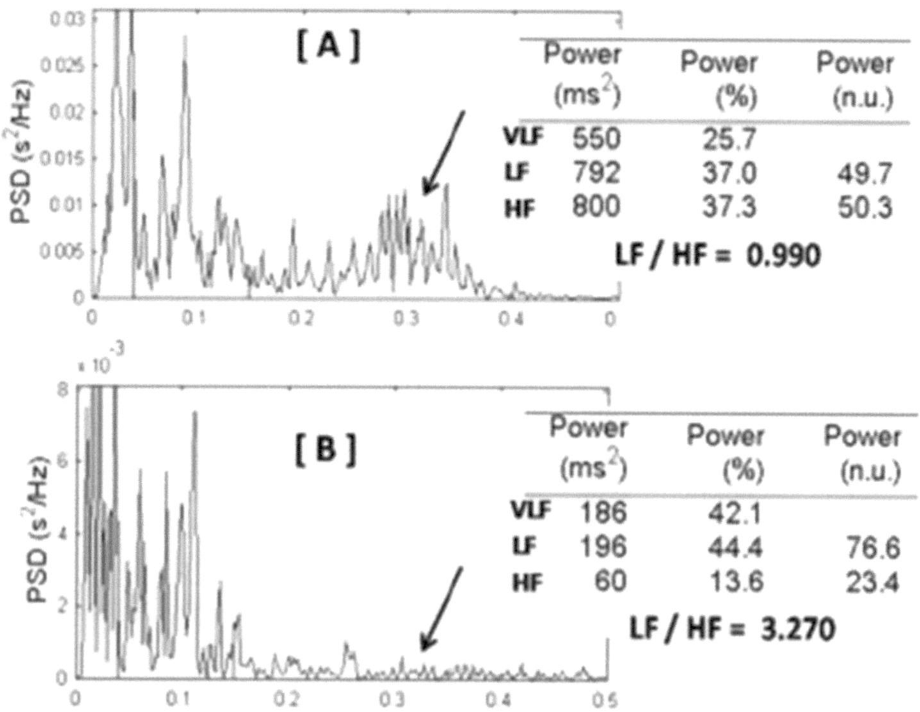

Figure 1. Spectral analysis of frequencies (Fast Fourier Transform) of a normal young adult (A) and a normal newborns (B). The high frequency (HF) component is proportionally smaller in the newborn (arrows) as well as the total power.

HRV is a physiologically grounded, theoretically explicated, empirically supported, computationally tractable measure of autonomic (dys)function (Ellis and Thayer, 2010). HRV may be recorded noninvasively, inexpensively, and with high fidelity via commercially available fitness watches (e.g., Polar RS800; www.polar.fi/en/) and analyzed with freeware (e.g., Kubios; http://kubios.uku.fi/).

Nevertheless, there have been relatively few empirical investigations of HRV and musical auditory stimulation compared to mean HR and musical auditory stimulation. HRV is not mentioned in either of the major literature reviews of musical auditory stimulation and physiological response. A majority of studies have been experimental rather than interventional, reporting significant changes in HRV as a function of musical auditory stimulational mood, genre, familiarity, or tempo (Bernardi et al, 2006; Ellis and Thayer, 2010). Only a few reports exist of musical auditory stimulational interventions that have included HRV as an index of autonomic function: in pediatric oncology patients, myocardial infarction patients, and geriatric patients (Okada et al, 2009).

According to the studies regarding musical auditory stimulation and autonomic nervous system, humans interact with musical auditory stimulation, both consciously and unconsciously, at behavioral, emotional, and physiological levels. James (1884) mused that the ANS "forms a sort of sounding-board, which every change of our consciousness, however slight, may make reverberate". While that sounding-board certainly reverberates to musical auditory stimulation, it is hoped that the present review begins to illustrate just how complex that interaction may be, and the associated implications for future research. With respect to experimental studies, it is important to explore how specific features of musical auditory stimulation (e.g., its beat, tempo, or pitch level) trigger neurophysiological, psychophysiological, emotional, and behavioral responses.

Skin conductance activity is a sensitive index of autonomic arousal, resulting from sympathetic innervation of the skin, and measured by alterations in the conductance of an applied current. During the surgical procedures, transient changes in SCA were recorded with Ag–AgCl electrodes on the distal palmar surface of the third and fourth fingers of the nondominant hand. Similarly, accelerative heart rate response (HRR), a less sensitive index of sympathetic and parasympathetic output, was monitored with single-lead chest ECG connected to the recording system (ADInstruments, Sydney, Australia). Digital event markings were used to identify stimulation intervals and target location for subsequent analysis (Gentil et al, 2009).

Measuring electrodermal activity is one technique that provides readily accessible autonomic indices, such as the skin conductance response (SCR). SCR is due to rapid fluctuations in eccrine sweat gland activity, which result from the liberation of acetylcholin by the sympathetic nervous system (Boucsein, 1992). This measure has the advantage over other measures of the autonomic nervous system such as heart rate, since SCR is under strict control of the sympathetic branch of the nervous system. Moreover, SCRs have been shown to be reliable measures of autonomic expressions of emotions, in domains other than musical auditory stimulation. For instance, in both visual (affective picture such as a beautiful landscape) and auditory (naturally occurring sounds such as crying baby) modalities, SCRs proved to be modulated by valence and to enhance with rated arousal (Bradley and Lang, 2000).

A previous study (Khalfa et al, 2002) indicated that event-related SCRs are sensitive measures of musical auditory stimulation-induced emotions. Moreover, results revealed that musical auditory stimulational excerpts could induce SCRs that differ according to underlying dimensions of emotion. Both fear and happiness were associated with higher SCR magnitudes than sadness and peace fulness. The fact that fear and happiness are strongly arousing emotions, as compared to sadness and peacefulness, suggests that arousal is the relevant emotional dimension as related to SCRs. This is in accordance with the literature showing that electrodermal activity is more sensitive to variations in emotional arousal rather than to valence (Bradley and Lang, 2000). The arousal effect obtained using musical auditory stimulational excerpts parallels the one obtained when slides of affective pictures or environmental sounds were employed (Bradley and Lang, 2000). In these previous experiments, larger SCR changes were significantly related to enhanced arousal ratings, but not to valence rating. In the present experiment, the pleasant emotion of happiness was not statistically differentiated from the unpleasant emotion of fear.

Another point raised by Khalfa et al (2002) is that SCR magnitudes do not parallel the corresponding clarity judgment of the emotion represented. Fearful excerpts eliciting the greatest SCRs were not rated as the most intense. Therefore, SCR was not a measure of the emotional category and clarity but was dependant upon arousal.

With respect to interventions with physiological targets (e.g., hypertension, tachycardia), it is important to consider that ANS dysfunction is mediated by the central nervous system (CNS), and that treatment of the former should be sensitive to the state of the latter. With respect to interventions with psychological targets (e.g., depression, anxiety), it is important to understand that ANS processes are not merely the downstream flotsam of activity in the CNS, but function as part of a sensitive feedback and feed-forward mechanism. Continued work within these different paradigms may reveal a common finding: that the ANS serves as the final common pathway by which musical auditory stimulation exerts a therapeutic effect on health and disease.

4. Physiological mechanisms

Based on Lee et al study (2010), white noise exposure above 50 dB enhances sympathetic activity. They also found strong correlation between LF/HF ratio (low frequency-high frequency ration) and noise intensity. LF/HF ratio corresponds to the sympathetic-vagal balance (Dias de Carvalho et al, 2011). Therefore, noise intensity was indicated to influence cardiac autonomic regulation. The cardiovascular responses to sound may be conducted through many pathways and one example is the startle response mediated by a brainstem circuit. The acoustic startle reflex, a well-known effect of loud sounds on cardiovascular system, is described as the abrupt response of the heart rate and blood pressure to a sudden loud sound stimulation. The typical intensity used to elicit a startle reflex is 110 dB, and the intensity is much louder than the environmental noise. However, the cardiac accelerative responses that habituated over trials were observed in the subjects evoked by repeated 60 dB and 110 dB white-noise stimuli. The responses were regarded as startle and defense response in humans or a fight/flight reaction in animals. The rise of blood pressure and heart rate to acoustic startle stimuli indicated an autonomic function responding to the acoustic stimuli (Samuels et al, 2007). Furthermore, cortical centers and also subcortical processing centers were thought to be involved in the cardiovascular and hormonal responses to a long-term stress activation by the environmental noises even though the noise intensity was as low as 53 dB26.

Indeed, Salimpoor et al (2011) found a temporal dissociation between distinct regions of the striatum while listening to pleasurable musical auditory stimulation. The combined psychophysiological, neurochemical and hemodynamic procedure that we used revealed that peaks of autonomic nervous system activity that reflect the experience of the most intense emotional moments are associated with dopamine release in the nucleus accumbens. This region has been implicated in the euphoric component of psychostimulants such as cocaine (Volkow et al, 1997) and is highly interconnected with limbic regions that mediate emotional responses, such as the amygdala, hippocampus, cingulate and ventromedial prefrontal cortex. In contrast, immediately before the climax of emotional responses there was evidence for relatively greater dopamine activity in the caudate. This subregion of the striatum is interconnected with sensory, motor and associative regions of the brain28 and has been typically implicated in learning of stimulus-response associations and in mediating the reinforcing qualities of rewarding stimuli such as food (Salimpoor et al, 2011).

Sutoo and colleagues (2004) hypothesize that musical auditory stimulation is effective for rectification of symptoms in various diseases that involve dopamine (DA) dysfunction. The loss of striatal DA accounts for most of the symptoms in Parkinson disease (PD), and treatment with L-DOPA, the immediate precursor of DA, improves some symptoms in PD. Therefore, some symptoms of PD might be rectified by musical auditory stimulation through enhanced calcium-dependent DA synthesis. Several studies have examined the effect of musical auditory stimulation therapy on symptoms of PD, and their clinical findings support this hypothesis (Paccheti et al, 1998). Pacchetti et al (1998) reported a significant improvement in motor function, emotional function, and activities of daily living after musical auditory stimulation therapy. It is possible that musical auditory stimulation enhances DA synthesis in the remaining DAergic nerve cells in the neostriatum and eases some symptoms of PD. In addition to PD, abnormally decreased neostriatal DAergic function has also been reported in epilepsy, dementia with Lewy bodies, or ADHD cases (Sidorenko, 2000). Therefore, musical auditory stimulation might attenuate symptoms of these diseases.

Previous reports demonstrate that exercise stimulates the calcium metabolic hormone and enhances blood calcium levels, thereby increasing DA synthesis in the brain, similar to the effect of musical auditory stimulation (Sutoo, 1996). Therefore, cardiovascular function in heart failure rats was decreased following exercise (Gao et al, 2007). The effect of exercise on blood pressure in spontaneously hypertensive rats was inhibited by pretreatment with EDTA, aMPT, or D2 receptor antagonists (Akiyama and Sutoo, 1999). In addition, some symptoms of PD or senile dementia are improved by exercise, and symptoms of epilepsy are improved by convulsions that have some resemblance to exercise with respect to movement (Sutoo and Akiyama, 2003). It is possible that the activities of daily life, such as musical auditory stimulation, exercise, or slight stress, enhance DAergic activity, and therefore subsequently regulate and/or affect various brain functions, and that this mechanism might underlie the improving effect of the activities of daily living on the symptoms in various diseases that involve DA dysfunction. Furthermore, unpublished data from our group showed in healthy women that acute musical auditory stimulational auditory stimulation with classical musical auditory stimulation (Mozart: Pachelbel, 70-80dB) decreased parasympathetic indices of HRV, such as NN50, pNN50 and RMSSD. Those responses are known as parasympathetic withdrawal, similar to the acute effects of exercise. Indicating that musical auditory stimulation acutely decreases parasympathetic activity and for long term enhance parasympathetic activity.

5. Brain aspects

As mentioned before, Nakamura and coworkers (2007) observed that musical auditory stimulational auditory stimulation decreases blood pressure and renal sympathetic nerve activity. This effect was based on the hypothalamic suprachiasmatic nucleus (SCN). It was previously reported that bilateral electrolytic lesions of the SCN eliminate changes in autonomic neurotransmission, blood glucose, and blood presurre caused by 2-deoxy-d-glucose (2DG), l-carnosine, and odors of grapefruit and lavender oil (Tanida et al, 2005). This implicates the SCN, a master circadian oscillator in mammals, in homeostatic control through autonomic nerves. The SCN sends multisynaptic sympathetic and parasympathetic projections to the pancreas, liver, and adrenal gland, as well as autonomic neural projections to peripheral tissues and organs, including the kidneys (Sly et al, 1999). These findings suggest that the SCN is a central regulator of autonomic nerve function. Nakamura and colleagues (2007) found that the changes in renal sympathetic activity and arterial blood pressure due to musical auditory stimulation stimulation disappeared after bilateral lesions of the SCN, suggesting that the SCN could mediate the effects of auditory stimulation with musical auditory stimulation on cardiac autonomic regulation. The multisynaptic efferent projections from the SCN to the medulla oblongata contain autonomic neurons that modulate blood pressure. Although the exact descending pathway responsible for the autonomic and cardiovascular effects of auditory stimulation with musical auditory stimulation remain to be determined, the histaminergic H3 receptor is likely to be a part of this pathway. The hypothalamic tuberomammillary nucleus (TMN) contains the cell bodies of histaminergic neurons, which release histamine and project to wide areas of the brain, including the SCN, which, like many areas of the brain, contains histaminergic H3 receptors38. Therefore, the neural connection between the TMN and the SCN could be part of the neural pathway between auditory stimulation with musical auditory stimulation and changes in cardiac autonomic regulation (Nakamura et al, 2007). However, the details of the mechanism are not certain, and further study will be needed.

In relation to electroencephalographic analysis, it is important to mention the Mozart effect. The "Mozart effect" refers to an enhancement of performance or change in neurophysiological activity associated with listening to Mozart's musical auditory stimulation. The effect can be found in the subsequently improved performance on spatial IQ tests (Rauscher et al, 1995). College students who had spent 10 minutes listening to Mozart's Sonata K 448 had Stanford-Binet spatial subtest IQ scores 8-9 points higher than students who had listened to a relaxation tape or listened to nothing. The IQ effects did not persist beyond the 10-15 min testing session. There have been several studies that replicated the Mozart effect, showing that exposure to Mozart produces an enhanced spatial performance (Rideout and Laubach 1996; Rideout and Taylor 1997. However, just as many, if not even more studies have failed to replicate the Mozart effect (Carstens et al, 1996; McCutchen 2000).

Neurophysiological changes while listening to Mozart were mainly observed using electroencephalographic (EEG) power and coherence measures. Changes in EEG power and coherence, especially on the right temporal area while listening to musical auditory stimulation were reported by Petsche and colleagues (Petsche et al. 1993). In another study it was found that in three of seven subjects right frontal and left temporal-parietal coherence activity induced by listening to the Mozart sonata (K.448) was carried over into the solution of the spatial-temporal tasks (Sarnthein et al, 1997). This carry-over effect was not present after listening to a text. It was further reported that listening to the Mozart sonata significantly decreased epileptiform activity in patients with seizures (Hughes et al. 2000). In a follow-up study analyzing the musical auditory stimulation of Haydn, Liszt, Bach, Chopin, Beethoven and Wagner it was found that Mozart's musical auditory stimulation continued to score significantly higher than the selections from the other six composers (Hughes 2000).

The brain is only part of all mechanism related to musical auditory stimulation-induced cardiovascular responses. From this viewpoint it seems reasonable that further research of the "Mozart effect" should to a greater extent focus on the influence that modulations in the frequency domain have on brain activity.

6. Concluding remarks

In this chapter we presented important studies which try to clarify the effects of auditory stimulation on cardiac autonomic regulation. Taking into consideration the potential of HRV as a clinical method to evaluate and identify health impairments of autonomic changes induced by auditory stimulus and is indicated to be used as a tool for early diagnosis and prognosis of autonomic dysfunction in subjects exposed to intense sounds for long term, it opens a wide path of research and clinical application of this method in individuals under that condition.

Author details

Vitor Engrácia Valenti and Heraldo L. Guida
Faculdade de Filosofia e Ciências, Universidade Estadual Paulista, UNESP, Marília, Brazil

Luiz Carlos de Abreu and Celso Ferreira
Faculdade de Medicina do ABC, Santo Andre, Brazil

Luiz Carlos M. Vanderlei and Lucas Lima Ferreira
Faculdade de Ciências e Tecnologia, Universidade Estadual Paulista,
UNESP, Presidente Prudente, Brazil

7. References

Akiyama, K., Sutoo, D. (1999). Rectifying effect of exercise on hypertension in spontaneously hypertensive rats via a calcium-dependent dopamine synthesizing system in the brain. *Brain Res,* Vol. 823, No. 2 (Feb) pp; 154– 160, ISSN 0006-8993.

Alvarsson, J.J., Wiens, S., Nilsson, M.E. (2010) Stress recovery during exposure to nature sound and environmental noise. *Int J Environ Rese Public Health,* Vol. 7, No. 9 (Sept) pp. 1036-46, ISSN 1661-7827.

Bernardi, L., Porta, C., Sleight, P. (2006). Cardiovascular, cerebrovascular, and respiratory changes induced by different types of music in musicians and non-musicians: the importance of silence. *Heart,* Vol. 92, No. 3 (March) pp. 445– 452, ISSN 1355-6037.

Bernardi, L., Porta, C., Casucci, G., Balsamo, R., Bernardi, N.F., Fogari, R., Sleight, P. (2009) Dynamic interactions between musical, cardiovascular, and cerebral rhythms in humans. *Circulation,* Vol. 119, No. 25 (Jun) pp. 3171-80. ISSN 0009-7322,

Boucsein, W. (1992). Electrodermal Activity, Plenum Press. New-York and London, p. 442.

Bradley, M.M., Lang, P.J. (2000). Affective reactions to acoustic stimuli. *Psychophysiology,* Vol. 37, No. 2 (Feb) pp. 204–215, ISSN 0048-5772.

Butler, R.A., Diamond, I.T., Neff, W.D. (1957). Role of auditory cortex in discrimination of changes in frequency. *J Neurophysiol.* Vol. 20, No. 1 (Jan) pp. 108–120, ISSN 1537-1603.

Carney, R.M., Freedland, K.E., Stein, P.K., Miller, G.E., Steinmeyer, B., Rich, M.W. (2007). Heart rate variability and markers of inflammation and coagulation in depressed patients with coronary heart disease. *J Psychosom Res,* Vol. 62, No. 4 (April) pp. 463-7, ISSN 0022-3999.

Carstens, C.B., Huskins, E., Hounshell, G.W. (1995). Listening to Mozartmaynot enhance performance on the Revised Minnesota Paper Form Board Test. *Psychol Reports,* Vol. 77, No. 1 (Jan) pp. 111-114, ISSN 0033-2941.

Colombari, E., Sato, M.A., Cravo, S.L., Bergamaschi, C.T., Campos, R.R. Jr., Lopes, O.U. (2001). Role of the medulla oblongata in hypertension. *Hypertension,* Vol. 38, No. 3 (September), pp. 549-54, ISSN 0950-9240

Chuang, C.Y., Han, W.R., Li, P.C., Song, M.Y., Young, S.T. (2011). Effect of Long-Term Music Therapy Intervention on Autonomic Function in Anthracycline-Treated Breast Cancer Patients. *Integrat Cancer Ther,* Vol 10, No. 3 (March) pp. 312-6, ISSN 1534-7354.

Clifton, T. (1983). Music as heard: A study in applied phenomenology. New Haven: Yale Univ. Press.

Davison, J.T.R. (1899). Music in medicine. *Lancet,* Vol. 154, No. 2 (Feb) pp. 1159–62, ISSN 0140-6736.

Dias de Carvalho, T., Marcelo Pastre, C., Claudino Rossi, R., de Abreu, L.C., Valenti, V.E., Marques Vanderlei, L.C. (2011). Geometric index of heart rate variability in chronic obstructive pulmonary disease. *Rev Port Pneumol,* Vol. 17, No. 2 (Feb) pp. 260-5, ISSN 0873-2159.

Ellis, R.J., Thayer, J.F. (2010). Music and Autonomic Nervous System (Dys)function. *Music Percept,* Vol. 27, No. 4 (Apr) pp. 317-326, ISSN 0730-7829.

Gao, L., Wang,W., Liu, D., Zucker, I.H. (2007). Exercise training normalizes sympathetic outflow by central antioxidant mechanisms in rabbits with pacing-induced chronic heart failure. *Circulation,* Vol. 115, No. 24 (June), pp. 3095-102, ISSN 0009-7322.

Gentil, A.F., Eskandar, E.N., Marci, C.D., Evans, K.C., Dougherty, D.D. (2009). Physiological responses to brain stimulation during limbic surgery: further evidence of anterior cingulate modulation of autonomic arousal. *Biol Psychiatry,* Vol. 66, No. 7 (Oct) pp. 695-701, ISSN 0006-3223.

Hughes, J.R., Fino, J.J. (2000). The Mozart effect: distinctive aspects of the music – a clue to brain coding? *Clin Electroencephalogr,* Vol. 31, No. 1 (Jan) pp. 94-103, ISSN 0009-9155..

Huron, D., Hellmuth Margulis, E. (2009). Musical expectancy and thrills. in Music and Emotion (eds. Juslin, P.N. & Sloboda, J.) (Oxford University Press, New York).

Hyde, I.M., Scalapino, W. (1918). The influence of music upon electrocardiogram and blood pressure. *Am J Physiol*, Vol. 46, No. 1 (Jan) pp.35–8, ISSN 1931-857X.

Khalfa, S., Isabelle, P., Jean-Pierre, B., Manon, R. (2002). Event-related skin conductance responses to musical emotions in humans. *Neurosci Lett*, Vol. 328, No. 2 (Aug) pp. 145-9, ISSN 0304-3940.

Koelsch, S., Siebel, W.A. (2005). Towards a neural basis of music perception. *Trends Cogn Sci*, Vol. 9, No. 4 (April) pp. 578–584, ISSN 1364-6613.

Lee, O.K., Chung, Y.F., Chan, M.F., Chan, W.M. (2005). Music and its effect on the physiological responses and anxiety levels of patients receiving mechanical ventilation: a pilot study. *J. Clin. Nurs.* Vol. 14, No. 4 (April) pp. 609–620, ISSN 1365-2702.

Lee, G.S., Chen, M.L., Wang, G.Y. (2010). Evoked response of heart rate variability using short-duration white noise. *Auton Neurosc*, Vol. 155, No. 1 (Jan) pp. 94-7, ISSN 1566-0702.

McCutcheon, L.E. (2000). Another failure to generalize the Mozart effect. *Psychol Rep*, Vol. 87, No. 2 (Feb) pp. 325-330, ISSN 0033-2941.

Nakamura, T., Tanida, M., Niijima, A., Hibino, H., Shen, J., Nagai, K. (2007) Auditory stimulation affects renal sympathetic nerve activity and blood pressure in rats. *Neurosci Lett*, Vol. 416, No. 1 (Jan) pp. 107-12 ISSN 0304-3940.

Okada, K., Kurita, A., Takase, B. (2009). Effects of music therapy on autonomic nervous system activity, incidence of heart failure events, and plasma cytokine and catecholamine levels in elderly patients with cerebrovascular disease and dementia. *Int Heart J*, Vol. 50, No. 1 (Jan) pp. 95-110, ISSN 1349-2365.

Pacchetti, C., Aglieri, R., Mancini, F., Martignoni, E., Nappi, G. (1998). Active music therapy and Parkinson's disease: methods, Funct. *Neurology*, Vol. 13, No. 1 (Jan) pp. 57– 67, ISSN 0893-0341.

Petsche, H., Richter, P., Stein, A., Etlinger, S.C., Filz, O. (1993). EEG coherence and musical thinking. *Music Percept*, Vol. 11, No. 1 (Jan) pp. 117-152, ISSN 1364-6613.

Rauscher, F.H., Shaw, G.L. Ky, K.N. (1995). Listening to Mozart enhances spatial temporal reasoning: towards a neurophysiological basis. *Neurosci Lett*, Vol. 195, No. 1 (Jan) pp. 44-47, ISSN 1364-6613.

Révész, G. (1953) Einführung in die Musikpsychologie. Bern: A.Frank Ag. Verlag.

Rideout, B.E., Laubach, C.M. (1996). EEG correlates of enhanced spatial performance following exposure to music. *Percept Motor Skill*, Vol. 82, No 3 (March) pp. 427-432, ISSN 0031-5125.

Rideout, B.E., Taylor, J. (1997). Enhanced spatial performance following 10 minutes exposure to music: A replication. *Percept Motor Skill*, Vol. 85, No. 1 (Jan) pp. 112-114, ISSN 0031-5125.

Sacks, O. (2007). Musicophilia: Tales of music and the brain. New York: Knopf.

Salimpoor, V.N., Benovoy, M., Longo, G., Cooperstock, J.R., Zatorre, R.J. (2009). The rewarding aspects of music listening are related to degree of emotional arousal. *PLoS ONE*, Vol. 4, No. 11 (Nev) pp. e7487, ISSN 1932-6203.

Salimpoor, V.N., Benovoy, M., Larcher, K., Dagher, A., Zatorre, R.J. (2011). Anatomically distinct dopamine release during anticipation and experience of peak emotion to music. *Nat Neurosc,* Vol. 14, No. 2 (Feb) pp. 257-62, ISSN 1097-6256.

Samuels, E.R., Hou, R.H., Langley, R.W., Szabadi, E., Bradshaw, C.M. (2007). Modulation of the acoustic startle response by the level of arousal: comparison of clonidine and modafinil in healthy volunteers. *Neuropsychopharmacol,* Vol. 32, No. 10 (Oct) pp. 2405-21, ISSN 0893-133X.

Sarnthein, J., von Stein, A., Rappelsberger, P., Petsche, H., Rauscher, F.H., Shaw, G.L. (1997). Persistent patterns of brain activity: an EEG coherence study of the positive effect of music on spatial-temporal reasoning. *Neurol Res,* Vol. 19, No. 1 (Jan) pp. 107-116, 0161-6412.

Särkämö, T., Tervaniemi, M., Laitinen, S., Forsblom, A., Soinila, S., Mikkonen, M., Autti, T., Silvennoinen, H.M., Erkkilä, J., Laine, M., Peretz, I., Hietanen, M. (2008). Music listening enhances cognitive recovery and mood after middle cerebral artery stroke. *Brain,* Vol. 131, No. 5 (May) pp. 866–876, ISSN 1460-2156.

Sidorenko, V.N. (2000). Effects of the medical resonance therapy music in the complex treatment of epileptic patients, Integr. *Physiol Behav Sci,* Vol. 35, No. 2 (Feb) pp. 212–217, ISSN 1053-881X.

Sly, J.D., Colvill, L., McKinley, J.M., Oldfield, J.B. (1999). Identification of neural projections from the forebrain to the kidney, using the virus pseudorabies. *J Auton Nerv Syst,* Vol. 77, No. 1 (Jan) pp. 73–82, ISSN: 1566-0702.

Sutoo, D., Akiyama, K. (1996). The mechanism by which exercise modifies brain function. *Physiol Behav,* Vol. 60, No. 2 (Feb) pp. 177–181, ISSN 0031-9384.

Sutoo, D., Akiyama, K. (2003). Regulation of brain function by exercise. *Neurobiol Dis,* Vol. 13, No. 1 (Jan) pp. 1 –14, ISSN 0969-9961.

Sutoo, D., Akiyama, K. (2004). Music improves dopaminergic neurotransmission: demonstration based on the effect of music on blood pressure regulation. *Brain Res.* Vol. 1016, No. 4 (April) pp. 255–262, ISSN 1432-1106.

Tanida, M., Niijima, A., Shen, J., Nakamura, T., Nagai, K. (2005). Olfactory stimulation with scent of essential oil of grapefruit affects autonomic neurotransmission and blood pressure. *Brain Res,* Vol. 1058, No. 1 (Jan) pp. 44–55 ISSN 0006-8993.

Task Force of the European Society of Cardiology and the North American Society of Pacing and Electrophysiology. (1996). Heart rate variability: standards of measurement, physiological interpretation and clinical use. *Circulation,* Vol. 93, No. 5 (May) pp.1043-65, ISSN 0009-7322.

Valenti, V. E., Sato, M.A., Ferreira, C., Abreu, L.C. (2007) Neural regulation of the cardiovascular system: Bulbar centers. Revista de Neurociências, Vol. 15, No. 4 (December), pp. 317-320, ISSN 0104-3579

Valenti, V.E., Ferreira, C., Meneghini, A., Ferreira, M., Murad, N., Ferreira Filho, C., Correa, J.A., Abreu, L.C., Colombari, E. (2009) Evaluation of baroreflex function in young spontaneously hypertensive rats. *Arquivos Brasileiros de Cardiologia,* Vol. 92, No. 3 (March), pp. 205-15, ISSN 0066-782X a

Valenti, V.E., Imaizumi, C., de Abreu, L.C., Colombari, E., Sato, M.A., Ferreira, C. (2009) Intra-strain variations of baroreflex sensitivity in young Wistar-Kyoto rats. Clinical and Investive Medicine, Vol. 32, No. 6 (December), pp.E251, ISSN 0147-958X b

Valenti, V.E., de Abreu, L.C., Sato, M.A., Fonseca, F.L., Pérez Riera, A.R., Ferreira, C. (2011). Catalase inhibition into the fourth cerebral ventricle affects bradycardic parasympathetic response to increase in arterial pressure without changing the baroreflex. *Journal of Integrative Neuroscience,* Vol. 10, No. 1 (March), pp. 1-14, ISSN 0219-6352 a

Valenti, V.E., Abreu, L.C., Sato, M.A., Ferreira, C. (2011). ATZ (3-amino-1,2,4-triazole) injected into the fourth cerebral ventricle influences the Bezold-Jarisch reflex in conscious rats. *Clinics,* Vol. 65, No 12 (December), pp. 1339-43, ISSN 807-5932 b

Valenti, V.E., De Abreu, L.C., Sato, M.A., Saldiva, P.H., Fonseca, F.L., Giannocco, G., Riera, A.R., Ferreira, C. (2011). Central N-acetylcysteine effects on baroreflex in juvenile spontaneously hypertensive rats. *Journal of Integrative Neuroscience,* Vol. 10, No. 2 (June), pp. 161-76, ISSN 0219-6352 c

Vanderlei, L.C., Pastre, C.M., Hoshi, R.A., Carvalho, T.D., Godoy, M.F. (2009) Basic notions of heart rate variability and its clinical applicability. Rev Bras Cir Cardiovasc, Vol. 24, No. 2 (Apr-Jun) pp. 205-17, ISSN 0102-7638.

Volkow, N.D., Wang, G.J., Fischman, M.W., Foltin, R.W., Fowler, J.S., Abumrad, N.N., Vitkun, S., Logan, J., Gatley, S.J., Pappas, N., Hitzemann, R., Shea, C.E. (1997). Relationship between subjective effects of cocaine and dopamine transporter occupancy. *Nature,* Vol. 386, No. 4 (Apr) pp. 827–830 ISSN, 1529-2908.

von Leupoldt, A., Taube, K., Schubert-Heukeshoven, S., Magnussen, H., Dahme, B. (2007). Distractive auditory stimuli reduce the unpleasantness of dyspnea during exercise in patients with COPD. *Chest,* Vol. 132, No. 10 (Oct) pp. 1506–1512, ISSN 0012-3692.

Chapter 7

Spiritual-Religious Coping – Health Services Empowering Patients' Resources

Marcelo Saad and Roberta de Medeiros

Additional information is available at the end of the chapter

http://dx.doi.org/10.5772/50445

1. Introduction

It is known that health is determined by physical, mental, social, and spiritual factors. During the last decades there has been a considerable increase in the number of studies showing positive associations between spirituality-religiosity and health. The most important works in that area began it be deeds in the 1980 decade and are increasing worldwide. Scientific literature have recorded that spiritual well-being is associated with better physical and mental health, according to psycho-neuro-immune models of health. Spirituality and religion can help patients, their families and caregivers dealing with illness and other stressful life events.

Concerning physical health, studies show that appropriate religiousness is related to better general health and longevity (due to better immunologic function and cardiovascular health) and less frequency to health services utilization [1]. In mental health, religiousness is related to less chance to develop and faster recovery of: marital disharmony, depression, suicide attempt, and drugs and alcohol abuse [1]. There are evidences that persons with a well developed spirituality tend to make ill less frequently, to have healthier habits of life and, when make ill, develop less depression and recover more quickly.

Many patients put their suffering into religious frameworks. Religion and spirituality are prevalent coping strategies both for physical and for mental illness. For many patients religion and spirituality play a significant role in their lives and may help them cope with their symptoms. Patients' personal beliefs may be fundamental to their sense of well-being and could help them to cope with negative aspects of illness or treatment. However, incorporating spirituality into medical practice continues to pose many challenges. Spirituality is often seen as a private and subjective area that lies outside of the therapeutic context, but patients' beliefs can have a substantial impact on construction of the meaning of illness, coping behavior, and preferences about treatment.

This chapter is intended to present evidences and discuss proposals on how health care services can empower spiritual-religious resources of patients in order to they can be used as an efficient coping strategy. Concepts will be discussed, such as faith, spirituality, religion, and the concept of spiritual-religious coping itself. The characteristics of the spiritual-religious coping structure will be described. The spiritual distress due to non-attended spiritual needs will be discussed, followed by a description of defensive behaviors that patients may adopt in these situations. The chapter ends proposing some suggestions for health care professionals and services to use these knowledge in practice.

2. Concepts

The terms faith, spirituality and religious beliefs have been used interchangeably but have significant conceptual differences which may be relevant in trying to understand their influence on medical treatment. While many people use the words spirituality and religion as synonyms, they are in fact very different. Although these terms are associated, they are not interdependent.

Faith: The concept of faith has never been defined fully and encompasses elements of both spirituality and religious beliefs, which may be further modified by culture and personal value systems [2]. Faith has a cognitive and an experiential aspect. The cognitive one associates "to have faith" with the profession of the learned doctrine. The experiential aspect is the inner courage that works as a shelter to help the person to endure difficulties of life.

Prayer may be defined as an intimate conversation with a higher being for the purpose of imploring or petitioning for something or someone. Prayer can be practiced as an individual or as a group. It can be practiced inside or outside of the presence of a spiritual healer or place of worship. You or your group can pray for yourself or pray for others, even people you don't know (intercession). You can pray near someone or at a distance (remote). You can pray with or without the knowledge of the recipient; and that is not to say who you are praying to and whether you consistently believe in a transcendent being.

Spirituality has many definitions on scientific literature. Perhaps the most complete associates spirituality to "the aspect of humanity that refers to the way individuals seek and express meaning and purpose, and the way they experience their connectedness to the moment, to self, to others, to nature, and to the significant or sacred" [3]. Spirituality is a complex and multidimensional part of the human experience, as an inner belief system. It helps individuals to search for the meaning and purpose of life, and it helps them to experience hope, love, inner peace, comfort, and support. Spirituality can be understood as the set of beliefs that brings vitality and meaning to the events of life. It is the human propensity for the interest for others and for himself. Spirituality can encompass both secular and religious perspectives.

Spiritual Well-Being: The World Health Organization has declared that spirituality is an important dimension of quality of life. How someone is faring spiritually affects that person's physical, psychological, and interpersonal states, and vice versa. All contribute to overall quality of life. Thus, it is particularly useful to try to measure spiritual well-being or its opposite, spiritual distress. [4]. Aspects of spirituality may have a beneficial effect on a variety of health-related physiological mechanisms. In particular, spirituality's emphasis on emotions, for example contentment, forgiveness, hope and love, may positively affect an individual's physical wellbeing. Furthermore spirituality may reduce feelings of negative emotions, such as anger, fear and revenge, reducing tension levels. [5]

Spiritual needs: they commonly identifies three basic concerns [6]: the need to find meaning in illness or disability; the need to affirm one's relationship or connect with others (including the Whole or a Supreme One); and the need to realize transcendent values, such as hope, faith, thrust, courage, love, and peace. Note that these needs are not necessarily religious. Before spiritual needs can be met, they must be recognized. Initially, it consists on documenting patient's religious affiliation, preferred religious practices and patient's beliefs on sources of hope and strength [6].

It is not always certain what the precise spiritual needs of a patient might be. Some might want help with specific religious rituals. Some might want to talk to members of their own faith communities about the meaning of suffering. Still others might want pastoral counseling regarding their fear of death. Defining the spiritual needs of patients is a matter that is being investigated empirically, but there are, at present, no well-validated research instruments for this purpose. Patients report a wide spectrum of spiritual needs, and meeting spiritual needs is correlated with patient satisfaction with care and their ratings of the quality of medical care [4].

Religion is an organized or institutionalized belief system that attempt to provide specific answers to mankind's general spiritual needs and questions [7]. Religion is a specific expression of spirituality, which involves elements as doctrine (structure of formal belief), myth (narrative religious), ethics (rules for life), ceremonial (organized practices), experience (personal commitment), and social institution (church, synagogue, etc.). Religion may be seen as multi-dimensional and it is divided it into a number of inner and outer dimensions. The inner ones include belief, non-organizational religiosity (private prayer), subjective religiosity (importance of religion in one's life), religious experience, religious knowledge and religious well being. The outer dimensions include affiliation or denomination, organizational religiosity (participation in church or synagogue activities), and religious commitment. The outer aspects may influence the construction of the inner ones.

Even if there are interfaces between religion and health, the primary goal of every religious life is beyond the matters of physical, mental, and social well-being. The goals are variously designated: salvation in Christianity; the elimination of avidya (mu-myung) to achieve the state of One-Mind (Il-shim) in Buddhism; the union of Yin and Yang in Tao in Taoism; and achieving the ability of ecstasy to combine the celestial and earthly worlds in shamanism [8].

Religiosity: it concerns the behaviors and attitudes a person has with respect to a particular religion. Measurable items include behaviors such as church attendance, prayer, the reading of sacred texts, and attitudes, such as strength of religious belief [4]. 'Religiosity' covers all measures of religious belief or religiousness as expressed in membership in religious communities, religious behavior and spiritual dimensions of religious belief. Religious beliefs represent a specific doctrine system shared by a group of people and defined by prescribed rules, value systems and practices of social participation that may mimic formal secular counseling, support and psychotherapeutic activities [2].

Relations between Spirituality and Religion: Many people find spirituality through religion; however, some people find spirituality through communing with nature, music, the arts, quest for scientific truth, or a set of values and principles [7]. Not everyone is religious, nor is religion a requirement for spiritual wellbeing. It is possible to have a well developed spirituality without being committed to a religion. The inverse is also true. Spirituality may be strong in persons of different religions, as well as in persons with individual beliefs that are not fitted in a formal religion. In the opposite sense, a person may have a strong religiosity (attending worships regularly), but have a low developed spirituality (by not deeply experiencing these aspects). Many people attend religious services diligently without relating to spirituality, and many who do not belong to a formal religion seek contact with the spiritual. To make this differentiation easier, table 1 confronts the main aspects that can be used to differentiate both concepts. Table 1: Confronting the main aspects that differentiate Religion and Spirituality (most based on Dein [9]):

RELIGION	SPIRITUALITY
Specific set of beliefs and practices	Feelings of peace and connectedness
Strongly determined by culture	Universal human characteristic
Community focused organization (from outside to inside)	Individualistic inner experience (from inside to outside)
Observable, measurable, objective	Less visible and measurable, more subjective
Formal, orthodox, organized	Less formal, less orthodox, less systematic
Behavior orientated, outward practices	Emotionally orientated, inward directed
Authoritarian in terms of behaviors	Not authoritarian, little accountability

Table 1. Confronting the main aspects that differentiate Religion and Spirituality (most based on Dein [9])

3. Spiritual-religious coping

Spiritual-Religious (S-R) coping is the use of religious beliefs, attitudes or practices to reduce the emotional distress caused by stressful events of life, such as loss or change, which gives suffering meaning and makes it more bearable. Religious beliefs and practices are used to regulate emotion during times of illness, change, and circumstances that are out of patients' personal control [1].

Spirituality has an impact on patients' ability to cope with illness. For many individuals, spiritual beliefs and practices provide a source of comfort, supply a font of wisdom to help make sense of what seems otherwise senseless, and prescribe a ritual pathway for addressing the basic spiritual questions of meaning, value, and relationship [4]. Aspects of religious coping include [7]:

- Cognitive aspects: the way we make sense of the world around us. They include questions such as: "Why do bad things happen to good people?" "What happens after death?"
- Experiential aspects have to do with connection and inner resilience. They encompass questions such as: "Am I alone or am I connected to something bigger?" "Can I find hope in this difficult situation?"
- Behavioral aspects have to do with ways in which a person's spiritual beliefs and inner spiritual state affect his or her behavior and life choices.

The response to life stressors may be directly mediated by S-R factors which provide a cognitive framework for providing meaning, which enables a healthier appraisal of those stressors through the provision of meaning and coherence. This may provide greater psychological resilience in the face of negative life events. Suffering is given a meaning in the world religions although there is marked variation in how this is done. It is not necessarily seen as destructive or humiliating, to be avoided at all cost [9].

Spirituality provides growth in several relationship fields. In the intrapersonal field (with himself), brings hope, altruism and idealism, purpose for life and for suffering. In the interpersonal field (with others) brings tolerance, unit, and the sense of belonging to a group. In the transpersonal field (with a supreme power), awakes the unconditional love, worship and the belief of not being alone [10].

Spiritual beliefs may assist people in providing a sense of control in understanding, coping with and interpreting events or experiences. Previous studies indicate that individuals who hold religious beliefs allow an individual to reduce the stressful reactions to events that they deem to be uncontrollable by reframing or reinterpreting those events, possibly gaining a new meaning and understanding from them [5].

It is important to have meaning or purpose in life. This sense of meaning is diminished by an illness. This loss and its associated rediscovery were central aspects of both depression and spirituality. Spirituality may provide such a sense of meaning through its emphasis on liturgy, worship and prayer found in the major religious traditions [9]. Adverse life events may be appraised in a different way. Religion provides a meaning context in which adversity can be understood.

Words such as spirituality and religion carry a variety of meanings for different people. Not all S-R coping is positive. S-R perceptions and rituality may well be a double-edged sword. Although much of the literature is suggestive of an overall positive effect of religion on health, at times religious practice might have a deleterious effect. What appears to be ultimately important in terms of health outcome is not religious involvement (e.g. church attendance) but how people actually deploy their religious beliefs to cope with adversity. Table 2 confronts some aspects of positive and negative S-R coping (based on [4];[7];[9])

	POSITIVE	NEGATIVE
What does it evoke	bring out the best in individuals, reinforcing active problem-solving behavior	encourage negative avoidance strategies based on the beliefs of abandonment and punishment
view of the deity	belief in a kind supportive God	distant and uncaring, or punishing for transgressions
effect on life adjustments and emotional health	lower levels of psychiatric symptoms; linked with improved health-care outcomes	associated with higher prevalence of psychiatric symptoms; worse medical outcomes

Table 2. Some aspects of positive and negative S-R coping

4. Effects of spirituality-religion over health

A relation between better health and religion or spirituality is found in studies covering heart disease, hypertension, cerebrovascular disease, immunological dysfunction, cancer, longevity, pain, disability, and less frequent health services utilization. Also higher religiousness affects behaviors and correlates such as taking exercise, smoking, substance misuse, alcohol abuse, burnout, and family and marital breakdown [11]. In mental health, higher religiousness is related to less chance to develop the following conditions, and faster recovery when they appear: marital disharmony, depression, anxiety, suicide attempt, and drugs and alcohol abuse [11]. The benefits are almost always threefold: aiding prevention, speeding recovery, and fostering equanimity in the face of ill health.

Studies on spirituality and mental health have looked at the mechanisms involved in spirituality, which may improve mental wellbeing. There is some evidence that positive coping styles can be very positive in terms of people's mental health [5]. Aspects of spirituality may have a beneficial affect on a variety of health-related physiological mechanisms. In particular, spirituality's emphasis on contentment, forgiveness, hope and love, may positively affect an individual's physical wellbeing. Furthermore spirituality may reduce feelings of negative emotions, such as anger, fear and revenge, reducing tension levels. [5]

The theories that can explain how S-R wellbeing may improve health are various. Some involved mechanisms may be the positive cognitive appraisal, the altered status of mind during prayer, and congregational benefits from the religious community.

Cognitive appraisal: Religion provides a source of hope. For instance, in Christianity and Judaism, no matter how bad the world is now, the current state will imminently change with the coming of a messianic age. The belief in an omnipotent God who supports a person through a crisis can be psychologically beneficial. Indirect benefits may surge from faith, such as relieving the fear of death among elderly people. Those who are religious often turn outwards towards others, away from self -reflection and this may have beneficial effects [9]. So, there are many healthy impacts from faith, hope and optimism.

Prayer: Some types of prayer may have a known biomedical explanation for their impact, based on the connection of body–mind–spirit, or even divine action. Prayer, like meditation, can invoke a relaxation response, where measurable impact on the human body can be gauged, such as the heart rate slowing, brain waves altering and respiration rates lowering. In addition to the relaxation response, psychological mechanisms that may impact a person's health through prayer may include increased social support, hope or decreased distress. Also there are psychological factors such as the emotional impact of worship. These mechanisms may explain the positive impact of praying for oneself or praying for another in their presence or with their knowledge.

Congregation and Cultural Effects: Religious congregations naturally supply favorable conditions for the promotion of physical and mental health, and are a powerful factor that modify the individual's attitudes toward life, death, happiness, and suffering. Many theories have been proposed in the literature to explain the reduced health risks amongst members of religious communities, including [5];[8];[12]: healthy and abstinent life style; religious fellowship protecting people from social isolation; strengthening family and social networks; providing individuals with a sense of belonging and self-esteem; and offering spiritual support in times of adversity. Individuals' mental health is often supported through engagement with members and leaders of religious congregations. Collective religious ceremonies have been been identified with higher community belonging, moral standards and self-esteem.

5. Spiritual distress and defensive behaviors

Human beings are complex, with physical, mental, and spiritual aspects. Suffering can result from issues pertaining to any of these aspects. Spiritual distress is a state of suffering due to spiritual causes. For example: a mother having difficulty understanding why a loving God would allow her child to die [7]. The spiritual distress refers to the existential anguish experienced by patients when their belief system cannot provide relief.

When patients suffer, they experience a sense of their own vulnerability and finitude, as well as a disruption and fracture of their own person and sense of community. As a result, the experience of suffering can be an opportunity to experience his own spirituality [13]. When well constructed, the belief structure is a source of comfort, welfare, security, meaning, idealism and force. Many patients use their beliefs when coping with its illnesses, and the cure can be influenced by the positivist reinforcement of the patient.

In contrast, a dysfunctional belief system may originate negative reactions that harm the healthcare evolution. If there is a disruption of the belief system, the spiritual distress can surge. It may be expressed by many ways, some of them are below described.

Attempt To Bargain For Recovery: The belief on the possibility to negotiate with deities, spirits, saints, or even God, to achieve a specific outcome results from certain parts of many scriptures where a worthy believer has his(her) plea attended. It is very common to see this behavior among patients, especially in life-threatening diseases. There is no problem when this attitude brings some hope to patient, but some people may exaggerate at a point of impair treatment.

Belief Of Being Deservedly Affected (Low Self Worth): Concepts associated with the idea of a fatalistic karma may put the patient in a "sell out" position, confounding submission to the will of God with apathetic waiver to all major happenings of life. An apparent resigned attitude may hide other negative values that are guiding the decisions of the patient.

Diminished Sense of Meaning and Purpose (Demotivation): It is important to have meaning or purpose in life. This sense of meaning is diminished by an illness. This loss and its associated rediscovery were central aspects of both depression and spirituality. Spirituality may provide such a sense of meaning through its emphasis on liturgy, worship and prayer found in the major religious traditions. The struggle to recover or sustain meaning, that is, the worthwhileness of living, is an expression of the patient's spirituality [14]. Religion provides a source of hope. Spiritual beliefs may assist people in providing a sense of control in understanding, coping with and interpreting events or experiences. Individuals with a dysfunctional religious beliefs system cannot reduce the stressful reactions to events that they deem to be uncontrollable by reframing or reinterpreting those events, possibly gaining a new meaning and understanding from them.

Guilt, Confusion, Religious Stigmas (Disruption): Some religious groups such as Orthodox Judaism and Catholicism may engender guilt and thus may be detrimental psychologically [9]. A constellation of confounding feelings may paralyze the individual and consume energy in a behavior similar to walk in circles. For example, some possible misconceptions from people with strong religious views [15]: (a) do not take pain medication (or don't take enough of it) for fear of becoming addicted; (b) pain should be dealt with only in spiritual terms, and taking medication for pain relief is relying on something other than God; (c) pain should not be relieved because it results in spiritual growth; (d) if you still have pain, then your faith is not strong enough.

Sorrow, Betrayal, Angry to God (Disappointment): The idea of a supportive God, who is with you in your suffering, the omnipotent God who supports a person through a crisis can be psychologically beneficial. This concept is sometimes linked to the idea of a reward due to past good actions. When a person's pray is not attended, a negative feeling of abandonment may surge.

Subtle Perception of Vulnerability and Finitude (Fear): When patients suffer, they experience a sense of their own vulnerability and finitude, as well as a disruption and fracture of their own person and sense of community [13]. The fear of loose something (a physical function, independence or even the life) may interfere with the emotional balance.

The consequent defensive behaviors patient can develop under spiritual distress may affect clinical treatment and quality of life. Below are described some manifestations of such behaviors.

Naïve Reliability on Religion Omnipotence: Religion would assist people in developing stronger coping styles. When religion is used as part of a wider approach to coping this typically provided a beneficial outcome for mental health and reduced mental distress. This is in direct contrast to those coping styles which used deferring (where the individual waits for God to intervene on their behalf) [5]. Excessive reliance on religious rituals or prayer may delay seeking necessary help for their mental health problems, leading to worsening the prognosis of psychiatric disorder. At the most extreme, strict adherence to a 'religious philosophy' might precipitate suicide as occurred in rare new religious movements. An example of a patient's thought inspired by negative coping is given by this phrase: "When the Lord wants to take me, He'll take me whatever I do. I don't see the need to bother with a bunch of new pills." [16].

Sudden Turn to Unusual Religious Practices: Since religious sentiment and sectarianism may rise during times of increased personal stress, unusual religious movements may sprung up during the times of rapid change and uncertainty. Individuals stressed by life or health shifts are more likely to get involved with unusual or innovative or charismatic religious movements [17]. The seek for reconnection with religious practices is positive only if it is not a desperate action to escape from reality.

Dependency on Religious Leaders Conduction: Long term involvement in a religious group may predispose to dependency on religious leaders. Patients have the legitimate right to consult a clergyman before forming an opinion about health issues. But it is dangerous to delegate decisions to a third part that represents only the religious view.

Obsessive Ritualistic Behavior: Formal religious organization and particularly religious rituals and religiously based moral or ethical reasoning can be considered as examples of the human cognitive capacity to order experience and to seek meaning. This tendency is also a healthy human capacity to be promoted. As with the attachment dimension, however, there are clinical excesses in the ordering of and attributing meaning or significance to experience [14]. Religions which emphasize rituals, such as Islam and Judaism, may predispose to obsessional behavior. [9]. Some pathologic expressions of attachment behavior that are desperate in nature, require therapeutic action that promotes modulation and containment. Therapeutic action encouraging containment of the expression of such attachment needs is important to avoid chaos in all aspects of such individuals' lives, including the religious dimensions of their lives. Faith-based efforts to order experience can hypertrophy to the degree that rituals lose their spiritual base. [14].

Sectarianism, Isolation, Fanaticism: Many devastating effects can be elicited by the over dominance of fanatic belief and consequent up rootedness from the instinctive foundation. Excessive devotion to religious practices might result in family break-up if the sole preoccupation of one spouse is towards religious practice. Differences in the levels of religiosity between spouses may result in marital disharmony. Religion can promote rigid thinking, overdependence on laws and rules, an emphasis on guilt and sin, and disregard for personal individuality and autonomy.

Refuse to Certain Kinds of Treatment: The beliefs system of the patient can affect clinical decisions when particular interpretation interfere with healthcare. Some religious assumptions can originate ideas that conflict with treatment, induce spiritual stigmas that create tension, and interfere with the adhesion to the diagnosis and to the treatment [18]. Religious views may influence a person's acceptance of various management approaches and her or his treatment goals. Koenig [11] lists four misconceptions about pain management that might be held by patients with strong religious views: 1) reluctance or refusal to take pain medication (or to take sufficient medication) because of addiction fears; 2) belief that pain should be dealt with only in spiritual terms, and taking medication for pain relief would be relying on something other than God; 3) belief that pain should not be relieved because pain may result in spiritual growth; 4) persistent pain may be regarded as a sign that the patient's faith is not strong enough.

6. Attitudes from health care professionals and services

To support the utilization of the spiritual resources by the patient, the Joint Commission on Accreditation of Healthcare Organizations suggests that each institution must [19]: understand and protect the cultural, psychosocial and spiritual values of each patient; prepare professionals to understand and respect beliefs and values of the patients; inform patients about their rights and how to regarding them; and lend aid that consider and respects the beliefs and values of the patient

Health Care Services must invest on some actions, in order to minimize conflicts between religious interests of patients and medical treatment. Some examples are given by the Multi-Faith Group for Healthcare Chaplancy [20]: training and development; appointments to chaplaincy posts; data protection; volunteers; worship and sacred spaces; and bereavement services.

Delgado [6] organized the lay spiritual interventions from health professionals in some categories, as: (a) Assessment: ask about faith, practices and symbols; (b) Communication: empathic and respectful listening, transmitting these findings to proper professionals; (c) Supporting emotionally: watch patients at spiritual suffering risk; empathic presence; be trustful; and (d) Supporting physically: create conditions to attend spiritual needs, as time, place, resources, privacy.

Obstacles to implementing spiritual care must not be underestimated, and include [21]: education (lack of training); economics (lack of staff or resources); environment (lack of space or privacy); personal (sensitivity or own belief systems). To achieve the benefits and overcome difficulties, the below discussions lists some suggestions for health care professionals and services. More systematically, we discuss a list of actions to promote the positive impact of spirituality and religiosity on the health treatment process, which would be followed by health care professionals and services (compiled from information from Saad [22] and Lucchetti [23])

Staff Training On Respect And Tolerance: Deriving from the writings of Freud in Totem and Taboo and The Future of an Illusion, clinicians have held religion to be a negative force in patients' lives, leading to guilt, dependency, obsessive behavior and illusory beliefs [9]. But health professionals are called both to cure and to care. Care involves recognition of the fragility and vulnerability of every human being as one who deserves our total commitment. Important values for this field are compassion, creativity, equanimity, honesty, hope, joy, patience and perseverance

It is important to know the basic precepts of the most prevalent religions in the hospital, especially about objections to suspension of treatments, to organs donation, to the necropsy and body cremation. Good clinical care includes sensitivity and curiosity about the cultural and religious values and beliefs of our patients. While substantial progress has been made in incorporating spirituality into the curriculum in a growing number of medical schools, the quality and depth of that instruction is quite varied [16].

The goal of staff training must be to develop an ability to understand better how one's patient engages illness and interprets therapeutic interventions, without prejudice and with an appreciation for the particular cultural and religious perspective brought to the clinical encounter by the patient. Even physicians who are not themselves religious can acknowledge and be sensitive to the spiritual dimensions of their work.

An example on how simple may be the training of healthcare professionals is this model adopted by our institution. A list of positive attitudes include: Empathy (being present, realist and honest); Respect to beliefs of the patient; Consider spirituality as component of the well-being; Remember the relation between illness and spiritual suffering; Inform the ways for spiritual support of the hospital. A list of negative attitudes: "To prescribe" religious activities for health improvement; To impose your religious beliefs to patient; To initiate prayers without know appreciation of the patient; To perform task proper of a priest; To give deep religious counseling.

Routine Religious Screening: It is crucial to examine the religious cultural background of the patient to understand the personality-particularly in respect to his or her value orientation. Always know the religious affiliation of the patient and try to determine the degree of observance regarding this religion. Inquiry about sources of hope, actual beliefs, personal practices, integration in a religious community, rituals, and importance in health care decisions. To ascertain a patient's spiritual beliefs, physicians may ask a set of questions that can be integrated into the patient's history. It may be done by asking a simple open-ended question, "What is your faith or belief? Do you consider yourself spiritual or religious? What role does spirituality or religion play in your life? What things do you believe in that give meaning to your life"? [24].

Treatment planning can usefully involve active attention to patient cues about their faith's importance, consideration of questions in the context of the patient's spiritual background, processing of questions to look for deeper spiritual questions or issues, and asking clarifying questions to assure accurate identification of spiritual development. It is important that the clinician have accurate information about the family's worldview to avoid prescriptions that might be offensive or undermine key precepts of the family's faith [25]. One way to begin is to ask the patient about what she or he finds meaningful or important in life and whether her or his spiritual views have relevance for these issues. It may be helpful to ensure that the patient has access to spiritual counselors as well as to a pastoral care team. It may also be beneficial to discuss with the patient and family how their spiritual practices can be incorporated into the care provided by the medical team.

Support Patient Religious Needs: Dein [9] called "The Religiosity Gap" the fact that clinicians are far less religious than the patients who consult them. Patients commonly use religious strategies to help them cope with their psychiatric symptoms. Clinicians must inquire about their patients religious lives in an attempt to facilitate self directed healing. Indeed, some studies indicate that patients are keen for their physicians to inquire about religion.

Trust and good communication are essential components of the doctor-patient relationship. Patients may find it difficult to trust you and talk openly and honestly with you if they feel you are judging them on the basis of their religion, culture, values, political beliefs or other non-medical factors [26]. By encouraging the family's continuance of healthy religious rituals such as prayer, communion, and anointing, the therapist can enhance family coping responses and possibly increase the efficacy of treatment [25]. Religion and spirituality are not confined to church attendance or affiliation, reading sacred writings, or celebrating Holy Days, or even to praying. There are also non-biblical inspirational literature, religious music, radio and television programming, books on tape and motivational recordings, religious parenting books, and religious books, tapes, and videos.

When the patient brings religious issues up, the physician should always acknowledge the spiritual concerns raised by the patient, respond to the patient, listen respectfully, and refer to pastoral or spiritual care when appropriate. Addressing patients' spirituality is warranted because it is associated with clinical outcomes and patient coping, because patients want it, and because it can affect their decision making. The spiritual concerns of patients affect them as whole persons and in their overall sense of well-being [4].

Spiritual approaches to pain management can take many forms, from prayer, to participation in religious services and rituals, to therapeutic touch, spiritual healing, mindfulness meditation, Reiki, and other strategies. Some of these strategies are explicitly religious, whereas others take a more secular spiritual approach. In some cases the strategy will have roots in religious tradition but will have been modified to make it more amenable to a diverse group of people. For example, mindfulness meditation has roots in Buddhism but is typically used in Western culture separately from its traditions within Buddhism.

Assisting the patient to engage in religious-spiritual activities involves [6]: referring to clergy; informing patient about resources; providing religious material; allowing for prayer, meditation and other practices; and helping the patient to attend religious services and related activities. Barriers to fulfill spiritual needs will always be in one of these groups [6]: personal, situational or knowledge related. Also there is the inability to differentiate psychological needs from spiritual needs. Many other spiritual activities may be proposed [5]:

- Belonging to a faith tradition, participating in associated community-based activities
- Ritual and symbolic practices and other forms of worship
- Pilgrimage and retreats
- Meditation and prayer

- Reading scripture
- Sacred music (listening to, singing and playing) including songs, hymns, psalms and chants
- Acts of compassion (including work, especially teamwork)
- Deep reflection (contemplation)
- Group or team sports, recreational or other activity involving a special quality of fellowship.

Guard Your Own Beliefs Discretely: All doctors have personal beliefs which affect their day-to-day practice. Some doctors' personal beliefs may give rise to concerns about carrying out or recommending particular procedures for patients [26]. The spiritual views of physicians and nurses may affect their beliefs about the pain management of their patients. For this reason, it may be useful for nurses to reflect on their own spiritual beliefs and values and what they mean to the nurse-patient relationship and to the nurse's beliefs about pain management. Some harm is possible if discussion about spirituality causes health professionals to defend or assert a particular religious perspective. The patient's spiritual views, whether secular, sacred, or religious, must be respected rather than challenged.

Health professionals should not normally discuss personal beliefs with patients unless those beliefs are directly relevant to the patient's care. They must not impose their beliefs on patients, or cause distress by the inappropriate or insensitive expression of religious, political or other beliefs or views. Equally, you must not put pressure on patients to discuss or justify their beliefs (or the absence of them) [26].

A helpful principle is to inform but not to recommend. For example, it is legitimate for a physician to inform patients of the potential health benefits of moderate consumption of alcohol, but it is ethically questionable to recommend moderate consumption to a patient who abstains from alcoholic beverages for religious reasons. Respect for autonomy requires that physicians leave it to such patients and their spiritual guides to determine whether a religious practice is worth an elevated health risk [14].

When the health professional has strong reservations about the religious or spiritual tradition to which the patient adheres and feels that such a referral would constitute a tacit endorsement of that religious or spiritual tradition, this fact should be disclosed to the patient. A patient's spirituality should be explored with an open-mindedness and neutrality that allows for tolerance of difference and avoids prejudice against (or for) particular spiritual or religious beliefs or practices.

Support from Religious Leaders: Spiritual care for a patient may be [7]:

- General spiritual care—bringing presence, compassion, understanding, and listening to each encounter. This can be provided by anyone at any time. It can traverse all cultural barriers by meeting a universal spiritual need without specific discussion about beliefs or God.
- Specific or specialized spiritual care—addressing the individual needs of the patient. Simple issues may be addressed by physicians. More complex issues will likely require

the expertise of well-trained spiritual care counselors such as chaplains trained in Clinical Pastoral Education.

It is important to assess and consider the value of consultation with or referral to clergy. Yet a well-timed religious or spiritual consultation with clergy is often necessary for effective and efficient treatment [25]. A chaplain may be seen as the legitimate person to whom spiritual issues may be addressed and can provide a model of 'holistic care'. But chaplains require a basic knowledge of health issues to ensure that they can pick up major mental illness and refer people for appropriate help.

Although all clinical settings do not have chaplains, most hospitals have chaplains on staff or available within the community. Chaplains who have completed clinical pastoral education training have a breadth of background to provide collegial and informed assistance in dealing with clinically relevant religious issues with most patients. Although chaplains are frequently consulted when approaching end-of-life issues with patients and their families, their potential for service is much broader [16].

For some traditions, it is vital that prayer and counsel come from fellow members of (or even authorities) in that tradition; for other traditions, this is unnecessary. These issues can often be avoided by referrals to appropriate persons within the patient's religious or spiritual tradition. Religious congregations are considered an important mechanism in molding people in terms of their mental health. Individuals' mental health is often supported through engagement with members and leaders of religious congregations. A spiritual community may provide a variety of support, including [5]:

- Protecting people from social isolation
- Providing and strengthening family and social networks
- providing individuals with a sense of belonging and self-esteem, and
- Offering spiritual support in times of adversity.

Physicians who anticipate conflicts between their own commitments and the requests of their patients (or their patients' families) should discuss with a chaplain or minister of the patient's religion the nature of the conflict, and should discuss with the patient or family about transference of care to a physician who will not experience such conflict.

Is This Treatment Really Necessary? Health professionals must honestly reflect to make distinction between ordinary versus extraordinary, proportionate versus disproportionate, and obligatory versus non-obligatory health care. Economic, social, psychological, and moral costs associated with treatment, or by the unlikelihood of achieving health [27]. Some little concessions may satisfy the patient and tranquilize the need to accomplish religious obligations. Many simple issues are common to practitioners of several religions, as the preference of the patient to be attended by a professional of the same sex. Also, patient may want to consult a religious leader of his-her denomination before to accept a procedure; this should be respected whenever possible.

For some patients, acknowledging their beliefs or religious practices may be an important aspect of a holistic approach to their care. Discussing personal beliefs may, when approached sensitively, help to work in partnership with patients to address their particular treatment needs. The staff must respect patients' right to hold religious or other beliefs and should take those beliefs into account where they may be relevant to treatment options [26]. It is important to assess whether the treatment plan is consistent with the family's religious beliefs. Clinicians have contact with families at life's critical transition points. By accurately identifying the family's beliefs, clinicians can work with families to accommodate the treatment for the best interest of everyone involved on it.

Should health professionals recommend that patients participate or cease participation in religion or spirituality for their well-being? Here, respect for the religious or spiritual adherence of the patient (or for his or her lack thereof) may conflict with what the professionals believes is in the therapeutic interest of the patient or with the religious or spiritual adherence (or lack thereof) of the professionals. The question is the degree of confidence with which a professional can determine that a religious belief, commitment, practice, or symbol is correlated with (or the cause of) a positive or negative condition that psychotherapy can affect [14].

Open discussion with the patient and her or his family about spiritual views and how they can be incorporated into the management plan will likely be beneficial for both the patient and the team. A person-centered approach is key to ensuring that the patient's spirituality is understood from her or his perspective. For some patients, the best health treatment will be that which is consistent with their spiritual or religious views.

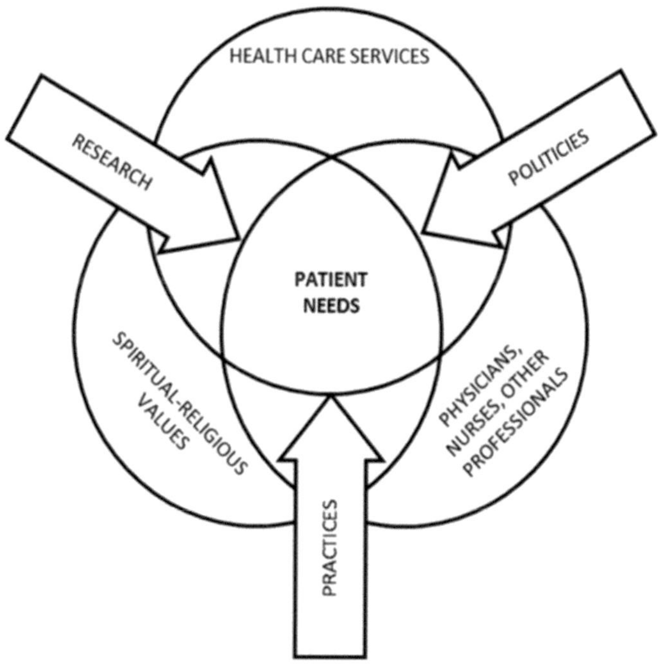

Figure 1. A scheme on how balancing the elements of attention to the special needs of patients to empower resources on spiritual-religious coping

Figure 1 illustrates how to solve the problem of meeting the special needs of patients by healthcare professionals and services. The elements that are at stake are the institutions (health care and rehabilitation), the people associated with the process (physicians, nurses, other professionals) and individual values of patient (religious and spiritual). The forces that bind these elements are the scientific research on the subject, the good practices adopted by institutions and government policies that support these achievements.

7. Conclusion

This chapter is intended to present evidences and discuss proposals on how health care services can empower spiritual-religious resources of patients in order to they can be used as an efficient coping strategy. It is known that a relation between better health and religion or spirituality is found in studies covering several physical and mental conditions. Spiritual-religious coping is the use of religious beliefs, attitudes or practices to reduce the emotional distress caused by stressful events of life, such as loss or change, which gives suffering meaning and makes it more bearable. Spiritual distress is a state of suffering due to spiritual causes. Generally it may be associated with unfulfilled spiritual needs. The consequent defensive behaviors patient can develop under spiritual distress may affect clinical treatment and quality of life. Health care services must invest on some actions, in order to minimize conflicts between religious interests of patients and medical treatment. We discussed a list of actions to promote the positive impact of spirituality and religiosity on the health treatment process, which would be followed by health care professionals and services. The elements that are at stake are the institutions (health care and rehabilitation), the people associated with the process (physicians, nurses, other professionals) and individual values of patient (religious and spiritual).

Author details

Marcelo Saad*
Hospital Israelita Albert Einstein, S. Paulo, SP, Brazil

Roberta de Medeiros
Centro Universitario S. Camilo, S. Paulo, SP, Brazil

8. References

[1] Koenig HG. Spirituality in patient care - Why, How, When, and What. Templeton Foundation Press, Pennsylvania, USA, 2002

[2] Kalra L. Faith Under the Microscope [editorial]. Stroke 2007, 38:848-849

[3] Puchalski, C.M., Ferrell, B., Virani, R., Otis-Green, S., Baird, P., Bull, J. (2009). Improving the quality of spiritual care as a dimension of palliative care: The Report of the Consensus Conference. J Palliat Med, 12(10), 885-904.

* Corresponding Author

[4] Sulmasy DP. Spirituality, Religion, and Clinical Care. Chest 2009;135; 1634-1642
[5] McCulloch A. Keeping the faith - Spirituality and recovery from mental health problems. ISBN 978-1-906162-08-5. Mental Health Foundation 2007 - www.mentalhealth.org.uk
[6] Delgado C. Meeting clients' spiritual needs. Nurs Clin North Am. 2007;42(2):279-93
[7] Anandarajah G. Doing a Culturally Sensitive Spiritual Assessment: Recognizing Spiritual Themes and Using the HOPE Questions. Virtual Mentor - Ethics Journal of the American Medical Association. May 2005, 7(5).
[8] Rhi BY. Culture, Spirituality, and Mental Health - The Forgotten Aspects of Religion and Health. The Psychiatric Clinics Of North America. September 2001, 24(3):569-79
[9] Dein S. The Faith of Patients. Presentation given at the Annual Meeting of the Royal College of Psychiatrists, Liverpool, June 2009
[10] McColl MA; Bickenbach J; Johnston J; Nishihama S; Schumaker M; Smith K; Smith M; Yealland B: Spiritual issues associated with traumatic-onset disability. Disabil Rehabil; 22(12):555-64, 2000
[11] Koenig HK, McCullough ME, Larson DB. Handbook of religion and health. Oxford: Oxford University Press, 2001.
[12] HOFF A, Johannessen-Henry CT, Ross L, Hvidt NC, Johansen C. Religion and reduced cancer risk – What is the explanation? A review. European Journal of Cancer 2008; 44(17):2573-2579
[13] Markwell H. End-of-life: a Catholic view. The Lancet. Volume 366, Issue 9491, 24-30 September 2005, Pages 1132-1135
[14] Lomax JW, Karff S, McKenny GP. Ethical considerations in the integration of religion and psychotherapy: three perspectives. Psychiatr Clin N Am 25 (2002) 547–559
[15] Unruh AM. Spirituality, Religion, and Pain. CJNR 2007, 39(2):66–86
[16] Meador KG. When Patients Say, "It's in God's Hands." . Virtual Mentor - American Medical Association Journal of Ethics. October 2009, Volume 11, Number 10: 750-754.
[17] Packer S. Religion and Stress. Encyclopedia of Stress (Second Edition), 2007, Pages 351-357
[18] Koenig HG. Religion, spirituality, and medicine – research findings and implication for clinical practice. Southern Med J 97(12):1194-1200, 2004
[19] Joint Commission on Accreditation of Healthcare Organizations. Evaluating your Spiritual Assessment Process. Joint Commission: The Source 2005:3(2):6-7
[20] Multi-Faith Group for Healthcare Chaplancy. Faith Requirements Resource Pack - A Guide for Hospital Staff to Improve Patient Care. Produced by the Department of Spiritual & Religious Care, Bradford Teaching Hospitals NHS Trust. 2003. Available at http://www.mfghc.com/resources/resources_74.pdf
[21] Culliford L. Spirituality and clinical care. BMJ 2002;325:1434–5
[22] Saad M, De Medeiros R. Alinhamento entre crenças religiosas do paciente e tratamento hospitalar. Einstein - Educ Contin Saúde. 2012;10(1):36-7
[23] Lucchetti G, Lucchetti ALG, Bassi RM, Vera AVD, Peres MFP. Integrating Spirituality into Primary Care. In Capelli O (Ed.): Primary Care at a Glance - Hot Topics and New Insights, ISBN: 978-953-51-0539-8, InTech Publisher, 2012

[24] Karff SE. Recognizing the Mind/Body/Spirit Connection in Medical Care. Virtual Mentor - American Medical Association Journal of Ethics. October 2009, Volume 11, Number 10: 788-792

[25] Moncher F.J., Josephson A.M. Religious and spiritual aspects of family assessment. Child Adolesc Psychiatric Clin N Am 13 (2004) 49–70

[26] General Medical Council. Personal Beliefs and Medical Practice. March 2008. http://www.gmc-uk.org/guidance/ethical_guidance/personal_beliefs.asp

[27] Engelhardt Jr HT, Iltis AS. End-of-life: the traditional Christian view. The Lancet. 2005,366(9490):1045-1049

Section 3

Therapeutic Resources

Botanical Species as Traditional Therapy: A Quantitative Analisys of the Knowledge Among Ranchers in Southeastern Brazil

Maria Franco Trindade Medeiros, Luci de Senna-Valle
and Regina Helena Potsch Andreata

Additional information is available at the end of the chapter

http://dx.doi.org/10.5772/50444

1. Introduction

Human communities around the world have developed health care practices based on their interaction with the components of their natural environment. Thousands of years of observation and experimentation have helped in developing different empirical medical systems that include the knowledge of plants [1-3]. Such knowledge is the subject of ethnobotany, which attempts to understand the perceptions, healing strategies, and natural resources used to fight diseases or maintain health in traditional medical systems.

Medical ethnobotany constitutes an important alternative among many other known therapies that are practiced worldwide. There is growing recognition that people in different parts of the world still use plant-based remedies as primary or complementary medicine (see, for example, [4-10]). Particularly in Latin America, Africa, and Asia, traditional medicine is part of the prevailing health care system [11]. Using plants for medicinal purposes is part of the body of traditional knowledge that is becoming increasingly more relevant to discussions on conservation biology, public health policies, and sustainable management of natural resources, biological prospection, and patents [12,13].

The present study explores the aspect of the empirical medicinal use of natural resources, including the cultural dimensions that influence the extraction of natural products. A quantitative analysis was performed based on the variables used in the study conducted with the ranchers who live in remnants of the Atlantic Forest in the State of Rio de Janeiro (Southeast, Brazil) [14, 15]. This area includes the so-called Rio das Pedras Reserve, which is situated on the Atlantic side of the Serra do Mar, in the Mangaratiba municipality. This study addressed the following questions. 1) Do people residing in preserved areas know about and/or use medicinal plants? Because these people reside in an environmental preservation area, it is expected that they use plant species therapeutically. 2) How will the triangulation of quantitative techniques be able to better assess the relative importance of plants in a culture? Considering that the wealth of knowledge/use of medicinal plants by a group of people is a complex system, it is believed that the data derived from different quantitative techniques may emphasize a plant's importance in relation to its versatility, quantify the percentage of informants claiming the use of a certain plant for the same major medicinal purpose, and indicate how homogenous the ethnobotanical information is among the informants.

2. Materials and methods

2.1. Study area

The Rio das Pedras Reserve is located in the western region of the State of Rio de Janeiro, in the Mangaratiba municipality on the Atlantic slope of the Serra do Mar, next to the Sepetiba Bay, between the coordinates 22º59' S and 44º05' W. The reserve has an area of 1,360 hectares (13 km^2). The access route to the Reserve is km 55 of the BR-101 highway (Rio/Santos), with a distance of 110 km from the city of Rio de Janeiro (Figure 1).

The area has an annual average temperature of 22ºC, an absolute maximum temperature of 38ºC, and a minimum of 12ºC. The highest rainfall index occurs in the months from December to February. The Grande River Basin is the main drainage basin; the Grande River is located in a valley with steep slopes (greater than 37º), and the elevations vary from 20 to 1,050 meters [16].

The current Reserve area corresponds to the former Goiabal Farm, an enterprise that focused on the cultivation and sale of bananas. The banana shipments were transported by boats bound for Rio de Janeiro. According to the report from the historian Alda Marília Cerqueira de Pinto (personal communication. 2000), after the death of Mr. Otacílio Cerqueira, the owner of the farm, his widow attempted to continue the operation; however, much of the banana production was diverted by the sharecroppers who sold their harvest directly. Therefore, to pay the debts acquired due to the maintenance of the farm and the lack of product requested by the banana buyers from Rio de Janeiro, the farm was sold to the French Club Méditerranée (Club Med) in 1986 for the construction of the Village Rio das Pedras at Praia Grande. Since then, the sharecroppers who planted the bananas and provided half of their production to the owner of the farm as payment for their occupation and use of the land became ranchers and have been paid indemnity to vacate the area.

As the property of Club Méditerranée, the Rio das Pedras Reserve was created in 1992 with the intention of preserving the Atlantic Forest from hunters and palm tree harvesters, in addition to providing ecological tours for its guests through the implementation of ecotourism in its trails [16]. Although Méditerranée Club intended to transform the area into a private natural history reserve, it was not officially included in this type of conservation unit. Many of the ranchers, who were sharecroppers before the implementation of the

Reserve, were compensated and left the region. However, there are still nine families that reside in the Reserve, mostly since birth (91%, with 11 men and 12 women in total), and they continue planting bananas as a form of subsistence.

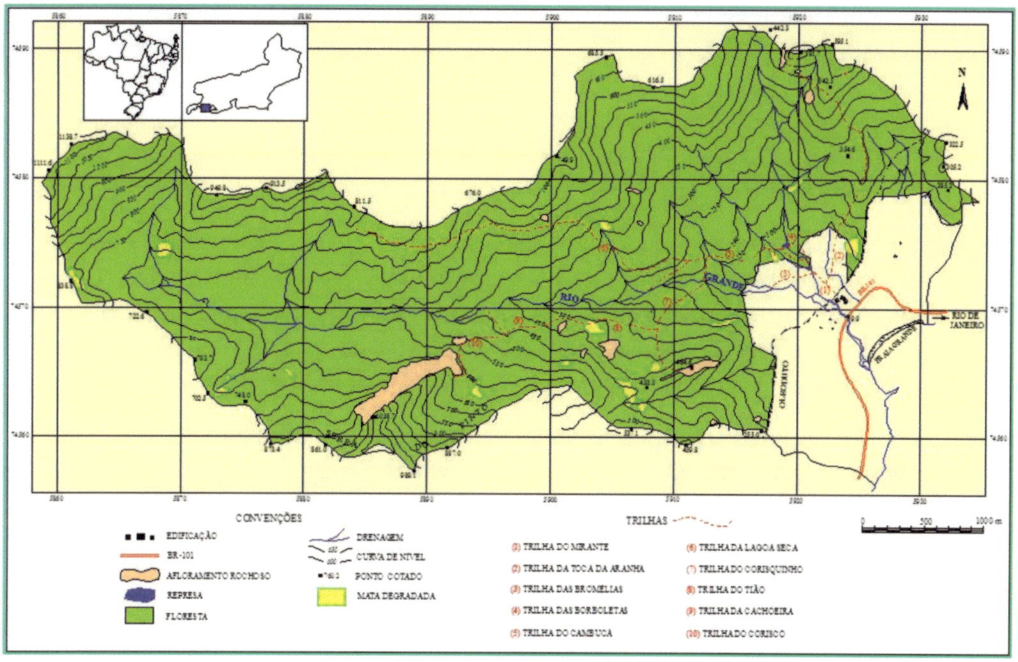

Figure 1. Location of the Rio das Pedras Reserve, Mangaratiba, RJ. Modified from a previous publication [17].

The ranchers from the Reserve are concentrated into two distinct areas: one where six families reside, with houses structurally made of bricks, and the other represented by three families who live in wattle and daub houses. There is no sewage system or electricity, and food is cooked using a wood stove. Water from the waterfall is transported to the houses through PVC pipes, but bathing occurs at the source of this water. The garbage produced is at times incinerated near the homes, as there is no specific location for this practice. Basic provisions, such as salt and sugar, are acquired in the supermarkets of Mangaratiba.

The banana cultivation is performed by the adults who receive R $3.00 to R $4.00 per box, comprising two to three bunches of bananas, and two of the individuals work in the Reserve, one as a guide and the other as a gardener.

2.2. Collection of data and botanical material

Field expeditions were conducted over one year and five months between November 1999 and August 2001 in the Rio das Pedras Reserve. During this period, the fieldwork was accomplished by visiting all of the resident ranchers in the area of the Rio das Pedras Reserve and included participant observation, the application of the free-listing technique, interviews, and guided tours. At the beginning of the study, the members of the community were informed about the purpose of the work proposed and were invited to participate in the study.

The free-listing technique helped with the initial approach of the research subject in which each collaborator was invited to list the medicinal plants for which they had knowledge/use. After this first survey, the key collaborators were intentionally selected because they were the "experts" in the use of plants with therapeutic purposes; these key collaborators had cited the largest number of plants during the free listing. A sample group composed of six collaborators, with an age range from 37 to 60 years of age, including two males and four females, was then selected.

Individual interviews were conducted to obtain greater detail about each of the plants mentioned in the free listing and with the possibility of other plants being included. Therefore, new meetings were arranged with the key collaborators for structured interviews using direct and closed questions and semi-structured interviews using open questions [18]. These events were focused on obtaining relevant information about the medicinal use of the plants.

At the end of each interview, the medicinal specimens were collected with the aid of the collaborators through a guided tour to the places where the specified plants grow. At this point, new plants could also be incorporated into the list of plants already mentioned during the interviews.

The collected botanical material was identified, herborized in accordance with the usual botanical techniques, and were deposited in the ICBA herbarium of the Santa Úrsula University (Universidade Santa Úrsula – RUSU), with duplicates in the Herbarium of the Botany Department of the National Museum (R), both located in the city of Rio de Janeiro (Brazil).

2.3. Data analysis

The quantitative techniques that were applied examined the importance of each use of plant species according to two principal categories: the total number of uses for each category and taxa and the informant consensus. For the total number of uses, the total number of species and the uses for each family cited by the ranchers were summed, according to a previous report [19]. The techniques included in the consensus among the informants are specified below.

The Relative Importance (RI) emphasizes a plant's importance in relation to its versatility. It was calculated based on the number of properties attributed to a species and the number of organ systems on which this species acts, as follows [20]: RI = NCS + NP, where 2 is the maximum value obtained by a species for RI (Relative Importance); NCS = the relative number of corporal systems, calculated by dividing the number of corporal systems treated by a given species [NCSS] by the total number of corporal systems treated by the most versatile species [NCSV]; and NP = the relative number of properties, calculated by dividing the number of properties attributed to a given species [NPS] by the number of properties attributed to the most versatile species [NPSV].

The therapeutic indications cited during the interviews were grouped by body systems according to the disease categories proposed by the International Classification of Diseases [21]. By means of the consensus of the informants, the importance of a species for a determined purpose and the categories that present greater importance to the ranchers could be obtained by the calculation of the Fidelity level (FL) and from the Informant Consensus Factor (FIC), respectively [19].

The Fidelity Level (FL) is calculated by the ratio of the number of informants that claim a use of a plant species to treat a particular disease (N_P) by the number of informants that use the plant as a medicine to treat any given disease (N), as expressed by the formula: FL(%) = $N_P/N x100$ [22].

The Informant Consensus Factor (ICF) is calculated as follows: ICF = $n_{ur} - n_t/n_{ur} - 1$, where 1 is the maximum value of the ICF when there is a complete consensus between the informants; n_{ur} = the number of use-reports in each category; and n_t = the number of taxa used [2].

3. Results and discussion

3.1. Plant resources known/used as therapy by ranchers residing in the conservation unit area

The pharmacopeia of the ranchers is composed of a list of 36 species of plants (Table 1). These species belong to 25 families of which five (Asteraceae, Lamiaceae, Araceae, Moraceae, and Rutaceae) comprise 46% of the total list (Figure 2). The Asteraceae, Lamiaceae, and Rutaceae families are among those with the greatest pharmacopeia representation in various regions of the world and include species with ample occurrence [20, 23, 24]. They also constitute important families from a cultural point of view and in relation to the chemical efficiency of their species; these are factors that, when combined, influence and determine the selection of species for medicinal purposes by the local populations [25].

A poorly differentiated overview can be observed when considering the sum of the medicinal uses for each family. A more significant ranking of families was obtained and included the following: Asteraceae, Lamiaceae, Caricaceae, Araceae, and Crassulaceae (Figure 2). From this perspective, the analysis shows that, although Caricaceae and Crassulaceae present only one cited species, these species are used for more than one medicinal purpose. These families can thus be considered more versatile with regard to the range of therapeutic applications, according to the indications from the ranchers.

Evaluating the medicinal flora in terms of the number of citations per species, the ranchers use a large number of species with only one citation (17 spp.) (Figure 3). Therefore, this fact can be an indicator that there are species with exclusive uses for certain therapeutic purposes, species that are not well known in the community, or even species that face the process of deletion from or insertion into the local pharmacopeia.

Taxon [Family]	Medicinal use	N_p	N	FL
Achyrocline satureioides (Lam.) DC. [Asteraceae]	for toothache during eruption	1	1	100
Alpinia zerumbet (Pers.) Burtt & Smith [Zingiberaceae]	as a sedative	1	3	33
	for high blood pressure	2	3	67
Baccharis trimera (Less.) DC. [Asteraceae]	for stomach ache	2	2	100
	for flu	2	2	100
Bidens pilosa L. [Asteraceae]	for hepatitis	2	2	100
Carica papaya L. [Caricaceae]	for bronchitis	1	2	50
	for flu	1	2	50
	for constipation	2	2	100
	for warts	2	2	100
Cecropia hololeuca Miq. [Moraceae]	for bronchitis	1	1	100
Chamaesyce prostrata (Aiton) Small [Euphorbiaceae]	for kidney stones	2	2	100
Chenopodium ambrosioides L. [Chenopodiaceae]	for a wound	1	5	20
Citrus aurantium L. [Rutaceae]	for flu	1	1	100
Citrus medica var. *limonum* L. [Rutaceae]	for cough	1	1	100
Coffea arabica L. [Rubiaceae]	for headache	1	1	100
Colocasia esculenta (L.) Schott [Araceae]	for anemia	2	2	100
Costus spiralis (Jacq.) Roscoe var. *spiralis* [Costaceae]	for kidney stones	2	2	100
Cymbopogon citratus (DC.) Stapf [Poaceae]	as a sedative	2	3	67
	for high blood pressure	1	3	33
	for flu	1	3	33
Desmodium triflorum (L.) DC [Leguminosae]	for internal inflammation	2	2	100
	for external inflammation	1	2	50
Elephantopus mollis Kunth. [Asteraceae]	for contusion	1	1	100
Eugenia uniflora L. [Myrtaceae]	for flu	4	4	100
Euterpe edulis Mart. [Arecaceae]	for stomach ache	1	1	100
Foeniculum vulgare L. [Apiaceae]	for diarrhea	2	2	100
Gossypium hirsutum L. [Malvaceae]	for internal inflammation	1	1	100
Jacaranda jasminoides (Thunb.) Sandwith [Bignoniaceae]	for itchiness	1	1	100
Kalanchoe brasiliensis Cambess. [Crassulaceae]	for bronchitis	1	3	33
	for flu	2	3	67
	for a wound	2	3	67
Matricaria chamomilla L. [Asteraceae]	as a sedative	1	1	100
Melissa officinalis L. [Lamiaceae]	as a sedative	1	1	100
	for high blood pressure	1	1	100
Mentha x *piperita* L. [Lamiaceae]	for flu	1	1	100
	as a dewormer	1	1	100
Mentha x *villosa* Huds. [Lamiaceae]	for bronchitis	1	2	50
	for flu	2	2	100
	as a dewormer	2	2	100
Musa paradisiaca L. [Musaceae]	for wound healing	3	3	100
Piper mollicomum Kunth. [Piperaceae]	for back pain	2	2	100
Pistia stratiotes (L.) Schott [Araceae]	as eye drops	2	2	100
Plectranthus barbatus Andr. [Lamiaceae]	for the liver	2	2	100

Taxon [Family]	Medicinal use	N_P	N	FL
Schinus terebinthifolius Raddi [Anacardiaceae]	as an antiseptic	1	1	100
Sechium edule (Jacq.) Sw. [Cucurbitaceae]	for high blood pressure	2	2	100
Solanum capsicoides All. [Solanaceae]	for skin boils	1	1	100
Sorocea guilleminiana Gaudich. [Moraceae]	for ulcers (gastritis)	1	1	100
Stachytarpheta cayennensis (Rich.) Vahl [Verbenaceae]	for stomach ache	1	1	100
	for toothache	1	1	100
Vernonia scorpioides (Lam.) Pers. [Asteraceae]	for bronchitis	1	1	100
	for flu	1	1	100
TOTAL: 25 families/36 taxa/28 therapeutic indications				

Table 1. Relationship of the taxa and their respective fidelity level values for medicinal use according to the pharmacopeia of the ranchers of the Rio das Pedras Reserve, in the Mangaratiba municipality, Rio de Janeiro state, Brazil. Legend: N_P = the number of informants that suggested the use of a species for the same purpose; N = the total number of informants that mentioned a plant for any use; FL = the fidelity level.

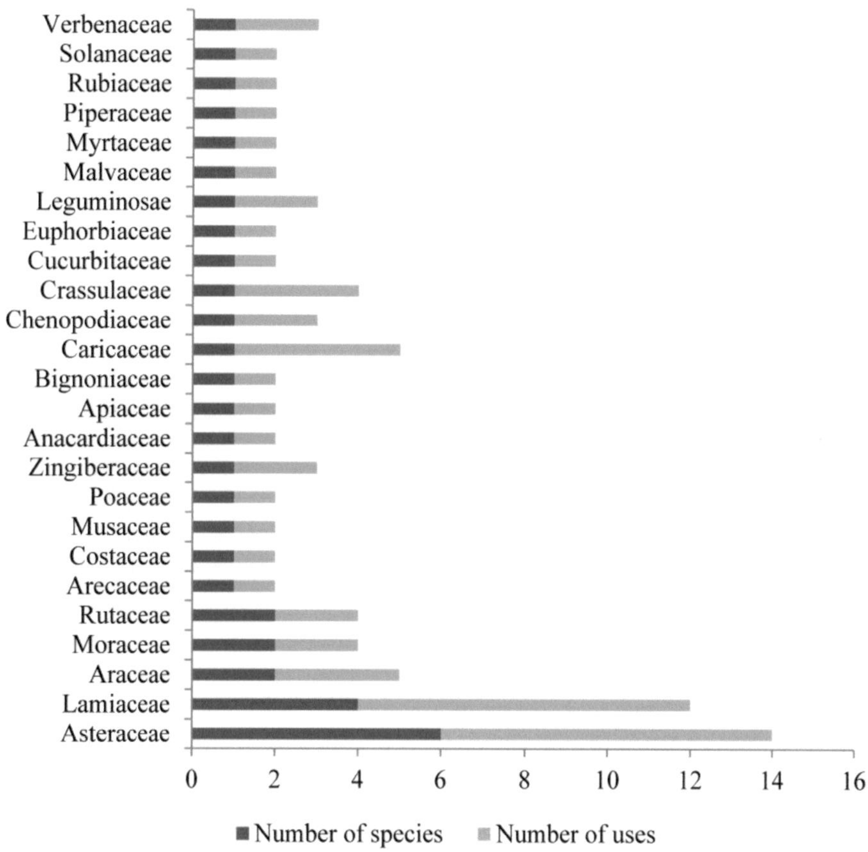

Figure 2. Distribution of the number of species and their respective therapeutic uses for each botanical family of the pharmacopeia of the Rio das Pedras Reserve ranchers, Mangaratiba municipality, Rio de Janeiro state, Brazil.

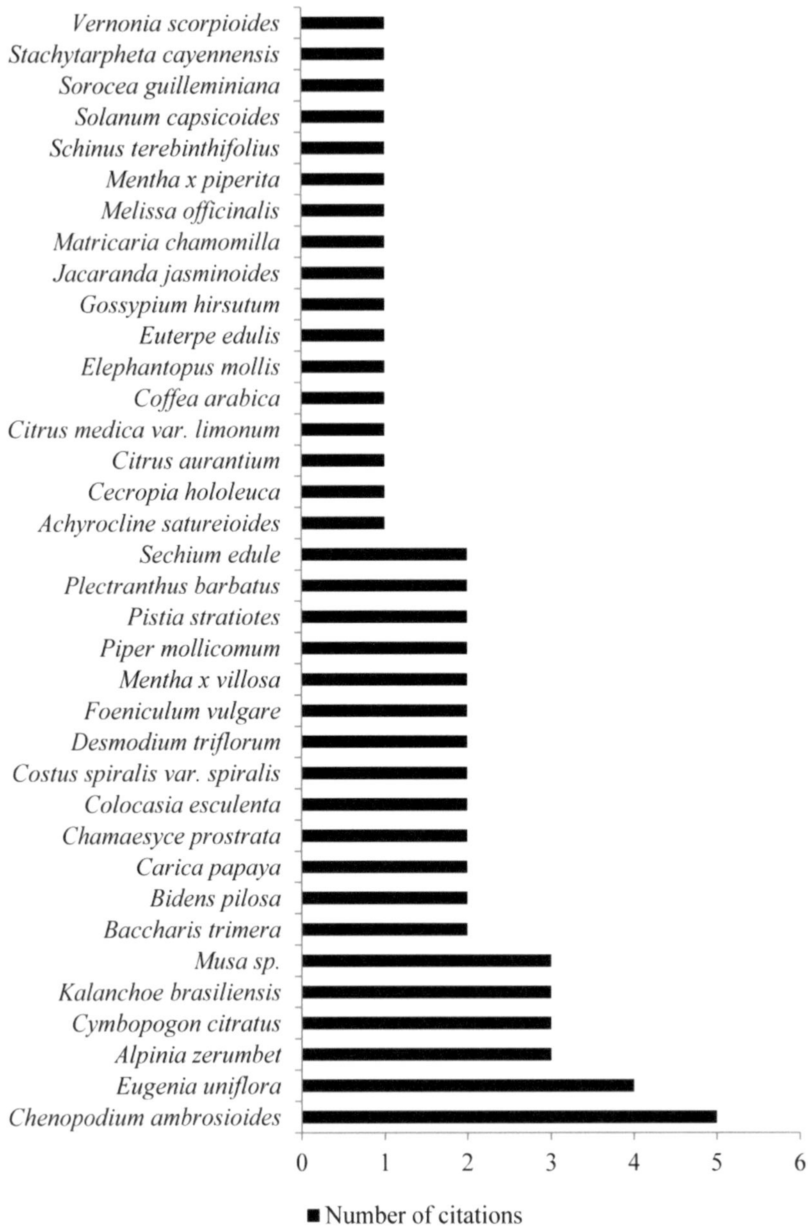

Figure 3. Number of citations per species of the pharmacopeia of the Rio das Pedras Reserve ranchers, Mangaratiba municipality, Rio de Janeiro state, Brazil.

In general, the species used by the ranchers are widely used even in other regions of Brazil, as indicated by such studies as those conducted in the Amazon Basin [26], Roraima State [27] the Maranhão Lowlands [28], Acre State [29], São Paulo State [30-32], Bahia State [33], and Rio de Janeiro State [10, 34]. These data reveal that, although the ranchers geographically inhabit the Atlantic Forest biome, their knowledge/use of species for medicinal purposes was formed based on the species cultivated in their backyards (around their houses). Furthermore, these plants, which primarily occur in anthropogenic zones, are characterized by species with ample occurrence and distribution in Brazil and have also reached different parts of the world in the most differentiated biogeographic regions of the Americas, Africa, Europe, Asia, and Oceania. Among these, there are some species that are not native to the Brazilian flora yet have a wide distribution in the Brazilian territory, for example, the *Mentha* species, *Citrus* species, *Arabian* Coffea L., *Colocasia esculenta* (L.) Schott, *Cymbopogon citratus* (DC.) Stapf, and *Matricaria chamomilla* L.

However, on the issue of the use of non-native species that have wide geographic distribution in detriment to the native species of Brazil, it is believed that this choice by the ranchers may be a consequence of the involuntary displacement and resettlement process that the families face when they leave the region as the result of the area becoming a conservation unit.

Within this context, the use of species in nearby locations would be adequate due to the lower energy expended for the collection of material and also due to the monitoring of the land use in the region. According to a previous report [35], the decrease in traditional botanical knowledge is related to the distancing of human populations from areas of native vegetation, which, in a way, is similar to the reality experienced by the ranchers, given that they were no longer able to move freely around the preserved forest areas.

Another factor to be considered is the proximity of the ranchers to the urban center of the city of Mangaratiba. In this sense, a previous report [36] affirms that it would not be the proximity to the native vegetation that would interfere with the knowledge and use of medicinal plants but the social factors, such as the proximity to urban centers, which would exert a negative influence on the knowledge and utilization. According to these authors, a proximity to urban centers permits a greater offering of western, academic medicine, which competes strongly with the use of plant resources and leads to the reduction of their use by traditional communities.

3.2. Triangulation of quantitative techniques as a tool to determine the relative importance of the plants used in traditional therapy

The medical system of the ranchers is composed of 28 therapeutic indications. The main therapeutic indications, i.e., those that constitute the greatest wealth of referred plants, are the use of plants for the flu and for bronchitis (Table 1). These medicinal applications are also among the main applications in certain previous studies [37-39].

The evaluation of the fidelity level (FL) showed that the species that obtained 100% agreement among the informants with regard to their use add up to 74%, which is equivalent to 39 reported uses for 30 species (Table 1).

Four species showed great versatility with regards to their use, with RI > 1; these plants are indicated for as many as four organ systems: *Carica papaya* L., *Cymbopogon citratus* (DC.) Stapf, *Kalanchoe brasiliensis* Cambess., and *Mentha x villosa* Huds. (Table 2). The use of these species also occurs in other locations, as is shown, for example, by the study of popular medicine [40] in the municipality of Rio Claro, State of São Paulo in which the authors cited the use of the male papaya (*Carica papaya* L.) against cough, flu, and catarrh.

Taxon	NCSS	NCS	NPS	NP	RI
Carica papaya	4	1	4	1	2
Cymbopogon citratus	3	0.75	3	0.75	1.5
Kalanchoe brasiliensis	3	0.75	3	0.75	1.5
Mentha x *villosa*	3	0.75	3	0.75	1.5
Alpinia zerumbet	2	0.5	2	0.5	1
Baccharis trimera	2	0.5	2	0.5	1
Chenopodium ambrosioides	2	0.5	2	0.5	1
Esculenta Colocasia	2	0.5	2	0.5	1
Desmodium triflorum	2	0.5	2	0.5	1
Melissa officinalis	2	0.5	2	0.5	1
Mentha x *piperita*	2	0.5	2	0.5	1
Stachytarpheta cayennensis	2	0.5	2	0.5	1
Vernonia scorpioides	2	0.5	2	0.5	1
Achyrocline satureioides	1	0.25	1	0.25	0.5
Pilosa Bidens	1	0.25	1	0.25	0.5
Cecropia hololeuca	1	0.25	1	0.25	0.5
Chamaesyce prostrata	1	0.25	1	0.25	0.5
Citrus aurantium	1	0.25	1	0.25	0.5
Citrus medicates to var. *limonum*	1	0.25	1	0.25	0.5
Arabian Coffea	1	0.25	1	0.25	0.5
Costus spiralis to var. *spiralis*	1	0.25	1	0.25	0.5
Elephantopus mollis	1	0.25	1	0.25	0.5
Uniflora Eugenia	1	0.25	1	0.25	0.5
Euterpe edulis	1	0.25	1	0.25	0.5
Foeniculum vulgare	1	0.25	1	0.25	0.5
Gossypium hirsutum	1	0.25	1	0.25	0.5
Jacaranda jasminoides	1	0.25	1	0.25	0.5
Matricaria chamomilla	1	0.25	1	0.25	0.5
Paradisiacal muse	1	0.25	1	0.25	0.5
Piper mollicomum	1	0.25	1	0.25	0.5
Pistia stratiotes	1	0.25	1	0.25	0.5
Plectranthus barbatus	1	0.25	1	0.25	0.5
Schinus terebinthifolius	1	0.25	1	0.25	0.5
Sechium edule	1	0.25	1	0.25	0.5
Solanum capsicoides	1	0.25	1	0.25	0.5
Guilleminiana Sorocea	1	0.25	1	0.25	0.5

Table 2. Values of the relative importance of each taxon used as medicine by the ranchers of the Rio das Pedras Reserve, Mangaratiba municipality, State of Rio de Janeiro, Brazil. Legend: NCSS= the number of corporal systems treated by a given species; NCS = the relative number of corporal systems; NPS = the number of properties attributed to a given species; NP = the relative number of properties; RI = the relative importance.

The organ systems that these plants act upon were observed by analyzing the contribution of plant species with regard to the functionality of the pharmacopeia of the ranchers. The medicinal species treat diseases grouped into eleven organ systems. Among these systems, six are the main systems with regard to the number of species cited: respiratory system disorders, infectious and parasitic diseases, digestive system disorders, skin and subcutaneous tissues diseases, nervous system disorders, and circulatory system disorders (Table 3). In a study conducted in the municipality of Barra do Piraí, Rio de Janeiro State, reference is made to plants used in rituals, for flu symptoms, and skin and healing problems as the most representative therapeutic indications in terms of the number of species [41]. In a study conducted in Santa Maria, Rio Grande Do Sul State, the flu, digestive problems, and anti-inflammatory uses are the most common indications [42]. In the semiarid region in Northeastern Brazil, a significant number of plants are also used to treat health problems, including circulatory, digestive, and respiratory disorders of organ systems [43-45]. Given that a larger number of species are used for the treatment of flu, bronchitis, skin diseases, and digestive system conditions, there is agreement between the present work and those by the above-mentioned authors.

According to the Informant Consensus Factor (ICF) in terms of the medicinal potential of the species cited by the ranchers of the Rio das Pedras Reserve, the organ system with the most consensus was related to respiratory system disorders (Table 3). Therefore, the results of the ICF point to this medicinal category as the one that the informants are the most confident about. All of the other categories obtained the minimum values expected, as the number of species was equivalent to the uses. In a previous study [44] in which the same index was calculated, respiratory diseases are also among the main disease categories.

Organ system	n_t	n_{ur}	ICF
Respiratory system disorders	11	15	0.29
Certain infectious and parasitic diseases	8	8	0
Diseases of the blood and hematopoietic organs	1	1	0
Nervous system disorders	5	5	0
Sensory system disorders [eyes]	1	1	0
Circulatory system disorders	4	4	0
Digestive system disorders	7	7	0
Skin and subcutaneous tissue diseases	7	7	0
Osteomuscular and connective tissue diseases	1	1	0
Genitourinary disorders	2	2	0
Injuries, poisoning, and other consequences of external causes	3	3	0

Table 3. Consensus for the therapeutic use of plant species among the ranchers of the Rio das Pedras Reserve, Mangaratiba municipality, Rio de Janeiro state, Brazil. Legend: n_{ur} = the sum of uses recorded by each informant for a category; n_t = the number of species indicated in the category; ICF = the informant consensus factor.

4. Conclusion

The ranchers have a knowledge of plant resources that point to a wealth of species that are mostly considered to be non-native to the biome in which they were found: the Atlantic Forest. These plants are generally collected in backyards, which can reinforce the importance of the environment upon the selection criteria of the species in a pharmacopeia. Moreover, when analyzing the list that compiles the pharmacopeia of the ranchers, another factor to be considered is the cultural influences that, throughout the history of this people, many have contributed to the adaptation of their pharmacopeia to the conditions in which they now live, after the creation of the conservation unit.

Considering the triangulation of quantitative techniques, it is important to emphasize that these analyses do not substitute for the careful qualitative analysis conducted with the ranchers from the Rio das Pedras Reserve, but they helped to demonstrate that *Carica papaya* L. is a species with the most effective pharmacological potential because it reached the maximum value for relative importance. With regard to the fidelity level, a large part of the indicated uses for each species achieved the maximum expected value.

The plants used by the ranchers that are included in the respiratory disease category, which is the category that obtained the greatest consensus with regard to use among the informants, are the species that deserves a proper pharmacological study. The following species fit into this category are: *Baccharis trimera* (Less.) DC., *Carica papaya* L., *Cecropia hololeuca* Miq., *Citrus aurantium* L., *Citrus medica* var. *limonum* L., *Cymbopogon citratus* (DC.) Stapft, *Eugenia uniflora* L., *Kalanchoe brasiliensis* Cambess., *Mentha* x *piperita* L., *Mentha* x *villosa* Huds., and *Vernonia scorpioides* (Lam.) Pers..

Finally, because of the value that such information held by the local populations about the plant kingdom represents for humanity, it is suggested that the application of quantitative indices will contribute to a deeper analysis and identification of new inferences in ethnobotany. This research highlights the importance of local perceptions and knowledge as potential information that can contribute to future applications and, therefore, as a new source of medicines from natural products.

Author details

Maria Franco Trindade Medeiros*

Applied Ethnobotany Laboratory, Biology Department, Federal Rural University of Pernambuco (Universidade Federal Rural de Pernambuco - UFRPE), Recife, PE, Brazil

Luci de Senna-Valle

Botany Departament, National Museum of the Federal University of Rio de Janeiro (Universidade Federal do Rio de Janeiro - UFRJ), Rio de Janeiro, RJ, Brazil

* Corresponding Author

Regina Helena Potsch Andreata
Angiosperm Laboratory, Santa Úrsula University (Universidade Santa Úrsula – RUSU), Rio de Janeiro, RJ, Brazil

Acknowledgement

The authors would like to thank the ranchers for their valuable participation in the research and the National Council for Scientific and Technological Development (Conselho Nacional de Desevolvimento Cientifico e Tecnológico-CNPq) for the research productivity scholarship awarded to Regina Helena Potsch Andreata.

5. References

[1] Arvigo R & Balick M (1998) Rainforest Remedies: One Hundred Healing Herbs of Belize. 2nd ed. Twin Lakes, US: Lotus Press. p. 219.
[2] Heinrich, M., Ankli, A., Frei, B., Weimann, C. & Sticher, O. 1998. Medicinal Plants in Mexico: Healers' Consensus and Cultural Importance. Social science & medicine 47(11): 1859-1871.
[3] Halberstein RA (2005) Medicinal Plants: Historical and Cross-cultural Usage Patterns. Annals of epidemiology 15(9): 686-699.
[4] Agelet, A. &Vallès, J. 2001. Studies on Pharmaceutical Ethnobotany in the Region of Pallars (Pyrenees, Catalonia, Iberian Peninsula). Part I. General Results and New or Very Rare Medicinal Plants. Journal of ethnopharmacology 77: 57-70.
[5] Camejo-Rodrigues, J., Ascensão, L., Bonet, M.À. & Vallès, J. 2003. An Ethnobotanical Study of Medicinal and Aromatic Plants in the Natural Park of "Serra de São Mamede" (Portugal). Journal of ethnopharmacology 89: 199-209.
[6] Ngoula MJ (2003) The Status of Medicinal and Aromatic Plants in Central and Southern Africa. In: ICS-UNIDO. Medicinal Plants and their Utilization. pp. 111-118.
[7] Akerreta S, Cavero RY, & Calvo MI (2007) First Comprehensive Contribution to Medical Ethnobotany of Western Pyrenees. Journal of ethnobiology and ethnomedicine 3: 26.
[8] Rigat M, Bonet MA, Garcia S, Garnatje T, & Vallès JJ (2007) Studies on Pharmaceutical Ethnobotany in the High River Ter Valley (Pyrenees, Catalonia, Iberian Peninsula). Journal of ethnopharmacology 113: 267-277.
[9] Parada M, Carrió E, Bonet MA, & Vallès J (2009) Ethnobotany of the Alt Empordà Region (Catalonia, Iberian Peninsula) - Plants Used in Human Traditional Medicine. Journal of ethnopharmacology 124: 609-618.
[10] Brito MR & Senna-Valle L (2011) Plantas Medicinais Utilizadas na Comunidade Caiçara da Praia do Sono, Paraty, Rio de Janeiro, Brasil [Medicinal Plants Used in the Caiçara Community of Praia do Sono, Paraty, Rio de Janeiro, Brazil]. Acta botanica brasilica 25: 363-372.
[11] World Health Organization (WHO) (2002) Traditional Medicine Strategy 2002-2005.

[12] Medeiros MFT, Senna-Valle L, Andreata RHP, & Fernandes LRRMV (2007) Informações Estratégicas Geradas através do Estudo de Patentes de Plantas Medicinais citadas pelos Sitiantes da Reserva Rio das Pedras, Mangaratiba RJ [Strategic Information Generated through the study of Medicinal Plant Patents cited by the Ranchers of the Rio das Pedras Reserve, Mangaratiba RJ]. Neotropical Biology Journal (Revista de biologia neotropical) 4: 139-147.

[13] Boscolo OH & Senna-Valle L (2010) An Ethnobotanical Survey as Subsidy for the Generation of Researches Related to Biotechnology. International journal of biotechnology 1(1):001-006.

[14] Medeiros MFT & Andreata RHP (2003) Cartilha sobre as Planas Medicinais Utilizadas pelos Sitiantes da Reserva Particular do Patrimônio Natural Rio das Pedras, Mangaratiba, RJ [Guidebook about Medicinal Plants used by the ranchers of the Rio das Pedras Natural Heritage private reserve, Mangaratiba, RJ]. In: Siqueira JC de, coordinator. Mangaratiba: Educação Ambiental – Resgate de Valores Socioambientais.. Rio de Janeiro: PUC–Rio; Petrobrás. pp. 49-66.

[15] Medeiros MFT, Fonseca VS, & Andreata RHP (2004) Plantas Medicinais e seus Usos pelos Sitiantes da Reserva Rio das Pedras, Mangaratiba, RJ, Brasil [Medicinal plants and their uses by the ranchers of the Rio das Pedras Reserve, Mangaratiba, RJ, Brazil]. Acta botanica brasilica 18(2): 391-399.

[16] Souza, R de (1997) Ecoturismo em Unidade de Conservação: Estudo de Caso da Reserva Rio das Pedras, Mangaratiba, Rio de Janeiro [Ecotourism in Conservation Units: Case Study of the Rio das Pedras Reserve, Mangaratiba, Rio de Janeiro]. Masters Thesis. Universidade Federal Rural do Rio de Janeiro, Rio de Janeiro.

[17] Agrofoto Aerofotografia S/A. (1999) Levantamento Planialtimétrico da RPPN-Reserva Rio das Pedras, km 445,5 da BR-101 (Rio-Santos). Escala 1:10.000, Município de Mangaratiba, estado do Rio de Janeiro [Planialtimetric survey of RPPN-Rio das Pedras Reserve, km 445.5 of BR-101 (Rio-Santos). 1:10.000 scale, Mangaratiba municipality, state of Rio de Janeiro].

[18] Alexiades MN (1996) Collecting Ethnobotanical Data: An Introduction to Basic Concepts and Techniques. In: Alexiades, MN, editor. Selected Guidelines for Ethnobotanical Research: A Field Manual. New York: Advances in economic botany. v.10. pp. 54-94.

[19] Phillips OL (1996) Some Quantitative Methods for Analyzing Ethnobotanical Knowledge. In: Alexiades MN, editor. Selected Guidelines for Ethnobotanical Research: A Field Manual. New York: Advances in Economic Botany. v. 10. pp. 171-197.

[20] Bennett BC & Prance GT (2000) Introduced Plants in the Indigenous Pharmacopoeia of Northern South America. Economic botany 54(1): 90-102.

[21] World Health Organization (WHO) (2006) International Statistical Classification of Diseases and Related Health Problems. 10th Revision.

[22] Friedman J, Yaniv Z, Dafni A, & Palewith D (1986) A Preliminary Classification of the Healing Potencial of Medicinal Plants, Based on a Rational Analysis of an Ethnopharmacological Field Survey among Bedouins in the Negev Desert, Israel. Journal of ethnopharmacology 16: 275-287.

[23] Rios M (1993) Plantas Utiles en el Noroccidente de Pichincha – Etnobotánica del Caserío Alvaro Pérez Intriago y la Reserva Forestal ENDESA. Quito: Hombre y Ambiente, número monográfico 26 [Useful Plants in Northwestern Pichincha – Ethnobotany of Caserío Alvaro Pérez Intriago and the ENDESA Forest Reserve. Quito: Man and Environment, monograph number 26]. 185 p.

[24] Albuquerque UP (2001) The Use of Medicinal Plants by the Cultural Descendants of African People in Brazil. Acta farm. bonaerense 20(2): 139-144.

[25] Heinrich M (2008) Ethnopharmacy and Natural Product Research - Multidisciplinary Opportunities for Research in the Metabolomic Age. Phytochemistry Letters 1(1): 1-5.

[26] Amorozo MCM & Gely A (1988) Uso de Plantas Medicinais por Caboclos do Baixo Amazonas, Barcarena, PA, Brasil [Use of Medicinal Plants by the Caboclos of the lower Amazonas, Barcarena, PA, Brazil]. Boletim do museu paraense emílio goeldi sér. bot. 4(1): 47-131.

[27] Berg ME & Silva MHL (1988) Contribuição ao Conhecimento da Flora Medicinal de Roraima [Contribution to the knowledge of the Medicinal Flora of Roraima]. Acta amazônica 18(1-2): 23-35.

[28] Rêgo TJAS (1988) Levantamento de Plantas Medicinais na Baixada Maranhense [Survey of Medicinal plants in the lowlands of Maranhão]. Acta amazônica 18(1-2): 75-88.

[29] Ming LC (1995) Levantamento de Plantas Medicinais na Reserva Extrativista "Chico Mendes" – Acre [Survey of Medicinal Plants in the Extractive Reserve "Chico Mendes" – Acre]. Doctoral Dissertation. Biosciences Institute, São Paulo State University (Universidade Estadual Paulista) "Júlio de Mesquita Filho", Botucatu.

[30] Begossi A, Leitão-Filho HF, & Richerson PJ (1993) Plant Uses in a Brazilian Fishing Community (Búzios Island). Journal of ethnobiology 13: 233-256.

[31] Begossi A, Figueiredo GM, & Leitão-Filho HF (1997) Ethnobotany of Atlantic Forest Coastal Communities: II. Diversity of Plant Uses at Sepetiba Bay (SE Brazil). Human ecology 25(2): 353-361.

[32] Begossi A, Hanazaki N, Tamashiro JY, Leitão-Filho HF (2000) Diversity of Plant Uses in two Caiçara Communities from the Atlantic Forest Coast, Brazil. Biodiversity and conservation 9: 597-615.

[33] Costa-Neto EM, Oliveira MVM (2000) The use of Medicinal Plants in the County of Tanquinho, State of Bahia, Northeastern Brazil. Revista brasileira de plantas medicinais 2(2): 1-6.

[34] Boscolo OH, Senna-Valle L (2008) Medicinal Use Plants in Quissamã, Rio de Janeiro, Brasil. Iheringia. Botanical Series 63: 263-278.

[35] Case RJ, Pauli GF, Soejarto DD (2005) Factors in Maintaining Indigenous Knowledge among Ethnic Communities of Manus Island. Economic botany 59: 356-365.

[36] Vandebroek I, Calewaert JB, De JonckheereStjin, et al. (2004) Use of Medicinal Plants and Pharmaceuticals by Indigenous Communities in the Bolivian Andes and Amazon. Bulletin of the World Health Organization 82: 243-250.

[37] Albuquerque UP, Oliveira RF (2007) Is the Use-impact on Native Caatinga Species in Brazil Reduced by the High Species Richness of Medicinal Plants? Journal of ethnopharmacology 113: 156-170.

[38] Barbosa JAA (2011) From Seeds to Fruit: Therapeutic Indications of Vegetables and their Parents in a Traditional Community from the Paraíba. Journal of biology and pharmacy 5: 48-63.
[39] Castro JÁ, Brasileiro BP, Lyra DH, Pereira DA, Chaves JL, Amaral CLF (2011) Ethnobotanical Study of Traditional Uses of Medicinal Plants: The Flora of Caatinga in the Community of Cravolândia, BA, Brazil. Journal of medicinal plants research 5: 1905-1917.
[40] Silva-Almeida MF, Amorozo MCM (1998) Popular Medicine in the Ferraz District, Rio Claro municipality, State of São Paulo. Brazilian journal of ecology 2(1): 36-46.
[41] Parente CET, Rosa MMT (2001) Commercialized plants as medicines in the municipality of Barra do Piraí, RJ. Rodriguésia 1(1): 47-59.
[42] Somavilla N, Canto-Dorow TS (1996) Survey of Medicinal Plants used in the Neighborhoods of Santa Maria, RS, Brasil. Science and Nature 18: 31-148.
[43] Albuquerque UP, Andrade LHC (2002) Traditional Botanical Knowledge and Conservation in an area of the Caatinga. Acta botanica brasilica 16: 273-285.
[44] Almeida CFCBR, Albuquerque UP (2002) Use and conservation of medicinal plants and animals in the state of Pernambuco (North east of Brasil): a case study. Interciência 27(6): 276-285.
[45] Cartaxo SL, Souza MMA, Albuquerque UP (2010) Medicinal Plants with Bioprospecting Potential Used in Semi-arid Northeastern Brazil. Journal of ethnopharmacology 131: 326-342.

Chapter 9

Hypocholesterolaemic Effects of Probiotics

Kalavathy Ramasamy, Zuhailah Mohd Shafawi,
Vasudevan Mani, Ho Yin Wan and Abu Bakar Abdul Majeed

Additional information is available at the end of the chapter

http://dx.doi.org/10.5772/50785

1. Introduction

There is growing interest in the use of nutraceutical products which includes probiotics, prebiotics and related metabolites with cholesterol-lowering properties to prevent cardiovascular diseases (CVDs) [1]. Probiotics are beneficial bacteria that influence the health of the host by improving their microbial balance. Modifications of intestinal flora have been shown to be beneficial on lipid metabolism in mice [2-6], rats [7-11], guinea pigs [12] and pigs [13]. In contrast, studies in humans [14,15] indicated that the role of fermented milk products as hypocholesterolaemic agents were inconsistent but more reliable effects were documented in the recent clinical studies [16-19]. The cholesterol-lowering effect of probiotics was found to be highly strain-specific as different strains exhibited different levels of cholesterol-lowering activity [20-22]. Therefore, it is important to identify probiotic strains that exhibit excellent cholesterol-lowering ability.

Cholesterol-reducing mechanism(s) by probiotics remain to be elucidated. Deconjugation of bile salt by the bile salt hydrolase (BSH) enzyme and subsequent co-precipitation of cholesterol at acidic pH is one of the models frequently used to explain hypocholesterolaemic effects of probiotics [21,23]. Other studies have shown reduction of cholesterol through assimilation of cholesterol into bacterial cell membrane [24-28], adhesion of cholesterol onto bacterial cell surface [28] and through the binding of bile acids to bacterial exocellular polysaccharides [29]. A recent study showed the ability of probiotics to be able to produce protein(s) with cholesterol-lowering effect [30]. Probiotics are able to grow in prebiotics (indigestible carbohydrate) producing short chain fatty acids (SCFAs). Butyrate, a SCFA has the ability to inhibit liver cholesterol synthesis [31]. The role of probiotics as hypocholesterolaemic agents should be further explored.

2. Cardiovascular disease and treatments

Hypercholesterolemia is the major cause of coronary diseases. Diseases related to hypercholesterolemia have been projected to be the number one leading cause of death in the world by 2020 [32]. In fact, Roth *et al.* [33] concluded that the global burden of CVDs requires immediate action based on analysis of health examination survey of eight countries. An ideal strategy to control this disease is to lower cholesterol through a combination of lifestyle and pharmacologic approaches.

Cholesterol-lowering drugs that are available have different mechanisms of actions. Statins (3-hyroxy-3-methylglutaryl coenzyme A reductase inhibitors) are generally able to inhibit cholesterol synthesis in the liver and peripheral tissues. They have been extensively studied and found to possess better therapeutic effects than other lipid lowering drugs [34]. A recent meta-analysis that involved 14 studies with over 90000 patients for 5 years showed that statins reduced the risks of major cardiovascular events and overall mortality [35]. Yet, another meta-analysis of 11 studies showed no reduction in mortality with the use of statins [36]. A similar conclusion was observed in the recent Cochrane review [37]. However, Blaha *et al.* [38] emphasize that statins are critical in patients with increased cardiovascular risk as opposed to low-risk patients. This is probably due to the adverse effects related to the use of this class of drugs, which include myopathy [39] and cognitive impairment [40-42]. Other pharmacological agents that are used in the management of hypercholesterolemia are bile acid sequestrants, cholesterol absorption inhibitors, niacin, and fibrates. Nevertheless, these drugs have also been associated with many adverse effects that limit treatment compliance as well as quality of life.

Non-pharmacological treatment serves as a supportive therapy to reduce cardiovascular risk in otherwise healthy people. The common recommendations are dietary modifications, exercise and weight control. Modification of diet will allow lower drug doses that will reduce the adverse effects of drugs. Clifton *et al.* [43] reported that although dietary intervention to lower cholesterol had been effective it was underutilized. The idea of preventing and lowering hypercholesterolemia using 'functional foods' has emerged recently. Functional foods are broadly defined as foods that provide additional physiological benefits to the consumer beyond basic nutrition [44]. Functional foods that are commercially available with health claims of reducing cholesterol levels include oat bran fibre, soy protein, fish oil fatty acids, plant sterols and stanols, probiotics and prebiotics [44].

3. Definitions of probiotics

Over the years, probiotics have been defined in several ways. The term probiotic was coined by Lily and Stillwell [45] to describe growth-promoting factors produced by microorganisms. Parker [46] subsequently defined it as organisms and substances, which contribute to intestinal microbial balance. However, Fuller [47] pointed out that this definition was too broad and redefined probiotic as a live microbial feed supplement, which beneficially affects the health of the host animal by improving its intestinal microbial balance. Havenaar *et al.* [48] considered the definition given by Fuller [47] to be restricted to feed supplements, animals and the intestinal tract, and described probiotics as mono or mixed cultures of live microorganisms which, when applied to animal or human, beneficially affected the host by improving the properties of the indigenous microflora. This definition does not restrict probiotic activities to intestinal microflora only, but also includes microbial communities at other sites of the body; the probiotic may consist of more than one bacterial species and that it can be applied to both human and animal. Salminen *et al.* [49] defined probiotics as microbial cell preparations or components of microbial cells that have a beneficial effect on the health and well-being of the host. This definition implies that probiotics do not necessarily need to be viable, and are limited to human only. Finally, FAO/WHO [50] described probiotics as live microorganisms which when administered in adequate amount confer a health benefit on the host.

4. Characteristics and health benefits of probiotics

Evidence is emerging that the intestinal flora does not exist as an entity by itself, but is constantly interacting with the environment, the central nervous system, the endocrine and the immune system [51-54]. There is growing scientific evidence to support the concept that maintenance of gut microflora may prevent or treat intestinal disorders [55-57]. Therefore, attempts have been made to improve health status by modulating the indigenous intestinal microbiota through probiotics [58,59]. However, for probiotics to be effective the selection of strains must be based on criteria that are coherent with the claim the probiotic is used for. Rational selection and validation of promising microbial strains should be based on scientific evidence obtained from *in vitro* models followed by *in vivo* studies. The important criteria that have been put forward by FAO/WHO [60] in the selection of food probiotics include identification of strains using state-of-the-art techniques, ability to tolerate gastric juice and bile, maintain stability and most importantly prove to be safe and beneficial to the consumer. The most common microorganisms in probiotic preparations that possess health benefits are lactic acid bacteria (LAB), mainly lactobacilli and bifidobacteria. Probiotics have been reported to improve intestinal tract health, enhance the immune system, reduce symptoms of lactose intolerance, decrease the prevalence of allergy, treat colitis and lower serum cholesterol levels [61-63].

5. Hypocholesterolaemic effects of probiotics

There has been considerable interest in the beneficial effects of lactobacilli and bifidobacteria on lipid metabolism since the discovery that fermented milk containing a wild *Lactobacillus* strain has hypocholesterolaemic effect in humans [64]. This study is often quoted as the basis for much of the animal and human studies subsequently carried out. The hypocholesterolaemic effects of probiotic *Lactobacillus* and *Bifidobacteria* strains on mice, rat, and human are summarised in Table 1. Taranto *et al.* [2,3] observed that administration of *L. reuteri* to mice reduced the serum total cholesterol (TC) by 20% and increased the ratio of HDL-C to LDL-C by 17%. Mice fed *L. plantarum* PH04 significantly ($P<0.05$) reduced serum

	Probiotic strains	Effects	References
Mice	*L. reuteri*	Serum TC lowered	Taranto *et al.* (1998, 2003)
		Serum TC lowered	Ngyuen *et al.* (2007)
		Serum LDL-C lowered	Jeun *et al.* (2010)
	L. fermentum SM-7	Serum TC and LDL-C lowered	Pan *et al.* (2011)
Rats	A mixture of probiotic microorganisms or *L. acidophilus*	Serum TC lowered	Fukushima and Nakano (1995, 1996, 1999)
	B. longum SPM1207	Serum TC and LDL-C lowered	Usman and Hosono (2000)
	B. longum SPM1207(sonication killed)	Serum TC and LDL-C lowered	Lee *et al.* (2009)
	L. plantarum Lp91	Plasma TC and LDL-C lowered	Shin *et al.* (2010)
	L. plantarum 9-41-A	Plasma HDL-C increased	Kumar *et al.* (2011)
		Serum TC and LDLC lowered	Xie *et al.* (2011)
Human	Probiotic-fermented milk product	Serum Total Cholesterol Variable data from 1974-1997	Taylor and Williams (1998)
		Variable data from 1988-1998	De Roos and Katan (2000)
	L. acidophilus L1	Serum TC lowered	Anderson & Gilliland, 1999
	B. longum BL1	Serum TC lowered	Xiao *et al.*, 2003
	L. acidophilus	No changes in blood lipid parameters	Lewis and Burmeister (2005)

Probiotic strains	Effects	References
L. fermentum	No changes in blood lipid parameters	Simons *et al.* (2006)
L. acidophilus and *B. lactis*	Serum TC	Ataie-Jafari et al (2009)
L. reuteri NCIMB 30242	Serum HDL-C increased Serum TC and LDL-C	Jones *et al.* (2012)

Table 1. Hypocholesterolaemic effects of probiotic *Lactobacillus* and *Bifidobacteria strains* in mice, rats and humans

cholesterol by 7% as compared to the control group [4]. The *L. plantarum* PH04 strain was isolated from infant faeces and reported to be able to produce bile salt hydrolase enzyme *in vitro*. In another study, Jeun *et al.* [5] demonstrated that LDL-C was significantly ($P < 0.05$) lower (by 42%) in mice fed *L. plantarum* KCTC3928 and fecal bile acid excretion was accelerated (45%). They also found expressions of the LDL-receptor and 3-hydroxy-3-methylglutaryl coenzyme A reductase were marginally affected by feeding *L. plantarum* KCTC3928 but interestingly the gene expression and protein levels of CYP7A1 were significantly upregulated [5]. The gene CYP7A1 encodes for cholesterol 7-α-hydroxylase, the rate-limiting enzyme in the bile acid biosynthetic pathway in liver and thus controls cholesterol and bile acid homeostasis [65]. The increase in cholesterol 7-α-hydroxylase may explain the increase in fecal bile excretion and low serum cholesterol level observed by Jeun *et al* [5] since bile acid formation is a major pathway of cholesterol excretion from the body. Recently, Pan *et al.* [6] isolated *L. fermentum* SM-7 from a fermented milk drink (koumiss) and it was found to exhibit acid and bile tolerance and exhibited antimicrobial activity against *E. coli* and *S. aureus in vitro*. In mice, *L. fermentum* SM-7 significantly reduced serum TC and LDL-C but did not increase HDL-C significantly [6]. The study also showed that there was no bacterial translocation in the liver, spleen, or kidney of the treated mice indicating safety of the *Lactobacillus* strain[6].

In a series of experiments in rats, Fukushima and Nakano [7,8], and Fukushima *et al.* [9] showed that *L. acidophilus* or a mixture of probiotic microorganisms consistently reduced the serum TC. Usman and Hosono [10] also observed a significant reduction in TC and LDL-C in rats fed *L. gasseri*. In a more recent study, *B. longum* SPM1207 isolated from healthy adult Koreans reduced serum TC and LDL-C significantly ($p < 0.05$), and slightly increased serum HDL-C in rats [11]. In another study, Shin *et al.* [10] demonstrated that *B. longum* SPM1207, although killed by sonication, could significantly reduce serum TC and LDL-C, but with no significant improvement in HDL-C when fed to rats for 3 weeks [66]. Kumar *et al.* [67] revealed a 23% reduction in plasma TC, 38% reduction in LDL-C and 19% increase in HDL-C of rats fed with L. plantarum Lp91, a bile salt hydrolase producing strain. The faecal excretion of cholic acid was also found to be significantly higher in the probiotic-fed rats [6].

The latest study also consistently showed significant reduction by about 25% and 33% of serum TC and LDL-C respectively in rats fed L. fermentum 9-41-A. This strain was also isolated from faeces of healthy adults and selected for its probiotic characteristics [6].

In contrast to animal models, studies in humans conducted between 1974 to 1997 (reviewed by Taylor and Williams [14]) and from 1988 to 1998 (reviewed by de Roos and Katan [15]) indicate that the role of fermented milk products as hypocholesterolaemic agents was equivocal, as the clinical studies performed gave variable results and no firm conclusions could be drawn. The contradictory results observed were mainly related to the experimental designs especially the use of inadequate sample size and variations in the baseline levels of blood lipids [68]. Anderson and Gilliland [16] conducted a randomised, placebo-controlled, crossover 10-week study that involved 48 hypercholesterolaemic subjects. The subjects consumed milk fermented containing *L. acidophilus* L1 twice daily. The serum TC of subjects who consumed the fermented milk was significantly reduced when compared to those who consumed placebo. Xiao *et al.* [17] used a randomised, single-blind, parallel study for 4 weeks amongst 32 subjects. Subjects who consumed yoghurt containing *B. longum* BL1 had significantly reduced serum TC and LDL-C as compared to those given placebo yoghurt. Lewis and Burmeister [69] however reported that freeze- dried *L. acidophilus* supplementation had no effect on elevated cholesterol subjects using a randomised, placebo-controlled, crossover 6-week study. Simons *et al.* [70] in a double blind, placebo-controlled, parallel design trial also reported once again no beneficial effects on blood lipids after supplementation of *L. fermentum* for 10 weeks in volunteers with TC of about 4 mmol/L. Ataie-Jafari *et al.* [18] reported that *L. acidophilus* and *B. lactis* exhibited cholesterol-lowering effect on hypercholesterolemic subjects. They used a placebo controlled, randomised, crossover trial for 6 weeks, in healthy subjects with serum TC of 5.17–7.76 mmol/l. The most recent study was that conducted by Jones *et al.* [19] on 114 hypercholesterolaemic adults who consumed yoghurt formulated to contain microencapsulated BSH-active *L. reuteri* NCIMB 30242 twice daily for 6 weeks. This double-blind, placebo-controlled, randomised, parallel, multi-centre study showed significant reductions in serum LDL-C (9%), TC (5%) and non–HDL-C (6%) over placebo but the serum concentrations of HDL-C remained unchanged.

A meta-analysis based on six studies was conducted by Agerhol-Larsen *et al.* [72] on the hyocholesterolaemic effect of fermented dairy product on plasma cholesterol levels. The short term intervention study showed reductions in TC (-8.51 mg/dL) and LDL-C (-7.74 mg/dL) in subjects who consumed the fermented dairy product when compared to the control [72]. Later, Guo et al. [71] conducted another meta-analysis of randomised controlled trials that evaluated the effects of probiotics consumption on blood lipids. Their study was based on 13 trials of 485 participants with high, borderline high and normal cholesterol levels. The results showed that subjects who received probiotics had significantly lower TC (-6.40 mg/dL) and LDL-C (-4.90 mg/dL) as compared to those taken placebo. Both the meta analyses resulted in a similar observation. It seems that the hypocholesterolaemic effects of probiotics in human clinical trials in the recent years have been more consistent.

6. Proposed mechanisms of cholesterol reduction by lactic acid bacteria *in vitro*

Although studies have shown that some lactic acid bacterial strains have a hypocholesterolaemic effect on the host, the mechanism(s) involved is not fully understood. Different hypotheses have been advanced to explain the hypocholesterolaemic effect of lactic acid bacteria *in vitro*. There was little or no information on the direct action of cultured milk products in reducing cholesterol until Gilliland *et al.* [24] and Walker and Gilliland [25] reported that cholesterol removal *in vitro* could be due to the active up-take or assimilation of cholesterol by the bacterial cell. From then on, the cholesterol assimilation model was frequently used to explain the *in vivo* hypocholesterolaemic effects.

Based on their findings, Gilliland *et al.* [24] proposed that the uptake of cholesterol by *Lactobacillus acidophilus* strains occurred only when the cultures were grown in the presence of bile under anaerobic conditions. They also found that uptake of cholesterol increased with increasing concentrations of bile salts in the media, and the uptake appeared to level off at oxgall concentrations greater than 0.4%. Noh *et al.* [26] noted that cholesterol removed from the culture supernatant of *L. acidophilus* incubated in the presence of bile salt was accompanied by an increase in the amount of cholesterol in the cell pellet. Noh *et al.* [26] noticed that cells that were grown in the presence of cholesterol micelles and bile salts were more resistant to lysis by sonication, suggesting that assimilation of cholesterol into the cellular membrane, resulted in sturdier bacterial cells. This lends support to the idea that cell membrane alteration occurred in the presence of both bile salts and cholesterol. They also observed that assimilation occurred both at pH 6.0 and without pH control. Similar results have been reported for bifidobacteria [73] and lactococci [28]. Kimoto *et al.* [28] observed that both live and heat-killed *Lactococcus lactis* subsp. *lactis* biovar *diacetylactis* N7 were able to remove cholesterol from growth media. However, the amount of cholesterol removed by live cells was significantly higher than that removed by dead cells. They found that cell density and dry weight were higher when the cells were grown in the presence of cholesterol, and the rate of cholesterol removal was more rapid during their exponential growth phase. Since only living cells can possibly uptake cholesterol into their membranes, they concluded that the mechanisms of cholesterol removal by the live strain were due to cholesterol assimilation and binding, while removal of cholesterol by dead cells was only due to binding onto bacterial cell surface. They also observed a difference in the fatty acid distribution pattern for *Lactococcus* grown with or without cholesterol. Later Taranto *et al.* [74] reported modifications in the lipid profile of *L. reuteri* grown with cholesterol, while Liong and Shah [75] also observed alteration in the fatty acid profiles of lactobacilli grown in the presence of cholesterol in the growth medium. Pigeon *et al.* [29] suggested that cholesterol removal by *L. delbrueckii* and *Streptococcus thermophilus* strains were due to binding of free bile acids to their cell membranes through exocellular polysaccharide (EPS). They found that the strains, which produced the most EPS, bound the greatest amount of bile acids, while the strains that produced the least amount of EPS only bound minimal amounts of bile acids and conjugated bile acids did not bind to the EPS. They hypothesized that the strains reduced serum cholesterol levels by binding to enhance excretion of free bile acids via the faeces. Tol and Aslim [76] also demonstrated a correlation between cholesterol removal and EPS production of *L. delbrueckii* spp.

However, Klaver and Van der Meer [23] proposed another mechanism of cholesterol reduction by lactic acid bacteria. They pointed out that the experimental set up to prove the cholesterol assimilation as hypothesized by Gilliland *et al.* [24] and Walker and Gilliland [25] did not take into account the effects of bacterial deconjugation of bile salts. They suggested that the removal of cholesterol was due to the disruption of the cholesterol micelles caused by bile salt deconjugation and co-precipitation of cholesterol with free bile salts as the pH of the medium dropped because of acid production during growth of lactobacilli and bifidobacteria. This conclusion was based largely on their observation that no cholesterol was removed when the growth medium was maintained at pH 6.0, a pH at which free bile acids would remain in solution and prevent the precipitation of free bile salts. They associated these results to the decreased solubility of free bile acids under acidic conditions which in turn reduced the solubility of cholesterol (thus termed co-precipitation of cholesterol). Taranto *et al.* [77] and Ahn *et al.* [21] also stressed that removal of cholesterol was closely related to bile salt deconjugation at low pH. Brashears *et al.* [27] demonstrated that strains of *L. acidophilus* were able to deconjugate bile salts and remove cholesterol when grown at both pH 6.0 and without pH control. On the other hand, strains of *L. casei* grown at pH 6.0 removed very little cholesterol compared to the same strains grown at uncontrolled pH. However, examination of cellular membranes of *L. casei* grown under both conditions revealed no cholesterol deposits. Therefore, the authors concluded that removal of cholesterol by *L. casei* was most likely due to co-precipitation of cholesterol with deconjugated bile salts at pH less than 6.0, while removal of cholesterol by *L. acidophilus* was due to assimilation of cholesterol into cellular membranes. Cholesterol reduction may be strain specific.

In an attempt to determine the validity of the hypothesis of assimilation and/or precipitation of cholesterol by *Lactobacillus* and *Bifidobacterium* species, Grill *et al.* [78] cultured a strain of each species in a medium containing different bile salts. They found that the cholesterol removing ability of bifidobacteria varied according to the type of bile salts. In the presence of taurocholic acid, the removal of cholesterol was due to bacterial uptake and co-precipitation, but in the presence of oxgall, only co-precipitation was observed. It seems that the composition of bile salt is another important factor in determining the amount of cholesterol removed through co-precipitation. Many studies, hypothesised that lactic acid bacterial strains are able to remove cholesterol through a combination of two or more mechanisms which includes, assimilation of cholesterol during growth, binding of cholesterol to cellular membrane and deconjugation of bile salts [27,75,79-86].

More recently, another mechanism was hypothesized by Kim *et al.* [30] who found the cell-free supernatant of *L. acidophilus* ATCC 43121 to contain proteins that were able to significantly reduce cholesterol levels even after heat-treated or controlled at pH 6.0. The extract exhibited greatest cholesterol-reducing activity when maintained at pH 4.0.

Subsequent analysis identified the up-regulated proteins to be associated with stress response, translation, and metabolic processes and also have functions related to the cell membranes. Huang and Zheng [87] reported that soluble factors produced by *L. acidophilus* have the ability to inhibit cholesterol absorption in Caco-2 cells by down-regulating the gene expression of Niemann-Pick C1-like 1 (NPC1L1). NCPC1L1 protein has been identified as a key player in cholesterol absorpstion and a promising target for cholesterol–lowering mechanisms [88]. These studies suggest the possibility to alter gut microbiota through supplementation of probiotics for reduction of cholesterol absorption. Lee *et al.* [89] investigated cholesterol reducing activity of lactobacilli using genetic and proteomic analysis and reported that ccpA which encodes the catabolite control protein to play an important role in cholesterol reducing activity of probiotics. They also hypothesized that membrane associated proteins play an important role in probiotic cholesterol reduction.

7. Cholesterol reduction by lactic acid bacteria *in vivo*

It has been suggested that assimilation of cholesterol during growth of probiotic lactic acid bacteria and binding of cholesterol to their cellular membrane would result in less cholesterol available for absorption, leading to reduced serum cholesterol of the host [24]. Fukushima and Nakano [7] suggested that the hypocholesterolaemic effects could also be due to the ability of probiotic organisms to inhibit hydroxymethylglutaryl coenzyme A (HMG CoA) reductase. It is well documented that suppression of HMG CoA reductase is correlated with the inhibition of cholesterol synthesis. Short chain fatty acids (SCFA) have also been implicated to be involved in the reduction of cholesterol. Hara *et al.* [90] observed that a dietary SCFA mixture and SCFA produced by the fermentation of sugar beet fibre significantly reduced plasma cholesterol levels in rats. They suggested that absorbed SCFA might have suppressed the cholesterol synthesis rate in the liver and were involved in the cholesterol-lowering effect. Fukushima *et al.* [9] also suggested that the lowering of cholesterol level in rats fed probiotics was probably due to specific SCFA metabolites such as propionic acid and butyric acid. Propionate and butyrate are able to reduce hepatic cholesterol synthesis [91]. However, researchers acknowledge that deconjugation of bile salts by probiotic strains could be an important factor in lowering serum cholesterol through interference with the enterohepatic absorption of bile salts and cholesterol.

8. Enterohepatic circulation of bile acids

Bile acids are synthesised from cholesterol in the liver and stored in the gall bladder. The steroid is conjugated with an amide bond at the carboxyl C_{24} position to one of two amino acids, glycine and taurine [92], before it is excreted into the small intestine. The conjugated bile salts are amphipathic in nature and form micelles that facilitate digestion, emulsification and absorption of lipids from the small intestine [93]. The conjugated bile salts are readily absorbed in the gastrointestinal tract by active transport mechanisms and are returned to the liver; this process is known as enterohepatic circulation. A large pool of bile acids accumulates and undergoes a number of enterohepatic cycles daily [94].

The conversion of cholesterol to bile acids is the major route by which cholesterol is metabolized. To date, only two studies have shown the ability of probiotics strains [5,95] to be able to up-regulate CYP7A1 an enzyme that catalyzes the conversion of cholesterol to bile acids. An increase in CYP7A1 leads to reduction in hepatic cholesterol levels [5,95] and increase fecal cholesterol [95] and bile acids [5] excretion in hamsters and mice respectively. However, in the intestine, the bile salts may also be deconjugated by probiotics strains through bile salt hydrolase activity resulting in free bile salts. Free bile salts are more likely to be excreted via the faeces than the conjugated ones [96-98].

9. Significance of bile salt deconjugation by probiotic strains

The peptide-like bond between the bile acid and taurine or glycine is not cleaved by most proteolytic enzymes, but it is by bile salt hydrolase (BSH), an intracellular enzyme [99]. Deconjugation of bile salts *in vitro*, has been demonstrated by intestinal bacteria, such as *Clostridium* [100], *Lactobacillus* [101], *Streptococcus* [101], and *Bifidobacterium* [100]. The BSH enzyme catalyses the hydrolysis of conjugated bile acid to produce free bile salt and the corresponding amino acid. The biological function of BSH in these microorganisms remains unclear. However, in recent years, BSH has received attention because of its potential therapeutic benefits for reducing cholesterol. Upon hydrolysis, the physico-chemical properties of bile salts change drastically. Deconjugated bile acids are less soluble at low pH and less absorbed in the intestine and are more likely to be excreted in the faeces [102]. Excretion of free bile acids via the faeces is the primary route of elimination of cholesterol from humans and other animals [5]. To maintain bile salt homeostasis, more bile acids need to be synthesised and this in turn will reduce cholesterol in the body pool as cholesterol is the precursor for bile acids. The hypocholesterolaemic effect of lactic acid bacteria in this manner is comparable with that of cholestyramine treatment, which like other bile salt sequestrants, binds bile salts and prevents them from being reabsorbed [97]. Intestinal microflora plays a major role in interfering with the reabsorption of bile acid from the intestine, thus, promoting their excretion [97]. Increased faecal bile acid concentrations have also been observed in probiotic-fed mice [5,10], rats [7,67] and in human [19]. These studies strongly suggest that the deconjugating activity of BSH-active lactic acid bacteria may be associated with the hypocholesterolaemic effect.

The significance of BSH activity other than its hypocholesterolaemic effect, is far from understood. However, it has been suggested that certain BSH-active bacteria are able to utilise the amino portion of the deconjugated bile salt. Van Eldere *et al.* [103] reported that bacteria that are able to produce BSH may be able to use the amino acid, taurine, as an electron acceptor which can improve growth. De Smet *et al.* [97] suggested that deconjugation may be a detoxification mechanism which is of vital importance to the *Lactobacillus* cell. It has also been suggested that BSH is a detergent shock protein that protects the bacteria from the toxicity of bile acids in the gastrointestinal tract [104]. Moser and Savage [105] reported that BSH activity may be important for the bacteria to survive and colonise the gastrointestinal tract. Given the potential importance of the enzyme, genes encoding it may be important targets for genetic manipulation. Although lactobacilli are able to deconjugate bile salts to unconjugated primary bile acids, they do not further transform the unconjugated bile acids into deoxycholate (secondary bile acids) [21]. This is a good probiotic trait because formation of secondary bile acids, which are usually produced by intestinal bacteria, may contribute to colon cancer and gallstones. Ooi and Liong [106] reported that there has been no study that specifically evaluated the detrimental effects of BSH of probiotics in humans and that further studies are required.

10. Conclusion

The consumption of probiotics is gaining popularity especially in the maintenance of health and prevention of disease. In particular, the role of probiotics as a hypocholesterolaemic agent has been explored extensively. Progress has been made in the recent years on the selection, identification and characterization of strains that actually fulfill the criteria of true probiotic microorganisms and that are able to exert cholesterol reducing effects *in vitro.* However, much remains to be done on the mechanism of action as it has not been very well understood. The potential of probiotics in reducing cholesterol levels in animal models have been quite consistent in the recent years but but larger and better controlled human trials with scientifically substantiated evidence of the benefits are required.

Author details

Kalavathy Ramasamy, Zuhailah Mohd Shafawi, Vasudevan Mani
Faculty of Pharmacy, Universiti Teknologi MARA (UiTM), Puncak Alam, Selangor, Malaysia

Abu Bakar Abdul Majeed*
Faculty of Pharmacy, Universiti Teknologi MARA (UiTM), Puncak Alam, Selangor, Malaysia
Research Management Institute (RMI), Universiti Teknologi MARA (UiTM), 40450 Shah Alam, Selangor, Malaysia

Ho Yin Wan
Institute of Bioscience, Universiti Putra Malaysia (UPM), Serdang, Selangor, Malaysia

11. References

[1] Sanz Y., Santacruz A., and Gauffin P. Gut Microbiota in Obesity and Metabolic Disorders. Proceeding of the Nutrition Society 2010;69(3):434-441.

[2] Taranto MP, Medici M, Perdigon G, Ruiz Holgado AP, Valdez GF. Evidence for Hypocholesterolemic Effect of *Lactobacillus reuteri* in Hypocholesterolemic Mice. Journal of Dairy Science 1998; 81: 2336-2340.

---

* Corresponding Author

[3] Taranto MP, Medici M, Perdigon G, Ruiz Holgado AP, Valdez GF. Effect of *Lactobacillus reuteri* on the Prevention of Hypercholesterolemia in Mice. Journal of Dairy Science 2003;83: 401-403.

[4] Nguyen TDT, Kang JH, Lee MS. Characterization of *Lactobacillus plantarum* PH04, a Potential Probiotic Bacterium with Cholesterol-lowering effects. International Journal of Food Microbiology 2007;113: 358-361.

[5] Jeun J, Kim S, Cho SY, Jun HJ, Park HJ, Seo JG, Chung MJ, Lee SJ. Hypocholesterolemic Effects of *Lactobacillus plantarum* KCT3928 by Increased Bile Excretion in C57BL/6 Mice. Nutrition 2010; 26: 321-330.

[6] Pan DD, Zeng XQ, Yan YT. Characterisation of *Lactobacillus fermentum* SM-7 Isolated from Koumiss, a Potential Probiotic Bacterium with Cholesterol-lowering Effects. Journal of the Science of Food and Agriculture 2011;91(3): 512-8.

[7] Fukushima M, Nakano M. The Effect of a Probiotic on faecal and Liver and Lipid Classes in Rats. British Journal of Nutrition 1995; 73: 701-710.

[8] Fukushima M, Nakano M. Effects of a Mixture of Organisms, *Lactobacillus acidophilus* or *Streptococcus faecalis* on Cholesterol Metabolism in Rats Fed on a Fat-and Cholesterol Enriched Diet. British Journal of Nutrition 1996;76: 857-867.

[9] Fukushima M, Yamada A, Endo T, Nakano M. Effects of A Mixture of Organisms, *Lactobacillus acidophilus or Streptococcus faecalis* on D6-Desaturase Activity in the Livers of Rats Fed a Fat- and Cholesterol-Enriched Diet. Nutrients 1999;15: 373-378.

[10] Usman and Hosono A. Effect of Administration of *Lactobacillus gasseri* on Serum Lipids and Fecal Steroids in Hypercholesterolemic Rats. Journal of Dairy Science 2000;83: 1705-1711.

[11] Lee DK, Jang S, Baek EH, Kim MJ, Lee KS, Shin HS, Chung MJ, Kim JE, Lee KO, Ha NJ. Lactic Acid Bacteria Affect Serum Cholesterol Levels, Harmful Fecal Enzyme Activity, and Fecal Water Content. Lipids in Health and Disease 2009; 8-21.

[12] Madsen CS, Janovitz E, Zhang R, Nguyen-Tran V, Ryan CS, Yin X, Monshizadegan H, Chang M, D'Arienzo C, Scheer S, Setters R, Search D, Chen X, Zhuang S, Kunselman L, Peters A, Harrity T, Apedo A, Huang C, Cuff CA, Kowala MC, Blanar MA, Sun CQ, Robl JA, Stein PD. The Guinea Pig as a Preclinical Model for Demonstrating the Efficacy and Safety of Statins. Journal of Pharmacology Experimental Therapeutics 2008;324(2): 576-86.

[13] Patterson JK, Lei XG, Miller DD. The Pig as an Experimental Model for Elucidating the Mechanisms Governing Dietary Influence on Mineral Absorption. Experimental Biology and Medicine 2008;233: 651-664.

[14] Taylor GR, Williams CM. Effects of Probiotics and Prebiotics on Blood Lipids. British Journal of Nutrition 1998;80: 225–230.

[15] de Roos NM, Katan MB. Effects of Probiotic Bacteria on Diarrhea, Lipid Metabolism, and Carcinogenesis: A Review of Papers Published Between 1988 and 1998. American Journal of Clinical Nutrition 2000;71(2): 405-11.

[16] Anderson JW, Gilliland SE. Effect of Fermented Milk (Yogurt) Containing *Lactobacillus acidophilus* L1 on Serum Cholesterol Hypercholesterolemic Humans. Journal of the American College of Nutrition 1999;18: 43-50.

[17] Xiao JZ, Kondo S, Takahashi N, Miyaji K, Oshida K, Hiramatsu A, Iwatsuki K, Kokubo S, Hosono A. Effects of Milk Products Fermented by *Bifidobacterium longum* on Blood Lipids in Rats and Healthy Adult Male Volunteers. Journal of Dairy Science 2003; 86: 2452-2461.

[18] Ataie-Jafari A, Larijani B, Alavi Majd H, Tahbaz F. Cholesterol-lowering Effect of Probiotic Yogurt in Comparison with Ordinary Yogurt in Mildly to Moderately Hypercholesterolemic Subjects. Annals of Nutrition and Metabolism. 2009;54(1): 22-7.

[19] Jones ML, Martoni CJ, Parent M, Prakash S. Cholesterol-lowering Efficacy of a Microencapsulated Bile Salt Hydrolase-active *Lactobacillus reuteri* NCIMB 30242 Yoghurt Formulation in Hypercholesterolaemic Adults. British Journal of Nutrition 2012;107(10):1505-13.

[20] Corzo G, Gilliland SE. Bile Salt Hydrolase Activity of Three Strains of *Lactobacillus acidophilus*. Journal of Dairy Science 1999;82: 472-480.

[21] Ahn YT, Kim GB, Lim KS, Baek YT and Kim HU, Deconjugation of Bile Salts by *Lactobacillus acidophilus* Isolates. International Dairy Journal 2003;13: 303-311.

[22] Mishra V, Prasad DN. Application of *In Vitro* Methods for Selection of *Lactobacillus casei* Strains as Potential Probiotics. International Journal of Food Microbiology 2005;103: 109-115.

[23] Klaver FAM, van der Meer R. The Assumed Assimilation of Cholesterol by Lactobacilli and *Bifidobacterium bifidum* is Due to Their BileSalt-Deconjugating Activity. Applied and Environmental Microbiology 1993;59: 1120-1124.

[24] Gilliland SE, Nelson CR, Maxwell C. Assimilation of Cholesterol by *Lactobacillus acidophilus*. Applied and Environmental Microbiology 1985;49: 377-381.

[25] Walker DK, Gilliland SE. Relationships Among Bile Tolerance, Bile Salt Deconjugation, and Assimilation of Cholesterol by *Lactobacillus acidophilus*. Journal of Dairy Science 1993;76: 956-961.

[26] Noh DO, Kim S H, Gilliland S E. Incorporation of Cholesterol into the Cellular Membrane of *Lactobacillus acidophilus* ATCC 43121. Journal of Dairy Science 1997;80: 3107-3113.

[27] Brashears MM, Gilliland SE, Buck LM. Bile Salt Deconjugation and Cholesterol Removal from Media by *Lactobacillus casei*. Journal of Dairy Science 1998;81: 2103-2110.

[28] Kimoto H, Ohmomo S, Okamoto T. Cholesterol Removal from Media by Lactococci. Journal of Dairy Science 2002; 85(12): 3182-3188.

[29] Pigeon RM, Cuesta EP, Gilliland SE. Binding of Free Bile Acids by Cells of Yogurt Starter Culture Bacteria. Journal of Dairy Science 2002;85: 2705-2710.

[30] Kim Y, Whang JY, Whang KY, Oh S, Kim SH. Characterization of the Cholesterol-reducing Activity in a Cell-free Supernatant of *Lactobacillus acidophilus* ATCC 43121. Bioscience Biotechnology Biochemistry 2008;72: 1483-1490.

[31] Trautwein EA, Rieckhoff D, Erbersdobler HF. Dietary Inulin Lowers Plasma Cholesterol and Triacylglycerol and Alters Biliary Bile Acid Profile in Hamsters. Journal of Nutrition 1998;128: 1937-1943.

[32] Labarthe DR, Dunbar SB. Global Cardiovascular Health Promotion and Disease Prevention: 2011 and Beyond. Circulation 2012;125(21): 2667-2676.

[33] Roth GA, Fihn SD, Mokdad AH, Aekplakorn W, Hasegawa T, Lim SS. High Total Serum Cholesterol, Medication Coverage and Therapeutic Control: An Analysis of National Health Examination Survey Data from Eight Countries. Bulletin of the World Health Organization 2011;89(2): 92-101.

[34] Martin SS, Metkus TS, Horne A, Blaha MJ, Hasan R, Campbell CY, Yousuf O, Joshi P, Kaul S, Miller M, Michos ED, Jones SR, Gluckman TJ, Cannon CP, Sperling LS, Blumenthal RS. Waiting for the National Cholesterol Education Program Adult Treatment Panel IV Guidelines, and in the Meantime, Some Challenges and Recommendation. American Journal of Cardiology. 2012 (In Press).

[35] Baigent C, Blackwell L, Emberson J, Holland LE, Reith C, Bhala N, Peto R, Barnes EH, Keech A, Simes J, Collins R. Efficacy and Safety of More Intensive Lowering of LDL Cholesterol: A Meta-Analysis of Data from 170,000 Participants in 26 Randomised Trials. Cholesterol Treatment Trialists' (CTT) Collaboration. Lancet 2010; 13: 376(9753):1670-81.

[36] Ray KK, Seshasai SR, Erqou S, Sever P, Jukema JW, Ford I, Sattar N. Statins and All-cause Mortality in High-Risk Primary Prevention: A Meta-analysis of 11 Randomized Controlled Trials Involving 65,229 Participants. Archives of International Medicine 2010;170)12): 1024-1031.

[37] Taylor F, Ward K, Moore TH, Burke M, Davey Smith G, Casas JP, Ebrahim S. Statins for the Primary Prevention of Cardiovascular Disease. Cochrane Database of Systematic Review 2011 Jan 19;(1): CD004816.

[38] Blaha MJ, Nasir K, Blumenthal RS. Statin Therapy of Healthy Men identified as "Increased Risk". Journal of the American Medical Association 2012;307(14): 1489-90.

[39] Redberg RF, Katz MH. Healthy Men Should Not Take Statins. Journal of the American Medical Association 2011;307(14): 1491-1492.

[40] Muldoon MF, Barger SD, Ryan CM, Flory JD, Lehoczky JP, Matthews KA, Manuck SB. Effects of Lovaststin on Cognitive Function and Psychological Well-being. American Journal of Medicine 2000;108(7): 538-546.

[41] Muldoon MF, Ryan CM, Sereika SM, Flory JD, Manuck SB. Randomized Trial of the Effects of Simvastatin on Cognitive Functioning in Hypercholesterolemic Adults. American Journal of Medicine 2004;117(11):823-9.

[42] Fernandez G, Spatz ES, Jablecki C, Phillips PS. Statin Myopathy: A Common Dilemma Not Reflected in Clinical Trials. Cleveland Clinical Journal of Medicine 2011;78(6): 393-403.

[43] Clifton P, Colquhoun D, Hewat C. Dietary Intervention to Lower Serum Cholesterol. Australian Family Physician 2009;38(6): 424-429.

[44] Jones PJ. Clinical Nutrition: Functional Foods – More Than Just Nutrition. Canadian Medical Association Journal 2002;166: 1555-1563.

[45] Lilly, DM, Stillwell, RH. Probiotics: Growth Promoting Factors Produced by Microorganisms. Science 1965;147: 747–748.

[46] Parker, RB. Probiotics: the Other Half of the Antibiotic Story. Animal Nutrition Health 1974;29: 4–8.

[47] Fuller, R. Probiotics in Man and Animals. Journal of Applied Bacteriology 1989;66: 365–378.

[48] Havenaar R, Ten Brink B, Huis in't Veld JHJ, In: Fuller, R. (Ed.), Probiotics, The scientific basis. Chapmann & Hall, London 1992 p. 209-224.

[49] Salminen S, Ouwehand A, Benno Y, Lee YK. Probiotics: How Should They be Defined? Trends in Food Science and Technology 1999;10: 107–110.

[50] FAO/WHO. (2002). Guidelines for the Evaluation of Probiotics in Food. Report of a Joint FAO/WHO Working Group on Drafting Guidelines for the Evaluation of Probiotics in Food. London, Ontario, Canada. ftp://ftp.fao.org/es/esn/food/wgreport2.pdf (June 3, 2012).

[51] Shanahan FA. Gut Reaction: Lymphoepithelial Communication in the Intestine. Science 1997;275, 1897–1898.

[52] Umesaki Y, Okada Y, Imaoka A, Setoyama H, Matsumoto S. Interactions Between Epithelial Cells and Bacteria, Normal and Pathogenic. 1997 Science; 276: 964–965.

[53] Wang J, Whetsell M, Klein JR. Local Hormone Networks and Intestinal T cell Homeostasis. Science 1997;275: 1937–1939.

[54] Holscher HD, Czerkies LA, Cekola P, Litov R, Benbow M, Santema S, Alexander DD, Perez V, Sun S, Saavedra JM, Tappenden KA. *Bifidobacterium lactis* Bb12 Enhances Intestinal Antibody Response in Formula-Fed Infants: A Randomized, Double-Blind, Controlled Trial. Journal of Parenteral and Enteral Nutrition, 2012;36 (1 Suppl): 106S

[55] Rolfe RD. The Role of Probiotic Cultures in the Control of Gastrointestinal Health. Journal of Nutrition 2000;130(2S Suppl): 396S-402S.

[56] De Vos. System Solutions by Lactic Acid Bacteria: From Paradigms to Practice. Microbial Cell Factories 2011; 10(Suppl 1): S2.

[57] Kolida S, Gibson GR. Synbiotics in Health and Disease. Annual Review of Food Science and Technology 2011;2: 373-393.

[58] Holzapfel, WH, Haberer P, Geisen R, Björkroth J, Schillinger U. Taxonomy and Important Features of Probiotic Microorganisms in Food and Nutrition. American Journal of Clinical Nutrition, 2001;73(Suppl.), 365S-373S.

[59] Rauch M, Lynch SV. The Potential for Probiotic Manipulation of the Gastrointestinal Microbiome. Current Opinion in Biotechnology 2012; 23: 192-201.

[60] FAO/WHO. Health and Nutritional Properties of Probiotics in Food Including Powder Milk with Live Lactic Acid Bacteria. Report of a joint FAO/WHO Expert Consultation On Evaluation of Health and Nutritional Properties of Probiotics in Food Including Powder Milk with Live Lactic Acid Bacteria. 2001.

[61] Sekhon SB , Jairath S. Prebiotics, Probiotics and Synbiotics: An Overview. Journal of Pharmceutical Education Research 2010;1(2).

[62] Khani S, Hosseini HM, Mohammad T, Nourani MR, Fooladi AAI. Probiotics as an Alternative Strategy for Prevention and Treatment of Human Disease: A Review. Inflammation and Allergy- Drug Target 2012;11, 79-89.

[63] Rauch M, Lynch SV. The Potential for Probiotic Manipulation of the Gastrointestinal Microbiome. Current Opinon in Biotechnology 2012;23(2):192-201.

[64] Mann GV, and Spoerry A. Studies of a Surfactant and Cholesteremia in the Maasai. American Journal of Clinical Nutrition 1974;27, 464-469.

[65] Li T, Matozel M, Boehme S, Kong B, Nilsson LM, Guo G, Ellis E, Chiang JY. Overexpression of Cholesterol 7α-hydroxylase Promotes Hepatic Bile Acid Synthesis and Secretion and Maintains Cholesterol Homeostasis. Hepatology 2011; 53(3): 996-1006.

[66] Shin HS, Shin YP, Lee, DK, Kim SA, An HM, Kim JR, Kim MJ, Cha MG, Lee SW, Kim KJ, Lee KO, Ha NJ. Hypocholesterolemic Effect of Sonication-killed *Bifidobacterium longum* Isolated from Healthy Adult Koreans in High Cholesterol Fed Rats. 2010 Archives of Pharmacal Research 2020; 33(9): 1425-1431.

[67] Kumar M, Nagpal R, Kumar R, Hemalatha R, Verma V, Kumar A, Chakraborty C, Singh B, Marotta F, Jain S, Yadav H. Cholesterol-lowering Probiotics as Potential Biotherapeutics for Metabolic Diseases. Experimental Diabetes Research 2012; 902-917.

[68] Pereira, DIA, Gibson GR. Effects of Consumption of Probiotics and Prebiotics on Serum Lipid Levels in Human. Critical Reviews in Biochemistry and Molecular Biology 2002;37 259-281.

[69] Lewis, SJ, Burmeister SA. Double-Blind Placebo-Controlled Study of the Effects of *Lactobacillus acidophilus* on Plasma Lipids. European Journal of Clinical Nutrition 2005; 59: 776-780.

[70] Simons LA, Amansec SG, Conway. Effect of *Lactobacillus fermentum* on Serum Lipids in Subjects with Elevated Serum Cholesterol. Nutrition Metabolism and Cardiovascular Diseases 2006;16: 531-535.

[71] Guo Z, Liu XM, Zhang QX, Shen Z, Tian FW, Zhang H, Sun ZH, Zhang HP, Chen W. Influence of Consumption of Probiotics on the Plasma Lipid Profile: A Meta-analysis of Randomised Controlled Trials. Nutrition, Metabolism and Cardiovascular Diseases 2011;21(11): 844-50.

[72] Agergolm-Larsen L, Bell ML, Grunwald GK, Astrup A. The Effect of a Probiotic Milk Product on Plasma Cholesterol: A Meta-analysis of Short Term Intervention Studies. European Journal of Clinical Nutrition 2000;54: 856-60.

[73] Rasic JL, Vujicic IF, Skrinjar M, Vulic M. Assimilation of Cholesterol by Some Cultures of Lactic Acid Bacteria and Bifidobacteria. Biotechnology Letters 1992;14: 39-44.

[74] Taranto MP, Fernandez M, Lorca M, de Valdez GF. Bile Salts and Cholesterol Induce Changes in the Lipid Cell Membrane of *Lactobacillus reuteri*. Journal of Applied Microbiology 2003;95: 86-91.

[75] Liong MT, Shah NP. Acid and Bile Tolerance and Cholesterol Removal Ability of Lactobacilli Strains. Journal of Dairy Science 2005; 88(1): 55-66.

[76] Tok E, Aslim B. Cholestrerol Removal by Some Lactic Acid Bacteria that can be Used as Probiotic. Microbiology Immunology 2010;54(5): 257-264.

[77] Taranto MP, Sesma F, de Ruiz Holgado AP, de Valdez GF. Bile Salt Hydrolase Plays a Key Role on Cholesterol Removal by *Lactobacillus reuteri*. Biotechnology Letters 1997;19(9): 845-847.

[78] Grill JP, Cayuela C, Antoine, JM, Schneider F. Effects of *Lactobacillus amylovorus* and *Bifidobacterium breve* on cholesterol. Letters in Applied Microbiology 2000; 31: 154-156.

[79] Marshall VM, Taylor. Ability of Neonatal Human *Lactobacillus* Isolates to Remove Cholesterol from Liquid Media. International Journal of Food Science and Technology 1995; 30: 571-577.
[80] Tahri K, Crociani J, Ballongue J, Schneider F. Effects of Three Strains of Bifidobacteria on Cholesterol. Letters in Applied Microbiology 1995; 21: 149-151
[81] Tahri K, Grill JP, Schneider F. Bifidobacteria Strain Behaviour Toward Cholesterol: Coprecipitation with Bile Salts and Assimilation. Current Microbiology 1996; 33: 187-193.
[82] Tahri K, Grill JP, Schneider F. Involvement of Trihydroxyconjugated Bile Salts in Cholesterol Assimilation by Bifidobacteria. Current Microbiology 1997; 34 79-84.
[83] Dambekodi PC, Gilliland SE. Incorporation of Cholesterol into the Cellular Membrane of *Bifidobaceterium longum*. Journal of Dairy Science 1998;81: 1818-1824.
[84] Lin MY, Chen TW. Reduction of Cholesterol by *Lactobacillus acidophilus* in Culture Broth. Journal of Food and Drug Analysis 2000;8(2): 97-102.
[85] Lye HS, Rahmat-Ali GR, Liong MT. Mechanisms of Cholesterol Removal by Lactobacilli Under Conditions that Mimic the Human Gastrointestinal Tract. International Dairy Journal 2010;20 169-175.
[86] Zeng XQ, Pan DD, Guo YX. The Probiotic Properties of *Lactobacillus buchneri* P2. Journal of Applied Microbiology 2010;108(6): 2059-2066.
[87] Huang Y, Zheng Y. The Probiotic *Lactobacillus acidophilus* Reduces Cholesterol Absorption Through the Down-regulation of Niemann-Pick C1-like 1 in Caco-2 cells. British Journal of Nutrition 2009; 1-6.
[88] Miura S, Saku K. Ezetimibe, a Selective Inhibitor of the Transport of Cholesterol. Internal Medicine. 2008;47(13):1165-70.
[89] Lee J, Kim Y, Yun HS, Kim JG, Oh S, Kim SH. Genetic and Proteomic Analysis of Factors Affecting Serum Cholestrol Reduction by *Lactobacillus acidophilus* A4. Applied and Environmental Microbiology 2010;76(14) 4829-4835.
[90] Hara H, Haga S, Aoyama Y, Kiriyama S. Short-chain Fatty Acids Suppress Cholesterol Synthesis in Rat Liver and Intestine. Journal of Nutrition 1999;129(5):942-8.
[91] Trautwein, EA, Rieckhoff D, Erbersdobler HF. Dietary Inulin Lowers Plasma Cholesterol and Triacylglycerol and Alters Biliary Bile Acid Profile in Hamsters. Journal of Nutrition 1998:28, 1937-1943.
[92] Savage DC, Lundeen SG, O'Connor LT. Mechanisms by which Indigenous Micoorganisms Colonise Epithelial Surfaces as a Reservoir of the Lumenal Microflora in the Gastrointestinal Tract. Microecology and Therapy 1995;21: 27-36.
[93] Elkin CA, Salvage DC. Identification of Genes Encoding Conjugated Bile Salt Hydrolase and Transport in *Lactobacillus johnsonii* 100-100. Journal of Bacteriology 1998;180(17): 4344-4349.
[94] Hofmann AF, Mysels KJ. Bile Acid Solubility and Precipitation *In vitro* and *In vivo*: The Role of Conjugation, pH, and Ca2+ Ions. Journal of Lipid Research 1992;33: 617-626.
[95] Wang CY, Wu SJ, Jong YF, Wang YP, Shyu YT. Cardiovascular and Intestinal Protection of Cereal Pastes Fermented with Lactic Acid Bacteria in Hyperlipidemic Hamsters. Food Research International 2012; In Press.

[96] Gilliland, SE and Speck ML. Antagonistic Action of *Lactobacillus acidophilus* Toward Intestinal and Foodborne Pathogens in Associative Cultures. Journal of Food Protein1977; 40: 12.

[97] De Smet, Van Hoorde, L. Vande Woestyne, M. Christiaens, H. Verstraete, W. Significance of Bile Salt Hydrolytic Activities of Lactobacilli. Journal of Applied Microbiology 1995; 79: 292-301.

[98] Corzo G, Gilliland SE. Bile Salt Hydrolase Activity of Three Strains of *Lactobacillus acidophilus*. Journal of Dairy Science 1999; 82: 472-480.

[99] Lundeen S, Savage D. Characterization and Purification of Bile Salt Hydrolase from *Lactobacillus Sp.* Strain 100-100. Journal of Bacteriology 1990;172(8): 4171-4177.

[100] Aries V, Hill MJ. Degradation of Steroids by Intestinal Bacteria. Biochimica and Biophysica Acta. 1970;202: 526-534.

[101] Gilliland SE, Speck ML. Deconjugation of Bile Acids by Intestinal Lactobacilli. Applied and Environmental Microbiology 1977;33(1): 15-18.

[102] Chickai T, Nakao H, Uchida K. Deconjugation of Bile Acids by Human Intestinal Bacteria Implanted in Germfree Rats. 1987;22: 669-974.

[103] Van Eldere J, Robben J, De Pauw G, Merckx R, Eyssen H. Isolation and Identification of Intestinal Steroid-desulfating Bacteria from Rats and Humans. Applied and Environmental Microbiology 1988; 54(8): 2112-7.

[104] Flahaut S, Frere J, Boutibonnes P, Auffray Y. Comparison of Bile Salts and Sodium Deodecyl Sulphate Stress Responses in *Entercoccus Faecalis*. Applied and Environmental Microbiology 1996;62(7): 1416-20.

[105] Moser AA, Savage D. Bile Salt Hydrolase Activity and Resistance to Toxicity and Conjugated Bile Salts are Unrelated Properties in Lactobacilli. Applied and Environmental Microbiology 2001;67(8): 3476-3480.

[106] Ooi LG, Liong MT. Cholesterol-lowering Effects of Probiotics and Prebiotics: A Review of *In vivo* and *In vitro* Findings. International Journal of Molecular Sciences 2010;11(6): 2499-2522.

Chapter 10

Traditional and Modern Medicine Harmonizing the Two Approaches in the Treatment of Neurodegeneration (Alzheimer's Disease – AD)

Bowirrat Abdalla, Mustafa Yassin, Menachem Abir,
Bishara Bisharat and Zaher Armaly

Additional information is available at the end of the chapter

http://dx.doi.org/10.5772/48558

1. Introduction

Neurodegenerative disorders, Primarily, are multifactorial diseases characterized by chronic and progressive loss of neurons in discrete areas of the brain, causing debilitating symptoms and globally decreasing cognitive function such as dementia, loss of memory, loss of sensory or motor capability, decreased overall quality of life and well-being, disability, and eventually, premature death. For most neurodegenerative diseases, there is little or no treatment; at best, treatments are symptomatic in nature and do not prevent or slow the progression of disease. Clearly, an understanding of pathological progression can help to identify points of intervention and lead to promising therapeutic approaches. A fundamental approach for reducing the burden of neurodegenerative diseases is thus to slow or halt progression, and ultimately, to prevent the onset of the disease process. Strategies for neurorescue, neurorepair, neuroprotection or treatment are being actively pursued by the basic, translational, and clinical research communities. As our population ages, the already enormous impact of neurodegeneration on society will become even larger without better prevention and treatment.

"Dementia" is an umbrella term describing a variety of diseases and conditions that develop when nerve cells in the brain die or no longer function normally. The death or malfunction of these nerve cells, called neurons, causes changes in one's memory, behavior and Ability to think clearly. In Alzheimer's disease (AD), these brain changes eventually impair an individual's Ability to carry out such basic bodily functions as walking and swallowing. As aged population dramatically increases in these decades, efforts should be made on the intervention for curing age-associated neurodegenerative diseases such as AD.

AD is considered to be the most widespread variety of dementia (57%-65%) or a condition typified by continuous decline of mental aptitudes (1,2).

AD affects about 5.4 million people in the United States alone, and that number is projected to reach 12-16 million by the year 2050 (3). Economically, AD is a major public health problem. In the United States in 2011, the cost of health care, long-term care, and hospice services for people aged 65 years and older with AD and other dementias was expected to be $183 billion, and this figure does not include the contributions of unpaid caregivers (3).

Currently, an autopsy or brain biopsy is the only way to make a definitive diagnosis of AD. In clinical practice, the diagnosis is usually made on the basis of the history and findings on Mental Status Examination.

Symptomatic therapies are the only treatments available for AD. The standard medical treatments include cholinesterase inhibitors and a partial *N*-methyl-D-aspartate (NMDA) antagonist. Psychotropic medications are often used to treat secondary symptoms of AD, such as depression, agitation, and sleep disorders.

2. Historical background

In 1901, a German psychiatrist named Alois Alzheimer observed a patient at the Frankfurt Asylum named Mrs. Auguste D. This 51-year-old woman suffered from a loss of short-term memory, among other behavioral symptoms that puzzled Dr. Alzheimer. Five years later, in April 1906, the patient died, and Dr. Alzheimer sent her brain and her medical records to Munich, where he was working in the lab of Dr. Emil Kraeplin. By staining sections of her brain in the laboratory, he was able to identify amyloid plaques and neurofibrillary tangles (4).

A speech given by Dr. Alzheimer on November 3, 1906, was the first time the pathology and the clinical symptoms of the disorder, which at the time was termed presenile dementia, were presented together. Alzheimer published his findings in 1907 (5).

In the past 15-20 years, dramatic progress has been made in understanding the neurogenetics and pathophysiology of AD. Four different genes have been definitively associated with AD, and others that have a probable role have been identified. The mechanisms by which altered amyloid and tau protein metabolism, inflammation, oxidative stress, and hormonal changes may produce neuronal degeneration in AD are being elucidated, and rational pharmacologic interventions based on these discoveries are being developed.

Rapid progress towards understanding the molecular underpinnings of neurodegenerative disorders such as AD is revolutionizing drug discovery for these conditions. Furthermore, the development of models for these disorders is accelerating efforts to translate insights related to neurodegenerative mechanisms into disease-modifying therapies.

AD or Alzheimer's-type dementia is a progressive degeneration of brain tissue that primarily strikes people over age 65. It is the most common cause of dementia and is marked by a devastating mental decline. Intellectual functions such as memory, comprehension, and speech deteriorate. Attention tends to stray, simple calculations become impossible, and ordinary daily activities grow increasingly difficult, accompanied by bewilderment and frustration.

AD characterized clinically by progressive memory deficits, impaired cognitive function, and altered and inappropriate behavior. AD places a considerable and increasing burden on patients, caregivers, and society. Aging represents the most important risk factor and dementia has become one of the major challenges in our societies due to the universal phenomenon of population aging in the world. Brain regions involved in learning and memory processes, including the temporal and frontal lobes as well as the hippocampus, are reduced in size in AD patients as the result of degeneration of synapses and death of neurons. AD is considered as a protein aggregation disorder, based on two key neuropathological hallmarks, namely the hyperphosphorylation of the tau protein resulting in the formation of neurofibrillary tangles (NFTs), and the increased formation and aggregation of amyloid-beta peptide (Aβ) derived from amyloid precursor protein (APP) (6).

Although the exact underlying cause initiating the onset of AD is still unclear, an imbalance in oxidative and nitrosative stress, intimately linked to mitochondrial dysfunction, characterizes already early stages of AD pathology.

3. Etiology of Alzheimer's Disease (AD)

The cause of AD is not entirely known, but is thought to include both genetic and environmental factors (Multifactorial). A diagnosis of AD is made when certain symptoms are present, and by making sure other causes of dementia are not present (DSM-IV criteria).

The only way to know for certain that someone has AD is to examine a sample of their brain tissue after death. The following changes are more common in the brain tissue of people with AD:

1. "Neurofibrillary tangles" (twisted fragments of protein within nerve cells that clog up the cell)
2. "Neuritic plaques" (Abnormal clusters of dead and dying nerve cells, other brain cells, and protein)
3. "Senile plaques" (areas where products of dying nerve cells have accumulated around protein).

When nerve cells (neurons) are destroyed, there is a decrease in the neurotransmitters. As a result, areas of the brain that normally work together become disconnected.

Healthy neurons have an internal support structure partly made up of structures called microtubules. These microtubules act like tracks, guiding nutrients and molecules from the body of the cell down to the ends of the axon and back. A special kind of protein, tau, binds to the microtubules and stabilizes them.

In AD, tau is changed chemically. It begins to pair with other threads of tau, which become tangled together. When this happens, the microtubules disintegrate, collapsing the neuron's transport system (see the image below). The formation of these neurofibrillary tangles (NFTs) may result first in malfunctions in communication between neurons and later in the death of the cells.

In addition to NFTs, the anatomic pathology of AD includes senile plaques (SPs; also known as beta-amyloid plaques) at the microscopic level and cerebrocortical atrophy at the macroscopic level (see the image below). The hippocampus and medial temporal lobe are the initial sites of tangle deposition and atrophy (7). This can be seen on brain magnetic resonance imaging early in AD and helps support a clinical diagnosis.

SPs and NFTs were described by Alois Alzheimer in his original report on the disorder in 1907 (5). They are now universally accepted as the pathological hallmark of the disease.

A continuum exists between the pathophysiology of normal aging and that of AD (8). Pathologic hallmarks of AD have been identified; however, these features also occur in the brains of cognitively intact persons. For example, in a study in which neuropathologists were blinded to clinical data, they identified 76% of brains of cognitively intact elderly patients as demonstrating AD (9).

AD affects the 3 processes that keep neurons healthy: communication, metabolism, and repair. Certain nerve cells in the brain stop working, lose connections with other nerve cells, and finally die. The destruction and death of these nerve cells causes the memory failure, personality changes, problems in carrying out daily activities, and other features of the disease.

The accumulation of SPs primarily precedes the clinical onset of AD. NFTs, loss of neurons, and loss of synapses accompany the progression of cognitive decline (8).

Considerable attention has been devoted to elucidating the composition of SPs and NFTs to find clues about the molecular pathogenesis and biochemistry of AD. The main constituent of NFTs is the microtubule-associated protein tau (see Anatomy). In AD, hyperphosphorylated tau accumulates in the perikarya of large and medium pyramidal neurons. Somewhat surprisingly, mutations of the tau gene result not in AD but in some familial cases of frontotemporal dementia.

Since the time of Alois Alzheimer, SPs have been known to include a starchlike (or amyloid) substance, usually in the center of these lesions. The amyloid substance is surrounded by a halo or layer of degenerating (dystrophic) neurites and reactive glia (both astrocytes and microglia).

One of the most important advances in recent decades has been the chemical characterization of this amyloid protein, the sequencing of its amino acid chain, and the cloning of the gene encoding its precursor protein (on chromosome 21). These advances have provided a wealth of information about the mechanisms underlying amyloid deposition in the brain, including information about the familial forms of AD.

Although the amyloid cascade hypothesis has gathered the most research financing, other interesting hypotheses have been proposed. Among these are the mitochondrial cascade hypotheses (10).

In addition to NFTs and SPs, many other lesions of AD have been recognized since Alzheimer's original papers were published. These include the granulovacuolar degeneration of Shimkowicz; the neuropil threads of Braak et al (11); and neuronal loss and synaptic degeneration, which are thought to ultimately mediate the cognitive and behavioral manifestations of the disorder.

3.1. Neurofibriliary tangles and senile plaques

Plaques are dense, mostly insoluble deposits of protein and cellular material outside and around the neurons. Plaques are made of beta-amyloid (Aβ), a protein fragment snipped from a larger protein called amyloid precursor protein (APP). These fragments clump together and are mixed with other molecules, neurons, and non-nerve cells.

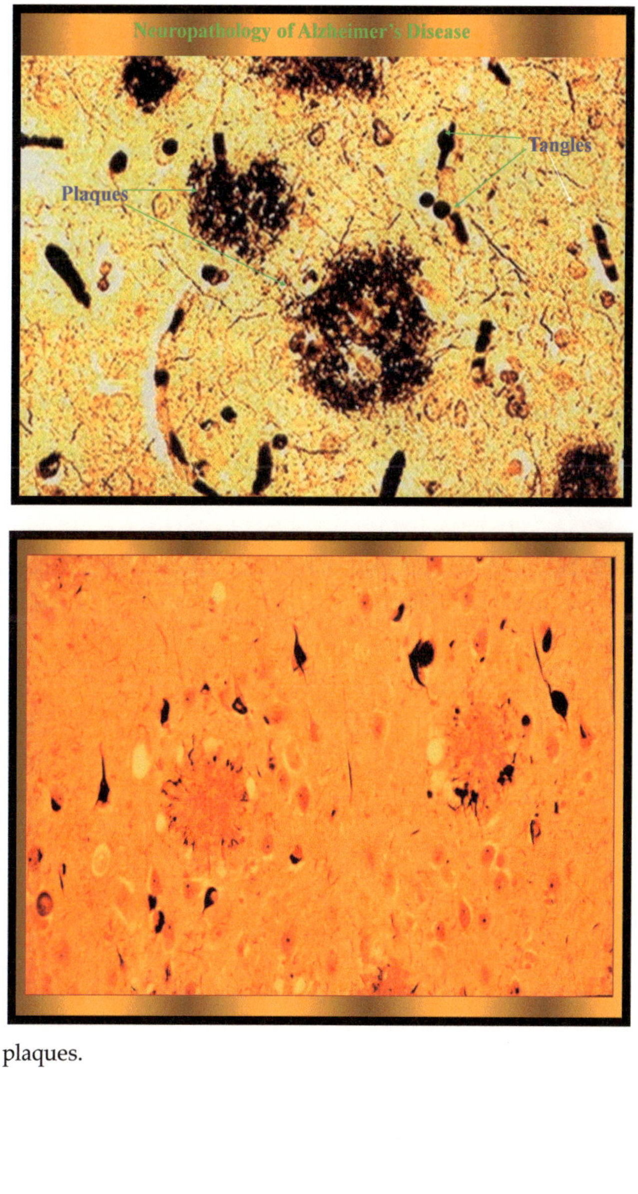

Figure 1. Amyloid plaques.

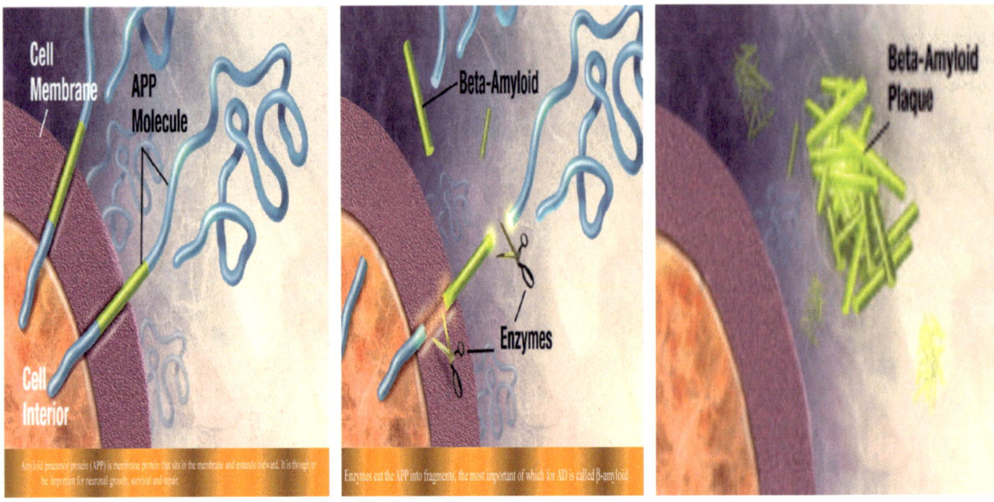

1 2 3

1. APP sticks through the neuron membrane.

2. Enzymes cut the APP into fragments of protein, including beta-amyloid.

3. Beta-amyloid fragments come together in clumps to form plaques.

Figure 2. Amyloid precursor protein (APP) is the precursor to amyloid plaque.

In AD, plaques develop in the hippocampus, a structure deep in the brain that helps to encode memories, and in other areas of the cerebral cortex that are used in thinking and making decisions. Plaques may begin to develop as early as the fifth decade of life (12). Whether Aβ plaques themselves cause AD or whether they are a by-product of the AD process is still unknown. It is known that changes in APP structure can cause a rare, inherited form of AD.

Tangles are insoluble twisted fibers that build up inside the nerve cell. Although many older people develop some plaques and tangles, the brains of people with AD have them to a greater extent, especially in certain regions of the brain that are important in memory. There are likely to be significant age-related differences in the extent to which the presence of plaques and tangles are indicative of the presence of dementia.

NFTs are initially and most densely distributed in the medial aspect and in the pole of the temporal lobe; they affect the entorhinal cortex and the hippocampus most severely (however, Braak et al found that in sporadic AD, tauopathy may appear first in the lower brainstem rather than in the transentorhinal region (12). As AD progresses, NFTs accumulate in many other cortical regions, beginning in high-order association regions and less frequently in the primary motor and sensory regions.

SPs also accumulate primarily in association cortices and in the hippocampus. Plaques and tangles have relatively discrete and stereotypical patterns of laminar distribution in the cerebral cortex, which indicate predominant involvement of corticocortical connections.

Although NFTs and SPs are characteristic of AD, they are not pathognomonic. NFTs are found in several other neurodegenerative disorders, including progressive supranuclear palsy and dementia pugilistica (chronic traumatic encephalopathy). SPs may occur in normal aging.

Therefore, the mere presence of these lesions is not sufficient to support the diagnosis of AD. These lesions must be present in sufficient numbers and in a characteristic topographic distribution to fulfill the current histopathologic criteria for AD. There is consensus that the presence of even low numbers of NFTs in the cerebral neocortex with concomitant SPs is characteristic of AD.

Some authorities believed that NFTs, when present in low densities and essentially confined to the hippocampus, were part of normal aging. However, the histologic stages for AD that Braak et al formulated include an early stage in which NFTs are present at a low density in the entorhinal and perirhinal (ie, transentorhinal) cortices (12). Therefore, even small numbers of NFTs in these areas of the medial temporal lobe may be abnormal.

4. Amyloid hypothesis versus tau hypothesis

A central but controversial issue in the pathogenesis of AD is the relationship between amyloid deposition and NFT formation. Evidence shows that abnormal amyloid metabolism plays a key pathogenic role. At high concentrations, the fibrillar form of Aβ has been shown to be neurotoxic to cultured neurons.

Cultured cortical and hippocampal neurons treated with Aβ protein exhibit changes characteristic of apoptosis (self-regulated cell destruction), including nuclear chromatin condensation, plasma membrane blebbing, and internucleosomal DNA fragmentation. The fibrillar form of Aβ has also been shown to alter the phosphorylation state of tau protein.

The identification of several point mutations within the APP gene in some patients with early-onset familial AD and the development of transgenic mice exhibiting cognitive changes and SPs also incriminate Aβ in AD. The apolipoprotein E (APOE) E4 allele, which has been linked with significantly increased risk for developing AD, may promote inability to suppress production of amyloid, increased production of amyloid, or impaired clearance of amyloid with collection outside of the neuron.

Autopsies have shown that patients with 1 or 2 copies of the APOE E4 allele tend to have more amyloid. Additional evidence comes from recent experimental data supporting the role of presenilins in Aβ metabolism, as well as findings of abnormal production of Aβ protein in presenilin-mutation familial AD.

Although very popular, the amyloid hypothesis is not uniformly accepted. On post-mortem analysis, amyloid plaques may be undetectable in the brains of patients who had severe AD but may be present in the brains of elderly patients who did not have dementia (13).

Dementia severity correlates better with the number of neocortical NFTs than with SPs. The tau protein stabilizes neuronal microtubules. Destabilization of the microtubular system is speculated to disrupt the Golgi apparatus, in turn inducing abnormal protein processing and increasing production of Aβ. In addition, this destabilization may decrease axoplasmic flow, generating dystrophic neurites and contributing to synaptic loss.

4.1. Granulovacuolar degeneration and neuropil threats

Granulovacuolar degeneration occurs almost exclusively in the hippocampus. Neuropil threads are an array of dystrophic neurites diffusely distributed in the cortical neuropil, more or less independently of plaques and tangles. This lesion suggests neuropil alterations beyond those merely due to NFTs and SPs and indicates an even more widespread insult to the cortical circuitry than that visualized by studying only plaques and tangles.

4.2. Cholinergic neurotransmission and Alzheimer disease

The cholinergic system is involved in memory function, and cholinergic deficiency has been implicated in the cognitive decline and behavioral changes of AD. Activity of the synthetic enzyme choline acetyltransferase (CAT) and the catabolic enzyme acetylcholinesterase are significantly reduced in the cerebral cortex, hippocampus, and amygdala in patients with AD.

The nucleus basalis of Meynert and diagonal band of Broca provide the main cholinergic input to the hippocampus, amygdala, and neocortex, which are lost in patients with AD. Loss of cortical CAT and decline in acetylcholine synthesis in biopsy specimens have been found to correlate with cognitive impairment and reaction-time performance. Because cholinergic dysfunction may contribute to the symptoms of patients with AD, enhancing cholinergic neurotransmission constitutes a rational basis for symptomatic treatment.

4.3. Oxidative stress and damage

Oxidative damage occurs in AD. Studies have demonstrated that an increase in oxidative damage selectively occurs within the brain regions involved in regulating cognitive performance (14).

Oxidative damage potentially serves as an early event that then initiates the development of cognitive disturbances and pathological features observed in AD. A decline in protein synthesis capabilities occurs in the same brain regions that exhibit increased levels of oxidative damage in patients with mild cognitive impairment (MCI) and AD. Protein synthesis may be one of the earliest cellular processes disrupted by oxidative damage in AD (15).

Oxidative stress is believed to be a critical factor in normal aging and in neurodegenerative diseases such as Parkinson disease, amyotrophic lateral sclerosis, and AD.

The apoptotic pattern of cellular death seen in oxidative stress is similar to that produced by Aβ peptide exposure, and Aβ neurotoxicity is attenuated by antioxidants such as vitamin E. Aβ may induce toxicity by engaging several binding sites on the membrane surface.

Several investigators now believe that converging environmental and genetic risk factors trigger a pathophysiologic cascade that, over decades, leads to Alzheimer pathology and dementia.

The following risk factors for Alzheimer-type dementia have been identified: Advancing age;Family history; APOE 4 genotype; Obesity; Insulin resistance; Vascular factors; Dyslipidemia; Hypertension; Inflammatory markers; Down syndrome and Traumatic brain injury (16-19).

In addition, epidemiologic studies have suggested some possible risk factors (eg, aluminum (20,21), previous depression) and some protective factors (eg, education (22, 23), long-term use of nonsteroidal anti-inflammatory drugs (24).

5. Genetics causes

Although most cases of AD are sporadic (ie, not inherited), familial forms of AD do exist. Autosomal dominant AD, which accounts for less than 5% of cases, is almost exclusively early onset AD; cases occur in at least 3 individuals in 2 or more generations, with 2 of the individuals being first-degree relatives (25).

Familial clustering represents approximately 15–25% of late-onset AD cases and most often involves late-onset AD. In familial clustering, at least 2 of the affected individuals are third-degree relatives or closer (25).

Mutations in the following genes unequivocally cause early-onset autosomal dominant AD:

The amyloid precursor protein (*APP*) gene on chromosome 21
The presenilin-1 (*PS1*) gene on chromosome 14
The presenilin-2 (*PS2*) gene on chromosome 1

Genetic alterations in AD and effects on APP metabolism.

Chromosome	Gene product	Age of onset	Effect
21	APP mutations	Early	Overproduction of Aβ
Trisomy C21	APP overproduction	Early	Overproduction of Aβ
14	Presenilin 1 mutations	Early	Increased production of Aβ (1-42)
1	Presenilin 2 mutations	early	Increased production of Aβ (1-42)
19	Apolipoprotein epsilon 4 allele (polymorphism)	late	Increased deposit of Aβ plaques and vascular deposits; earlier onset of AD

All 3 of these genes lead to a relative excess in the production of the stickier 42-amino acid form of the Aβ peptide over the less sticky 40-amino-acid form.

This beta-pleated peptide is postulated to have neurotoxic properties and to lead to a cascade of events (as yet incompletely understood) that results in neuronal death, synapse loss, and the formation of NFTs and SPs, among other lesions. Nonetheless, the mutations that have been found to date account for less than half of all cases of early-onset AD.

Other than the apolipoprotein E epsilon 4 (APOE E4) genotype, no polymorphisms in other genes have been consistently found to be associated with late-onset AD. However, genome-wide association studies have identified the following additional susceptibility loci (26).

6. APP mutations

The observation that patients with Down syndrome (trisomy 21) develop cognitive deterioration and typical pathological features of AD by middle age led to the discovery of the *APP* gene on chromosome 21. Simultaneously, a locus segregating with a minority of early-onset familial AD kindreds was mapped to this chromosome, in the same region as the *APP* gene.

Subsequently, several missense mutations within the *APP* gene that resulted in amino acid substitutions in APP were identified in these familial AD kindreds. Such mutations appear to alter the previously described proteolytic processing of APP, generating amyloidogenic forms of Aβ.

Skin fibroblasts from individuals carrying *APP* mutations produce increased Aβ 42/43. Increased plasma concentration of Aβ 42/43 is also seen in these patients, regardless of age, sex, or clinical status. Interestingly, some patients with sporadic AD may exhibit similar elevations of plasma Aβ 42/43.

7. PS1 and PS2 mutations

Approximately 50-70% of early-onset autosomal-dominant AD cases appear to be associated with a locus (AD3) mapped by genetic linkage to the long arm of chromosome 14 (14q24.3). Numerous missense mutations have been identified on a strong candidate gene, called *PS1*.

At the same time, another autosomal dominant locus responsible for early-onset AD was localized to chromosome 1. Two mutations were identified on the candidate gene, designated *PS2*. The physiological role of presenilins and the pathogenic effects of their mutations are not yet well understood.

7.1. APOE

The gene encoding the cholesterol-carrying apolipoprotein E (*APOE*) on chromosome 19 has been linked to increased risk for AD, principally late-onset but also some early-onset cases. The gene is inherited as an autosomal codominant trait with 3 alleles. The APOE E2 allele, the least prevalent of the 3 common APOE alleles, is associated with the lowest risk of developing AD (27), with a lower rate of annual hippocampal atrophy and higher cerebrospinal fluid Aβ and lower phosphotau, suggesting less AD pathology (28).

The E3 allele confers intermediate risk of developing AD, with less risk than the E4 allele. The E3 allele, which is more common than the E2 allele, may protect tau from hyperphosphorylation, and the E2 allele's effect on tau phosphorylation is complex.

APOE E4 gene "dose" is correlated with increased risk and earlier onset of AD (29). Persons with 2 copies of the APOE E4 allele (4/4 genotype) have a significantly greater risk of developing AD than persons with other APOE subtypes. Mean age at onset is significantly lower in the presence of 2 APOE E4 copies. A collaborative study has suggested that APOE E4 exerts its maximal effect before the age of 70 years.

Many APOE E4 carriers do not develop AD, and many patients with AD do not have this allele. Therefore, the presence of an APOE E4 allele does not secure the diagnosis of AD, but instead, the APOE E4 allele acts as a biological risk factor for the disease, especially in those younger than 70 years.

8. Treatment of Alzheimer's disease – From medical chemistry to plants

The worldwide population and especially the wesearn and U.S. population is getting older, and as it ages, AD is becoming an increasingly bigger concern. Within the next 50 years, the incidence of Alzheimer's is expected to quadruple, affecting one in 45 Americans.

Today, there is still no cure for Alzheimer's. People with the disease progressively lose memory and the ability to function as Alzheimer's advances.

Several different types of medications are used to treat the memory loss, behavior changes, sleep problems, and other symptoms of AD. These medications won't stop the disease, but they can slow down the symptoms for a few months or even years. All of these medications can have side effects, which can be even more pronounced in the elderly.

Early diagnosis and treatment allows AD patients to maintain the highest levels of cognitive and functional ability possible.

Today main pharmacological treatment of AD is Cholinesterase inhibitors (ChEIs), and mental exercises are used in an attempt to prevent or delay the deterioration of cognition in patients with AD. Here, we will try to shed lights on the important available pharmacological treatments and complementary therapies such as Herbal medicine utilized on the treatment of AD:

9.1. Pharmacological treatment

A. Cholinesterase inhibition

Numerous lines of evidence suggest that cholinergic systems that modulate information processing in the hippocampus and neocortex are impaired early in the course of AD. These observations have suggested that some of the clinical manifestations of AD are due to loss of cholinergic innervation to the cerebral cortex.

Centrally acting ChEIs prevent the breakdown of acetylcholine. Four such agents have been approved by the FDA for the treatment of AD, as follows:

Tacrine
Donepezil (Aricept, Aricept ODT)
Rivastigmine (Exelon, Exelon Patch)
Galantamine (Razadyne, Razadyne ER)

Of note, tacrine has potential hepatotoxicity and hence requires frequent blood monitoring. Since the other ChEIs have become available, tacrine has rarely been prescribed.

All ChEIs have shown modest benefit on measures of cognitive function and activities of daily living. Patients on ChEIs have shown slower declines on cognitive and functional measures than patients on placebo. However, ChEIs do not address the underlying cause of the degeneration of cholinergic neurons, which continues during the disease. The ChEIs may also alleviate the noncognitive manifestations of AD, such as agitation, wandering, and socially inappropriate behavior (30).

Although the usefulness of ChEIs was originally expected to be limited to the early and intermediate stages of AD (because the cholinergic deficit becomes more severe later in disease and because fewer intact cholinergic synapses are present), they are also helpful in advanced disease (31). ChEIs are also helpful in patients with AD with concomitant infarcts and in patients with dementia with Lewy bodies. Frequently, AD and dementia with Lewy bodies occur in the same patient; this is sometimes called the Lewy body variant of AD.

The ChEIs share a common profile of adverse effects, the most frequent of which are nausea, vomiting, diarrhea, and dizziness. These are typically dose related and can be mitigated with slow up-titration to the desired maintenance dose. In addition, gastrointestinal side effects may be reduced by using the transdermal patch rather than the oral form of the drug. As antimuscarinic drugs are used for the treatment of incontinence, logically, ChEIs might exacerbate incontinence. One brief report has supported this hypothesis (32).

ChEIs prescribed to treat dementia can provoke symptomatic bradycardia and syncope and precipitate fall-related injuries, including hip fracture. In a study of older adults with dementia who were taking cholinesterase inhibitors, hospital visits for syncope were found to be more frequent in patients receiving ChEIs than in control patients (31.5 vs 18.6 events per 1000 person-years (33). Other syncope-related events, including hospital visits for bradycardia, permanent pacemaker insertion, and hip fracture, were also found to be more common in patients receiving cholinesterase inhibitors. ChEI use in older adults with dementia is associated with increased risk of syncope-related events; these risks must be weighed against the benefits of taking ChEIs (33).

Anecdotal reports exist of acute cognitive and behavioral decline associated with the abrupt termination of ChEIs. In several of these cases, restarting the ChEI did not lead to substantial improvement. These reports have implications concerning the best practice when switching a patient from one ChEI to another in this class. Reasons for switching might include undesirable side effects or an apparent lack of efficacy. Nonetheless, no published data are available to help clinicians know when it would be helpful to switch to another ChEI.

The common practice of tapering a patient off one CNS-active medication before starting a new one should not be followed when changing ChEIs. For example, a patient who was taking 10 mg of donepezil should be started the next day on galantamine at a dose of at least 8 mg/day and possibly 16 mg/day. No current evidence supports the use of more than 1 ChEI at a time. Centrally acting anticholinergic medications should be avoided.

It is not uncommon for patients to receive both ChEIs and anticholinergic agents, which counteract each other. Medications with anticholinergic effects, such as diphenhydramine, tricyclic antidepressants (eg, amitriptyline, nortriptyline), and oxybutynin (commonly used for bladder spasticity), can cause cognitive dysfunction. Therefore, a careful listing of the patient's medications is important so that the physician can reduce the doses of, or ideally eliminate, all centrally acting anticholinergic agents.

Cholinesterase inhibitors (ChEIs) are used to palliate cholinergic deficiency. All 4 currently approved ChEIs (ie, tacrine, donepezil, rivastigmine, galantamine) inhibit acetylcholinesterase (AChE) at the synapse (specific cholinesterase). Tacrine was the first agent that was approved for AD, but because of its potential to cause hepatotoxicity, it is now rarely used.

Tacrine and rivastigmine also inhibit butyrylcholinesterase (BuChE). Although BuChE levels may be increased in AD, it is not clear that rivastigmine and tacrine have greater clinical efficacy than donepezil and galantamine.

Galantamine has a different second mechanism of action; it is also a presynaptic nicotinic modulator. No data exist to indicate that this second mechanism is of clinical importance.

Donepezil (Aricept, Aricept ODT)

Donepezil is indicated for the treatment of dementia of the Alzheimer type. Donepezil has shown efficacy in patients with mild to moderate AD, as well as moderate to severe AD. It selectively inhibits acetylcholinesterase, the enzyme responsible for the destruction of acetylcholine, and improves the availability of acetylcholine. Donepezil's long half-life provides a long duration of drug availability for binding at the receptor sites. There is no evidence to suggest that the underlying disease process of dementia is affected by administration of donepezil.

Dosing recommendations for mild to moderate AD are 5-10 mg given once daily. Patients with moderate to severe AD can be given 10 or 23 mg once daily.

Rivastigmine (Exelon, Exelon Patch)

Rivastigmine is indicated for the treatment of mild to moderate dementia of the Alzheimer type. Initial dosing recommendations are 1.5 mg given twice daily, with a maximum dose of

12 mg/day. Rivastigmine is a potent, selective inhibitor of brain AChE and BChE. Rivastigmine is considered a pseudo-irreversible inhibitor of AChE.

While the precise mechanism of rivastigmine's action is unknown, it is postulated to exert its therapeutic effect by enhancing cholinergic function. This is accomplished by increasing the concentration of acetylcholine through reversible inhibition of its hydrolysis by cholinesterase.

Galantamine (Razadyne, Razadyne ER)

Galantamine is indicated for the treatment of mild to moderate dementia of the Alzheimer type. It enhances central cholinergic function and likely inhibits AChE. There is no evidence that galantamine alters the course of the underlying dementing process. The dosing recommendation for the immediate-release formulation is 4 mg twice daily. The extended-release formulation is given at a dose of 8 mg once daily. The maintenance dose after dose titration is 16-24 mg/day.

Tacrine

Tacrine was the first agent approved for AD. It is indicated in patients with mild to moderate dementia. It is associated with hepatotoxicity and is no longer commonly used. Tacrine inhibits AChE, the enzyme responsible for the destruction of acetylcholine, and improves the availability of acetylcholine. Tacrine inhibits both AChE and BChE; however, it is more selective for AChE.

N-Methyl-D-Aspartate Antagonists

The only drug in the *N* -methyl-D-aspartate (NMDA) antagonist class that is approved by the US Food and Drug Administration is memantine. This agent may be used alone or in combination with AChE inhibitors.

Memantine (Namenda, Namenda XR)

Namenda is approved for the treatment of moderate to severe dementia in patients with AD. The initial dose for the immediate-release formulation is 5 mg once daily, and it can be titrated to a maximum dose of 20 mg/day. The initial dose for the extended-release formulation is 7 mg once daily, and it can be titrated to a maximum dose of 28 mg/day. Side effects include dizziness, confusion, headache, constipation, nausea, and agitation.

B. Treatment of moderate to severe disease

The partial *N* -methyl-D-aspartate (NMDA) antagonist memantine (Namenda, Namenda XR) is believed to work by improving the signal-to-noise ratio of glutamatergic transmission at the NMDA receptor. Blockade of NMDA receptors by memantine is thought to slow the intracellular calcium accumulation and thereby help prevent further nerve damage. This agent is approved by the FDA for treating moderate and severe AD.

Several studies have demonstrated that memantine can be safely used in combination with ChEIs. The combination of memantine with a ChEI has been shown to significantly delay institutionalization in AD patients (34). Studies suggest that the use of memantine with donepezil affects cognition in moderate to severe AD (35) but not in mild to moderate AD (36, 37). Dizziness, headache, and confusion are some of the most common side effects of memantine.

A variety of behavioral and pharmacologic interventions can alleviate clinical manifestations of AD, such as anxiety, agitation, depression, and psychotic behavior. The effectiveness of such interventions ranges from modest and temporary to excellent and prolonged. No specific agent or dose of individual agents is unanimously accepted for the wide array of clinical manifestations. At present, the FDA has not approved any psychotropic agent for the treatment of AD.

C. Antidepressants and mood modulators

- Antidepressants, such as citalopram (Celexa), fluoxetine (Prozac), paroxetine (Paxil), and sertraline (Zoloft) treat irritability and mood.
- Anxiolytics, such as lorazepam (Ativan) and oxazepam (Serax) treat anxiety and restlessness.
- Antipsychotic medications, such as aripiprazole (abilify), clozapine (Clozaril), haloperidol (Haldol), and olanzapine (Zyprexa) treat hallucinations, delusions, agitation, and aggression.

Antidepressants have an important role in the treatment of mood disorders in patients with AD. Depression is observed in more than 30% of patients with AD, and it frequently begins before AD is clinically diagnosed. Therefore, palliation of this frequent comorbid condition may improve cognitive and noncognitive performance.

Nyth found citalopram to be beneficial in mood and other neuropsychiatric symptoms in patients in the moderate stage of AD (38). Because citalopram can cause dose-dependent increases in the QT interval, the FDA recommends using a maximum of 40 mg a day and considering 20 mg a day in the elderly (39).

Weintraub et al (40) and Petracca et al (41) found sertraline and fluoxetine to have no short- or long-term benefit in mood over placebo. Similarly, Banerjee et al found that treatment of depression with sertraline or mirtazapine provided no benefit compared with placebo and increased the risk of adverse events (42).

Other mood modulators, such as valproic acid, can be helpful for the treatment of disruptive behaviors and outbursts of anger, which patients with moderately advanced or advanced stages of AD may have.

Results of several studies indicate that anticonvulsants (eg, gabapentin, valproic acid) may have a role in the treatment of behavioral problems in patients with Alzheimer disease. However, a trial of 313 patients with moderate AD found that 24 months of treatment with valproate did not delay emergence of agitation or psychosis, did not slow cognitive or functional decline, and was associated A variety of experimental therapies have been proposed for AD. These include antiamyloid therapy, reversal of excess tau phosphorylation, estrogen therapy, vitamin E therapy, and free-radical scavenger therapy. Studies of these therapies have yielded mostly disappointing results.

In the past 10 years, numerous antiamyloid therapy studies have been conducted to decrease toxic amyloid fragments in the brain, including studies of the following:

- Vaccination with amyloid species
- Administration of monoclonal antiamyloid antibodies
- Administration of intravenous immune globulin that may contain amyloid-binding antibodies
- Selective amyloid-lowering agents
- Chelating agents to prevent amyloid polymerization
- Brain shunting to improve removal of amyloid
- Beta-secretase inhibitors to prevent generation of the A-beta amyloid fragment

To date, no phase III study of antiamyloid therapies has shown a combination of acceptable efficacy and side effects.

Growing awareness that tau is a central player in AD pathogenesis has suggested that this protein may offer an avenue for therapeutic intervention. Studies are ongoing with agents that may prevent or reverse excess tau phosphorylation and thereby diminish formation of neurofibrillary tangles (43).

Free-radical scavenger therapy has also attracted attention, because excess levels of free radicals in the brain are neurotoxic. Nonetheless, no study has demonstrated efficacy of free-radical scavengers in the treatment of the cognitive symptoms of AD.

Various studies indicate that oxidative stress may be a part of the pathogenesis of AD. In the AD, high-dose vitamin E (2000 units per day of alpha-tocopherol) for 2 years slowed the progression of disease in patients with moderate AD (44). This benefit presumably resulted from the antioxidant effects of vitamin E.

Subsequent studies, however, have suggested that vitamin E supplementation may increase risk of adverse cardiovascular outcomes. Therefore, use of vitamin E is not currently recommended.

Transcranial magnetic stimulation (TMS) has been used to identify therapeutic targets in AD and to monitor the effects of pharmacologic agents, and both TMS and transcranial direct current stimulation are being explored for a possible therapeutic role in AD. However, evidence of therapeutic benefit from these modalities is highly preliminary (45).

10. Herbal medicine is the bridge between complementary therapies & conventional treatment

In all cultures, the origins of herbal medicine are lost in the mists of time. There is little doubt that humans used herbs for healing well before anything could be written about them. At some point in an advancing culture, written documents become the repository for knowledge that had been passed on from one generation to the next. Among the earliest such documents are those describing the religious beliefs of the people and those describing the medical practices. Medical foods are dietary supplements intended to compensate specific nutritional problems caused by a disease or condition.

Effective pharmacological drugs for treating AD are still to be discovered. Current western pharmacological approaches against neurodegeneration in dementia develop symptom-relieving and disease-modifying drugs. Current integrative and holistic approaches of Chinese medicine to discovering drugs for neurodegeneration in dementia include (1) single molecules from the herbs, (2) standardized extracts from a single herb, and (3) herbal formula with definite composition. At present, acetylcholinesterase inhibitors (AChEI) are the first group of drugs approved by the FDA to treat mild to moderate Alzheimer's disease. Most of these drugs such as huperzine and galanthamine are originally isolated from plants. However, AChE inhibitors have limited success as they only improve memory in mild dementia but cannot stop the process of neurodegeneration; while memantine possesses neuroprotective effects only with a little ability in memory enhancement. There has been a major rush among neuroscience research institutions and pharmaceutical firms worldwide to search for safer and more effective therapeutic agents for AD.

However, mounting evidence obtained *in vitro* and *in vivo*, suggests that various traditionally used plants significantly affect key metabolic alterations culminating in AD-typical neurodegeneration.

Beside synthetic drugs, a variety of AD related medicine originates from traditionally used plants. In this respect, *Ginkgo biloba* and galantamine represent the most famous cases.

Indeed, the majority of recent reports on plants with traditional uses and activities relevant for AD originate from the traditional Chinese and Oriental Medicine, as well as from Kampo Ayurveda and Mediterranean traditional knowledge.

11. *Ginkgo Biloba* – From traditional Chinese medicine to a standardized drug

Originally, *Ginkgo biloba* (Coniferae) has been traditionally used for respiratory disorders in China and to improve memory loss associated with blood circulation abnormalities in Iran. This herb has been subjected to numerous investigations regarding its potential in cognitive disorders. Standardized extracts, particularly EGb 761, derived from the plants' leaves are successfully used as herbal drug for the improvement of cognitive and memory impairment. EGb 761 represents a prototype of plant extracts for attenuating Central Nervous System disorders, due to the fact that both flavonoids and terpenic lactones, which are partly also present in numerous other plant extracts, have been identified as the active principles in *Ginkgo* extracts as well as the ample experimental evidence on EGb 761's protective efficiency *in vitro* and *in vivo*. The potential of EGb 761 to attenuate the cytotoxic effects of Alzheimer's related neurotoxic amyloid peptides when added to the culture medium was demonstrated not only in neuronal-like cell lines but also primary neurons, though with different efficiency. The impact of *Ginkgo* extract has been largely attributed to its antioxidant activity. The effects of oxidative stress were reduced in lymphocytes and brain cells derived of EGb 761-treated AD-transgenic and non-transgenic mice. Recent data, however, indicate that *Ginkgo biloba* extract-761 (Gbe-761) also affects the production of neurotoxic beta-amyloid peptides (Aβ), for example, by up-regulating α-secretase activity both in cells and animals.

We speculate that metabolic alterations, mediated by vasodilatory and tropic effects of EGb 761, might be responsible for this finding.

Ginkgo biloba extract (Gbe) and two ingredients, bilobalide and ginkgolide B, are presented to the CSWG as part of a review of botanicals being used as dietary supplements in the United States. (1 of 3 adults in the United States is now taking dietary supplements). Sweeping deregulation of botanicals now permits GBE to be sold as a dietary supplement to a willing public eager to "improve brain functioning" or "promote radical scavenging activity.".

Gbe is a well defined product, and it or its active ingredients, the ginkgolides, especially ginkgolide B, and bilobalide, has clearly demonstrated biological activity. It can be consumed in rather large doses for an extended period of time. Under the Dietary Supplement Health and Education Act of 1994, Gbe can be sold legally if it is not labeled or accompanied by any therapeutic or health claims. Herbal remedies can be labeled with descriptions of their role in affecting physiological structure or function, but must be labeled with a disclaimer that the product has not been evaluated by the FDA for cure, prevention, or treatment of a disease.

12. Standardized ingredients of Gbe

The extract utilized in medicine is standardized in a multi-step procedure designed to concentrate the desired active principles from the plant. These extracts contain approximately 24% flavone glycosides (primarily composed of quercetin, kaempferol, and isorhamnetin) and 6% terpene lactones (2.8-3.4% ginkgolides A, B, and C, and 2.6-3.2% bilobalide). Ginkgolide B accounts for Aβout 0.8% of the total extract and bilobalide accounts for Aβout 3% of the extract. Other constituents include proanthocyanadins, glucose, rhamnose, organic acids, D-glucaric acid and ginkgolic acid (at most 5 ppm ginkgolic acids). Much of the curative properties of Gbe are due to the activities of these flavonoids.

Human Exposure: There is potential for ingestion of Gbe to a widespread consumer population, since this product is readily available without prescription at a cost highly competitive with prescription medications. The recommended dose of Gbe is 120 to 160 mg daily for persons with intermittent claudication and 240 mg daily for cerebrovascular insufficiency, early stage Alzheimer's disease, resistant depression, and impotence.

13. Galantamine

Galantamine is an alkaloid known form several members of the *Amaryllis* family (Amaryllidaceae), and the idea for developing a medical product for AD from these species seems to be based on the local use of one of these species in a remote part of Europe. It has become an important therapeutic options used to slow down the process of neurological degeneration in AD. Its development from little known observational studies in the Caucasus Mountains (Southern Russia), to the use of this drug in Eastern European countries (esp. Bulgaria) in the treatment of poliomyelitis and ultimately to the recent introduction onto Western markets in the treatment of AD. Galantamine was first isolated from snowdrop (*Galanthus* spp.) but today it is obtained from *Narcissus* spp. and *Leucojum* spp. as well as synthetically. According to unconfirmed reports, in the 1950s, a Bulgarian pharmacologist noticed the use of the common snowdrop growing in the wild by people who were rubbing it on their foreheads to ease nerve pain. Also, some of the earlier publications indicate the extensive use of snowdrop in Eastern Europe, such as Romania, Ukraine, the Balkan Peninsula, and in the Eastern Mediterranean countries. However, Mashkovsky and Kruglikova-Lvov published the first work that establishes the acetylcholine esterase inhibiting properties of galantamine isolated from *Galanthus woronowii*. Poliomyelitis was one of the first indications for galantamine, especially in the Eastern and Central European, since the compound enhances nerve impulse transmission at the synapse. Studies indicating blood–brain barrier penetration of the alkaloid pioneer the development of CNS-related indications. Based on the knowledge of galantamine in both the peripheral and central nervous system, many countries in Eastern Europe used it as an acknowledged treatment in *Myasthenia gravis* and muscular dystrophy, residual poliomyelitis paralysis symptoms, trigeminal neurologica, and other forms of neuritis. A crucial step for the success of galantamine as a medicine against AD was based on the synthesis developed in the mid-1990s. The scientific rationale for using cholinesterase inhibitors in the management of AD is based on the cholinergic hypothesis. Impairment of the central cholinergic system represents one hallmark of AD, which is characterized by loss of cholinergic neurons in the forebrain and a marked decrease in the activity of choline acetyltransferase. Overall, galantamine represents an example for the successful ethnobotany-driven development of a natural product into a clinically important drug.

In the last years, focus on AD drug discovery is shifting away from AChE inhibitors and a large number of other targets are currently being explored.

Ginseng products are popularly referred to as "adaptogen," which connotes that these products purportedly increase to physical, chemical, and biological stress and builds up general vitality, including physical and mental capacity for work. *Panax ginseng* roots are traditionally taken orally as adaptogens, aphrodisiacs, nourishing stimulants, and in the treatment of sexual dysfunction in men. The fresh root, can be directly chewed, or soaked in various wines for a period of time before drinking or chewing. Ginseng is most often availble either in whole or sliced dried form. However, usually ginseng is used at subclinical doses for a short period and as such; it does not produce measurable medicinal effects. *Panax notoginseng* is widely used in traditional Chinese medicine (TCM) to improve learning and memory. Moreover, protective actions against cerebral ischemia, beneficial effects on the cardiovascular system, and haemostatic, antioxidant, hypolipidemic, hepatoprotective, renoprotective, and estrogen-like activities.

14. *Galanthus woronowii* (snowdrop-Galantamine)

The delicate white flower and the Bulb of *Galanthus woronowii*

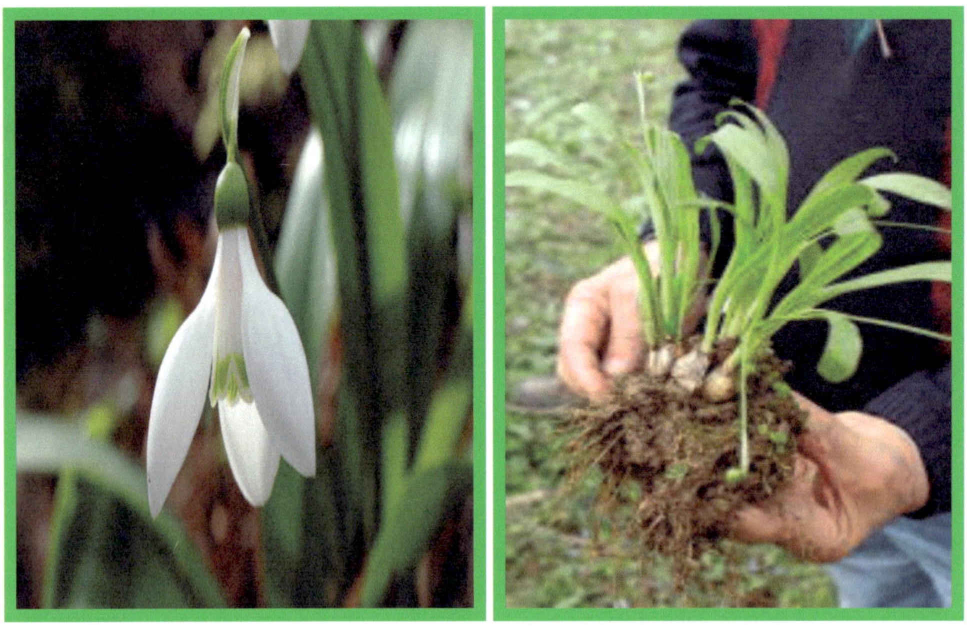

Figure 3. About this species

A snowdrop native to Turkey, Russia and Georgia, *Galanthus woronowii* was named in honour of the Russian botanist and plant collector Georg Woronow (1874–1931). It is popular in cultivation in Europe, and valued for its wide, green, shiny leaves, whicht provide good ground-cover and contrast with the leaves of the commonly grown snowdrop *G. nivalis*. *Galanthus woronowii* occurs from northeastern Turkey to the western and central Caucasus (Georgia and Russia). It is primarily found around the eastern Black Sea coast in the ancient provinces of Colchis and Lazistan (the Euxine Province). It occurs at 70–1,400 metres above sea level, in stony and rocky spots (on calcareous rocks, in gorges, on stony slopes and on scree), on river banks, in scrub and at forest margins, and sometimes as an epiphyte or on fallen tree trunks, rooting in moss (46-48).

15. Cannabinoid therapy

The scientific literature indicates that cannabinoid therapy may provide symptomatic relief to patients afflicted with AD while also moderating the progression of the disease.

The intracerebroventricular administration of the synthetic cannabinoid prevented cognitive impairment and decreased neurotoxicity in rats injected with amyloid-beta peptide (49).

Additional synthetic cannabinoids were also found to reduce the inflammation associated with AD in human brain tissue in culture. In the results of Ramirez et al. 2005 indicate that cannabinoids succeed in preventing the neurodegenerative process occurring in the AD,"(50). Follow up studies by investigators demonstrated that the administration of the nonpsychotropic plant cannabinoid cannabidiol (CBD) also mitigated memory loss in a mouse model of the disease (51). Investigators at the Scripps Research Institute in California in 2006 reported that THC (Tetrahydrocannabinol (THC) is the active chemical in cannabis and is one of the oldest hallucinogenic drugs known) inhibits the enzyme responsible for the aggregation of amyloid plaque — the primary marker for AD — in a manner "considerably superior" to approved Alzheimer's drugs such as donepezil and tacrine. The investigators's results provide a mechanism whereby the THC molecule can directly impact AD pathology," researchers concluded. "THC and its analogues may provide an improved therapeutic option for AD by simultaneously treating both the symptoms and the progression of the disease (52).

More recently, investigators at Ohio State University, reported that older rats administered daily doses of synthetic cannabinoid [WIN 55,212-2 ($C_{27}H_{26}N_2O_3.CH_3SO_3H$)] for a period of three weeks performed significantly better than non-treated controls on a water-maze memory test. Marchalant et al. 2007, reported that rats treated with the compound experienced a 50 percent improvement in memory and a 40 to 50 percent reduction in inflammation compared to controls (53).

Previous preclinical studies have demonstrated that cannabinoids can prevent cell death by anti-oxidation. Some experts believe that cannabinoids' neuroprotective properties could also play a role in moderating AD (54). Campbell and Gowran. 2007, reported that "Cannabinoids offer a multi-faceted approach for the treatment of AD by providing neuroprotection and reducing neuroinflammation, whilst simultaneously supporting the brain's intrinsic repair mechanisms by augmenting neurotrophin expression and enhancing neurogenesis. Manipulation of the cannabinoid pathway offers a pharmacological approach for the treatment of AD that may be efficacious than current treatment regimens (55).

In addition to potentially modifying the progression of AD, clinical trials also indicate that cannabinoid therapy can reduce agitation and stimulate weight gain in patients with the disease. Most recently, investigators at Berlin University (2006), reported that the daily administration of 2.5 mg of synthetic THC over a two-week period reduced nocturnal motor activity and agitation in AD patients in an open-label pilot study (56).

Clinical data presented at the 2003 annual meeting of the International Psychogeriatric Association previously reported that the oral administration of up to 10 mg of synthetic THC reduced agitation and stimulated weight gain in late-stage Alzheimer's patients in an open-label clinical trial (57). Improved weight gain and a decrease in negative feelings among AD patients administered cannabinoids were previously reported by Volicer et al. 1997 (58).

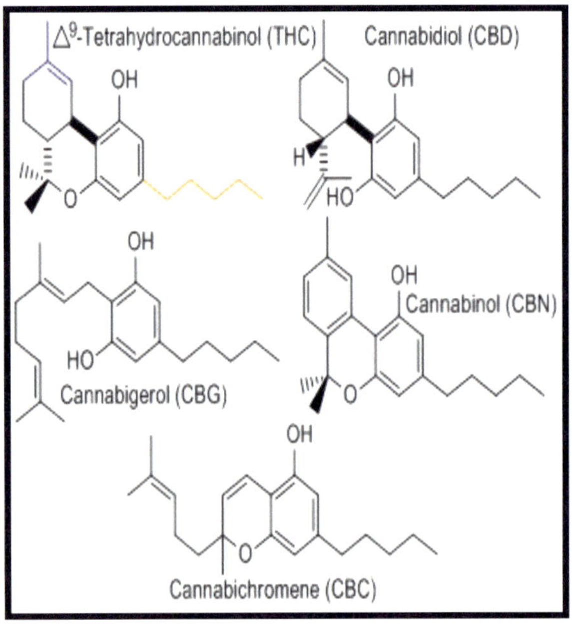

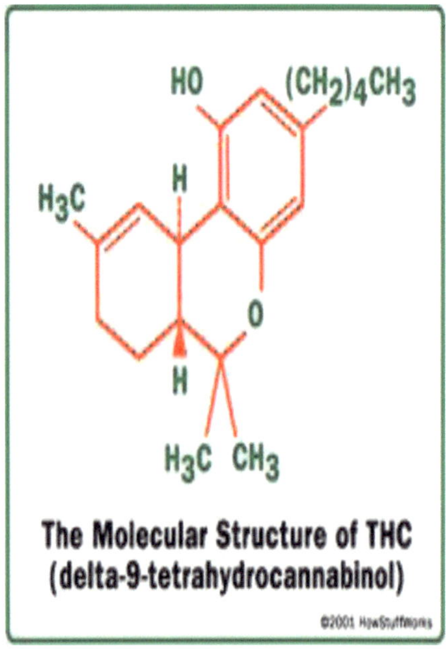

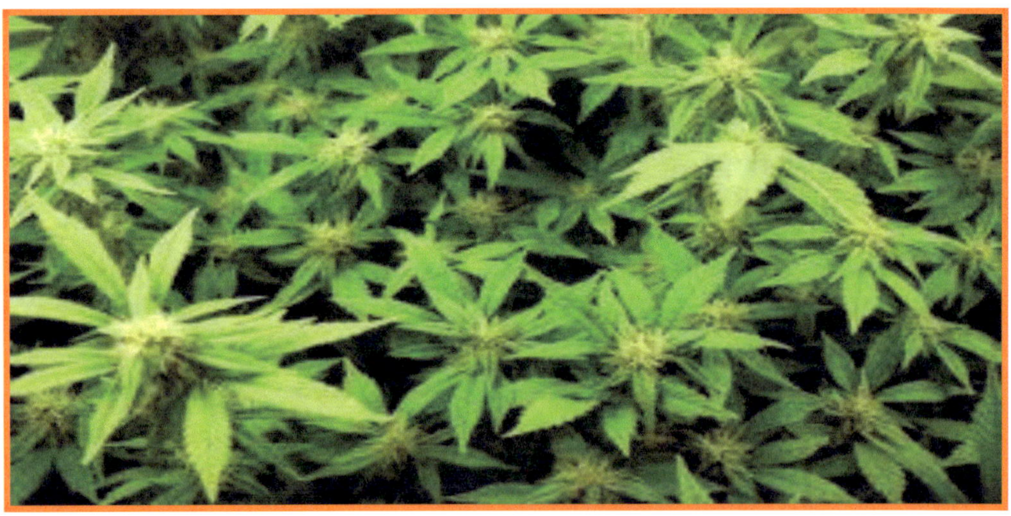

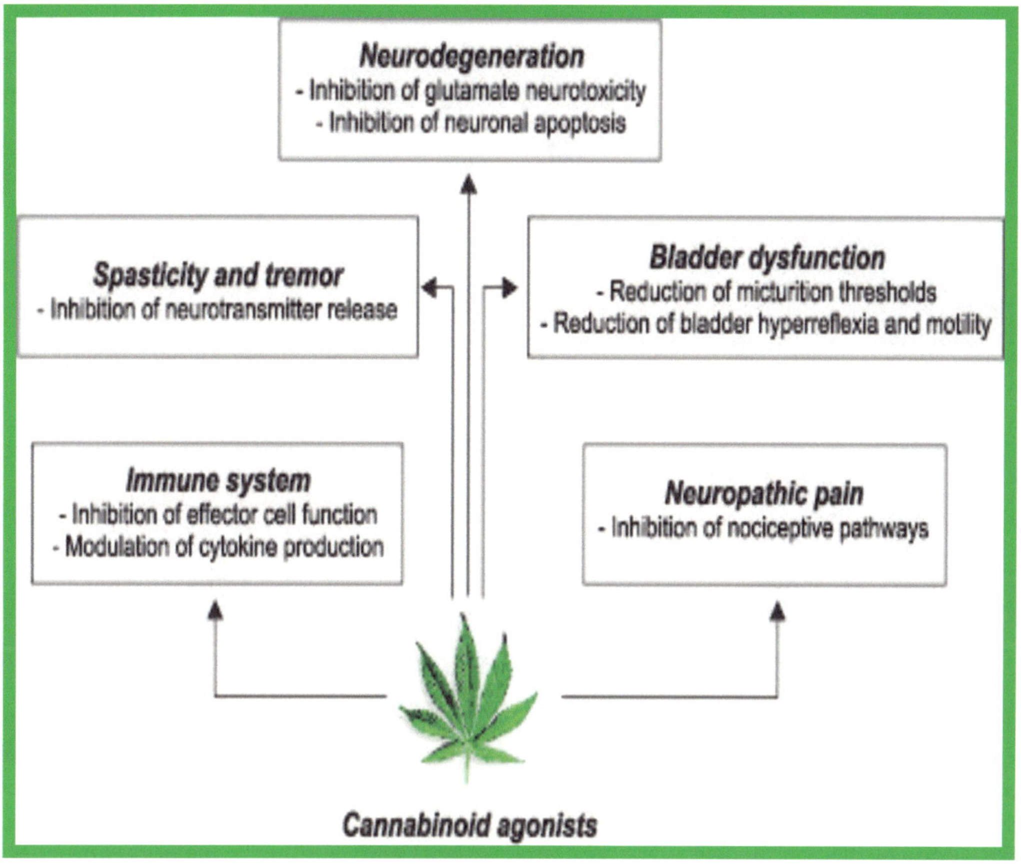

16. Curcumin (diferuloylmethane)

Curcumin (diferuloylmethane), a polyphenol compound responsible for the bright yellow color of turmeric, is believed to be the principal pharmacological agent. It is prepared from the roots of *Curcuma longa (59).* In addition to curcumin, turmeric contains the curcuminoids atlantone, bisdemethoxycurcumin, demethoxycurcumin, diaryl heptanoids, and tumerone. Turmeric also contains sesquiterpenoids and the constituent ar-tumerone (60). Other constituents include sugars, resins, proteins, vitamins, and minerals (including iron and potassium).

Due to various effects of curcumin, such as decreased Beta-amyloid plaques, delayed degradation of neurons, metal-chelation, anti-inflammatory, antioxidant and decreased microglia formation, the overall memory in patients with AD has improved (61).

Researchers found that curcumin may help the macrophages to clear the amyloid plaques found in Alzheimer's disease. Macrophages play an important role in the immune system. They help the body to fight against foreign proteins and then effectively clear them. Curcumin was treated with macrophages in blood taken from nine volunteers: six AD patients and three healthy controls. Beta amyloid was then introduced. The AD patients, whose macrophages were treated with curcumin, when compared with patients whose macrophages were not treated with curcumin, showed an improved uptake and ingestion of the plaques. Thus, curcumin may support the immune system to clear the amyloid protein (61,62).

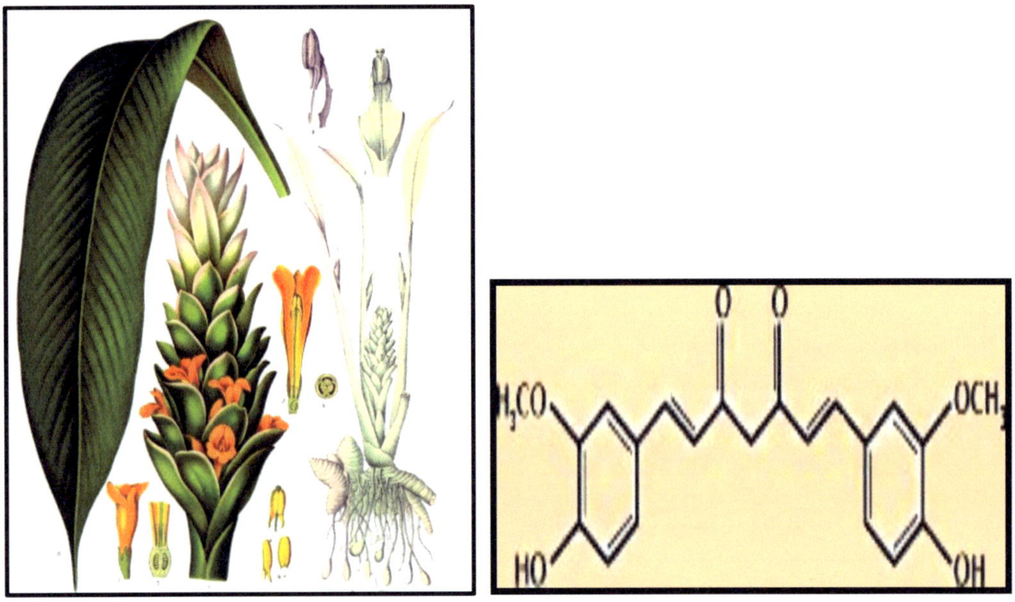

Figure 4. Curcumin (diferuloylmethane).

In addition, Curcumin has powerful antioxidant and anti-inflammatory properties; according to the scientists, these properties believe help ease Alzheimer's symptoms caused by oxidation and inflammation (63). It is well known that Aβ induced oxidative stress which is a well-established pathway of neuronal cell death in AD (64). Three curcuminoids from turmeric (*Curcuma longa* L.), including curcumin, demethoxycurcumin, and bisdemethoxycurcumin, were found to protect PC12 rat pheochromocytoma and normal human umbilical vein endothelial (HUVEC) cells from beta A(1-42) insult. These compounds may protect the cells from beta A(1-42) insult through antioxidant pathways. Other animal studies of AD also suggest that curcumin may reduce levels of amyloid and oxidized proteins and prevent cognitive deficits (65). One alternative mechanism of action for these effects suggested by Baum et al (65), is metal chelation, which may reduce amyloid aggregation or oxidative neurotoxicity. Since curcumin more readily binds the redox-active metals and than the redox-inactive, curcumin might exert a net protective effect against beta toxicity or might suppress inflammatory damage by preventing metal induction of NF-kappaB. Mouse studies that evaluated the effects of dietary curcumin on inflammation, oxidative damage, and plaque pathology demonstrated that both low and high doses of curcumin significantly lowered oxidized proteins and interleukin-1beta, which is a proinflammatory cytokine elevated in the brains of these mice (66). Low-dose but not high-dose curcumin treatment has been shown to reduce the astrocytic marker GFAP and significantly decrease insoluble (Aβ), soluble Abeta, and plaque burden by 43-50%. However, levels of amyloid precursor (APP) in the membrane fraction were not reduced.

17. Huperzine A (Qian Ceng Ta)

Huperzine A, shows promise for enhancing memory and protecting cognitive functions and may improve cognition in AD.

Huperzine-A is a new supplement derived from an ancient traditional Chinese herbal medicine that offers hope to those suffering from AD and other age-related mental conditions (67).

Existing evidence suggests that patients with AD who have taken *Huperzine A* have improved general cognitive function, global clinical status, functional performance and reduced behavioural disturbance compared to patients taking placebos. In addition to benefiting patients suffering from Alzheimer's, Huperzine's memory-enhancing properties suggest that it may be an effective agent for improving memory and learning in healthy humans as well. Huperzine A is a natural compound derived from an ancient Chinese remedy, *Qian Ceng Ta*. This traditional herbal medicine was prepared from *Huperzia serrata*, a clubmoss that grows on the ground in damp forests and rock crevices. Brewed as an herbal tea, Qian Ceng Ta has been used in China to treat fever, inflammation, and irregular menstruation, and has been used as a diuretic.

In the late 1980's, researchers in China discovered that a purified alkaloid extracted from Huperzia, Huperzine A, was a potent, reversible inhibitor of acetylcholinesterase (AChE). Huperzine A readily crosses the blood-brain barrier to prevent acetylcholinesterase (AchE) from destroying acetylcholine. Indeed, part of the damage involved in AD is a loss of acetylcholine-containing neurons in the basal forebrain. This suggests that drugs that could inhibit cholinesterase, which breaks down acetylcholine, could increase the ability of remaining cholinergic neurons. Scientists know that Huperzine A can block acetyl cholinesterase and that it can work both in the peripheral and central nervous systems (68).

Scientists had previously learned that AchE inhibitors such as tacrine and donepezil worked by sliding into the AChE molecule to "jam up" its molecular machinery and impair its ability to degrade acetylcholine (69,70).

In summary, Huperzine A is rapidly absorbed when taken orally, and possesses a very slow rate of dissociation from the enzyme and a longer duration of action. Studies in rodents show that AChE remains inhibited by 33% after 6 hours. Huperzine A has a strong specificity for AChE, and is exceptionally well-suited to its new role, fitting into the active sites of acetylcholinesterase much like a key slipping into a lock. "Hup-A appears to bind more tightly and specifically to acetylcholinesterase than the other AChE inhibitors". This makes it a promising agent for treating various forms of dementia including AD (71-73).

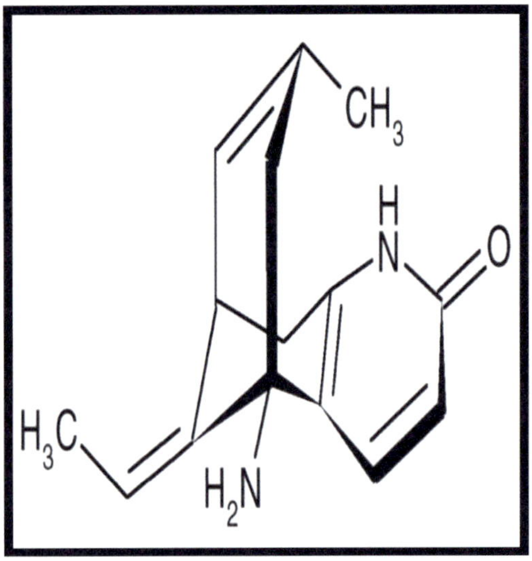

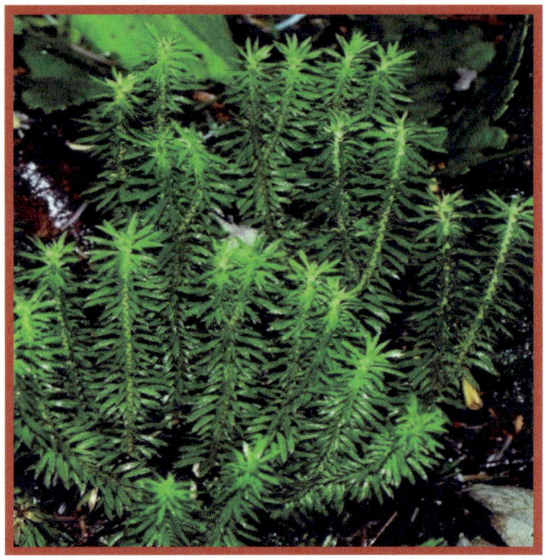

18. Rosemary (Rosmarinus officinalis) - used as Aromatherapy

Aromatherapy uses essential oils from plants, either applied in a *lotion and absorbed by the skin or inhaled and absorbed into* the lungs and nasal passages, to improve physical and mental health. Aromatic oils from plants have been used for over 5,000 years: To protect against stroke and other neurodegenerative diseases such as Alzheimer's and Lou Gehrig's disease. Rosemary contains carnosic acid, a powerful antioxidant, which helps to fight off free radicals in the brain. Carnosic acid stimulates the synthesis of Nerve Growth Factor (NGF) which may help prevent nerve cell deterioration in Alzheimer's (74).Rosmarinus officinalis is a woody evergreen native to the Mediterranean and a universal symbol of remembrance used to honor those who have passed on. The tradition of laying sprigs of rosemary across the coffin or upon a tombstone dates back to ancient Egypt. This custom continued well into the medieval period and beyond. For instance, Shakespeare's Juliet was bestowed with rosemary upon her untimely death. In Australia, where Anzac Day is celebrated in remembrance of one's family ancestors, it is still customary to wear sprigs of rosemary today. Rosemary is also associated with enhancing memory and recall. Shakespeare's Ophelia petitions Hamlet with, "There's rosemary, that's for remembrance, pray you love, remember." Scholars of ancient Greece wore wreaths of rosemary about the brow to help improve recall while taking exams. This reputation has earned the herb a place among traditional wedding herbs used to grace the bride's bouquet, headpiece, and dress. Wedding guests are also given sprigs of rosemary to wear to help them remember the occasion. It was also once common to add rosemary to the couple's wine to help them remember their sacred vows to each other. At one time, it was customary for the bride and groom to plant rosemary near the marital threshold on their day of matrimony. However, the old saying "where rosemary flourished, the woman ruled," prompted some husbands to pluck the plant from the ground lest anyone should think he wasn't fit to rule the roost. Perhaps this is why the practice fell out of favor by the late 15th century. Rosemary takes its name from the

Latin ros maris, which means "dew of the sea." This is likely in reference to the herb's preference for growing along the seashore of its indigenous domain. The Spanish began to call the plant Romero because they believed that another Mediterranean native took refuge beneath a large rosemary bush to shelter herself and her young son as they fled to Egypt to escape Herod. In honor of this brave, young woman, the plant came to be known as Rose of Mary, which was eventually shortened to the modern name familiar to us today.

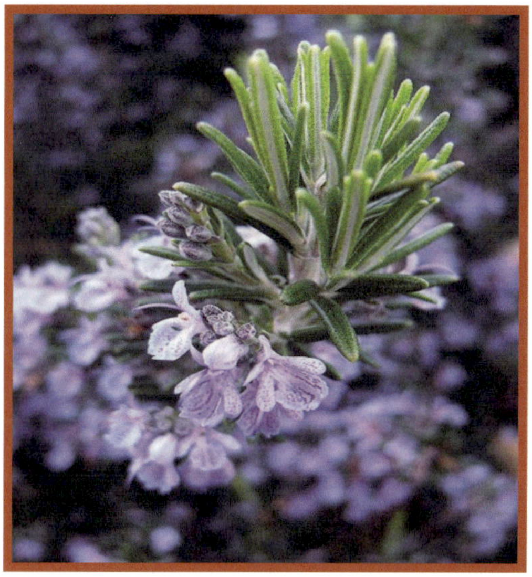

During the Middle Ages, rosemary was thought to be capable of dispelling negativity. As such, it was tucked under pillows to thwart nightmares and visits from evil spirits. It was also burned in the house to keep the black plague from entering. Perhaps this association with protection is why rosemary is still a common ingredient in incense used to cleanse sacred spaces. It was also thought to promote prosperity. In fact, 16th century merchants would often hire perfumers to infuse their shops with spirits of rosemary. The herb was also a popular addition to nosegays, wreaths, and other floral displays to encourage happiness of home and hearth.

Medicinally, rosemary has a wealth of uses, both old and new. In one of the earliest herbals known to be printed in England, Rycharde Banckes recommended that one gather leaves of rosemary and "...boyle them in fayre water and drinke that water for it is much worthe against all manner of evils in the body." Indeed, rosemary was once thought to be a cure for poor digestion, migraine, joint disorders, and muscle aches. In fact, Queen Elizabeth of Hungary was reputedly cured of semi-paralysis when she sipped a concoction of rosemary to ease her painful joints. Hence, this formula came to be known as the infamous Hungary Water. Today, rosemary is recognized as possessing several medicinal properties. For one thing, the plant contains salicylic acid, the forerunner of aspirin. This may explain why massaging the oil of rosemary into joints effectively eases arthritic or rheumatic pain. It also contains antibacterial and antimicrobial agents, and is used by modern herbalists to treat a variety of skin disorders, including dandruff. Rosemary is also being studied for its potential anti-cancer effects since initial studies indicate that its compounds inhibit carcinogenic chemicals from binding to cellular DNA. Rosemary may also become useful in preventing and treating Alzheimer's disease in the near future. Researchers have discovered that certain phytochemicals in the herb prevent the degradation of acetylcholine, an important brain chemical needed for normal neurotransmission. A deficiency of this chemical is commonly seen in Alzheimer's patients.

The majority of recent reports on plants with traditional uses and activities relevant for AD originate from the traditional Chinese and Oriental Medicine, as well as from Kampo Ayurveda and Mediterranean traditional knowledge. They are many plants useful for the treatment of Neurodegenerative diseases and they are many athor still to be discovered.

Author details

Bowirrat Abdalla, Mustafa Yassin, Menachem Abir, Bishara Bisharat and Zaher Armaly
EMMS Nazareth-The Nazareth Hospital, Nazareth

19. References

[1] Bowirrat A, Friedland RP, Farrer L, Baldwin C, Korczyn A. Genetic and Environmental Risk factors for Alzheimer's disease in Israeli Arabs. Journal of Molecular Neuroscience. 2002; 19(1-2):239-245.
[2] Bowirrat A, Treves TA, Friedland RP, Korczyn AD. Prevalence of Alzheimer's Type Dementia in an elderly Arab population. European Journal of Neurology 2001; 8(2):119-123.
[3] Alzheimer's Association. 2010 Alzheimer's disease facts and figures. *Alzheimers Dement*. 2010;6(2):158-94.
[4] Maurer K, Maurer U. *Alzheimer: The Life of a Physician and Career of a Disease*. New York: Columbia University Press; 2003.
[5] Alzheimer A. Uber eine eigenartige Erkangkung der Hirnrinde. In: *Allgemeine Zeitschrift fur Psychiatrie und Psychisch-Gerichtliche Medizin*. 64. 1907:146-148.
[6] Haass C, Selkoe DJ. Soluble protein oligomers in Neurodegeneration: lessons from the Alzheimer's amyloid |[beta]|-peptide. Nature Reviews Molecular Cell Biology. 2007; 8, 101–112.
[7] Braak H, Braak E. Neuropathological stageing of Alzheimer-related changes. *Acta Neuropathol*. 1991;82(4):239-59.
[8] Serrano-Pozo A, Frosch MP, Masliah E, Hyman BT. Neuropathological alterations in Alzheimer disease.Cold Spring Harb Perspect Biol. 2011;3(9):a006189.
[9] Brayne C, Richardson K, Matthews FE, et al. Neuropathological correlates of dementia in over-80-year-old brain donors from the population-based Cambridge city over-75s cohort (CC75C) study. J Alzheimers Dis. 2009;18(3):645-58.
[10] Swerdlow RH, Khan SM. The Alzheimer's disease mitochondrial cascade hypothesis: an update. Exp Neurol. 2009;218(2):308-15.

[11] Braak H, Thal DR, Ghebremedhin E, Del Tredici K. Stages of the pathologic process in Alzheimer disease: age categories from 1 to 100 years. J Neuropathol Exp Neurol. 2011;70(11):960-9.

[12] Braak H, Braak E, Grundke-Iqbal I, Iqbal K. Occurrence of neuropil threads in the senile human brain and in Alzheimer's disease: a third location of paired helical filaments outside of neurofibrillary tangles and neuritic plaques. Neurosci Lett. 24 1986;65(3):351-5.

[13] Davinelli S, Intrieri M, Russo C, Di Costanzo A, Zella D, Bosco P, et al. The "Alzheimer's disease signature": potential perspectives for novel biomarkers. Immun Ageing. 2011;8:7.

[14] Higgins GC, Beart PM, Shin YS, Chen MJ, Cheung NS, Nagley P. Oxidative stress: emerging mitochondrial and cellular themes and variations in neuronal injury. *J Alzheimers Dis*. 2010; Suppl 2:S453-73.

[15] Ding Q, Dimayuga E, Keller JN. Oxidative damage, protein synthesis, and protein degradation in Alzheimer's disease. Curr Alzheimer Res. 2007;4(1):73-9.

[16] Rocchi A, Orsucci D, Tognoni G, Ceravolo R, Siciliano G. The role of vascular factors in late-onset sporadic Alzheimer's disease. Genetic and molecular aspects. Curr Alzheimer Res. 2009;6(3):224-37.

[17] S Roriz-Filho J, Sá-Roriz TM, Rosset I, Camozzato AL, Santos AC, Chaves ML, et al. (Pre)diAβetes, brain aging, and cognition. Biochim Biophys Acta. 2009;1792(5):432-43.

[18] Naderali EK, Ratcliffe SH, Dale MC. Obesity and Alzheimer's disease: a link between body weight and cognitive function in old age. Am J Alzheimers Dis Other Demen. 2010;24(6):445-9.

[19] de la Monte SM. Insulin resistance and Alzheimer's disease. BMB Rep. 2009;42(8):475-81.

[20] Perl DP. Relationship of aluminum to Alzheimer's disease. Environ Health Perspect. 1985;63:149-53.

[21] Perl DP, Moalem S. Aluminum and Alzheimer's disease, a personal perspective after 25 years. J Alzheimers Dis. 2006;9(3 Suppl):291-300.

[22] Goldbourt U, Schnaider-Beeri M, Davidson M. Socioeconomic status in relationship to death of vascular disease and late-life dementia. J Neurol Sci. 2007;257(1-2):177-81.

[23] McDowell I, Xi G, Lindsay J, Tierney M. Mapping the connections between education and dementia. J Clin Exp Neuropsychol. 2007;29(2):127-41.

[24] Szekely CA, Zandi PP. Non-steroidal anti-inflammatory drugs and Alzheimer's disease: the epidemiological evidence. CNS Neurol Disord Drug Targets. 2010;9(2):132-9.

[25] Goldman JS, Hahn SE, Catania JW, LaRusse-Eckert S, Butson MB, Rumbaugh M, et al. Genetic counseling and testing for Alzheimer disease: joint practice guidelines of the American College of Medical Genetics and the National Society of Genetic Counselors. Genet Med. 2011;13(6):597-605.

[26] Hollingworth P, Harold D, Sims R, et al. Common variants at ABCA7, MS4A6A/MS4A4E, EPHA1, CD33 and CD2AP are associated with Alzheimer's disease. Nat Genet. 2011;43(5):429-35.

[27] Caselli RJ, Dueck AC. APOE varepsilon2 and presymptomatic stage Alzheimer disease: how much is not enough?. Neurology. 2010;75(22):1952-3.
[28] Chiang GC, Insel PS, Tosun D, et al. Hippocampal atrophy rates and CSF biomarkers in elderly APOE2 normal subjects. Neurology. 2010;75(22):1976-81.
[29] Finch CE, Morgan TE. Systemic inflammation, infection, ApoE alleles, and Alzheimer disease: a position paper. Curr Alzheimer Res. 2007;4(2):185-9.
[30] Kavanagh S, Gaudig M, Van Baelen B, et al. Galantamine and behavior in Alzheimer disease: analysis of four trials. Acta Neurol Scand. 2011;124(5):302-8.
[31] Farlow M, Veloso F, Moline M, et al. Safety and tolerAβility of donepezil 23 mg in moderate to severe Alzheimer's disease. BMC Neurol. 2011;11:57.
[32] Starr JM. Cholinesterase inhibitor treatment and urinary incontinence in Alzheimer's disease. J Am Geriatr Soc. 2007;55(5):800-1.
[33] Gill SS, Anderson GM, Fischer HD, Bell CM, Li P, Normand SL, et al. Syncope and its consequences in patients with dementia receiving cholinesterase inhibitors: a population-based cohort study. Arch Intern Med. 2009;169(9):867-73.
[34] Lachaine J, Beauchemin C, Legault M, Bineau S. Economic evaluation of the impact of memantine on time to nursing home admission in the treatment of Alzheimer disease. Can J Psychiatry. 2011;56(10):596-604.
[35] Schmitt FA, van Dyck CH, Wichems CH, Olin JT. Cognitive response to memantine in moderate to severe Alzheimer disease patients already receiving donepezil: an exploratory reanalysis. Alzheimer Dis Assoc Disord. 2006;20(4):255-62.
[36] Porsteinsson AP, Grossberg GT, Mintzer J, Olin JT. Memantine treatment in patients with mild to moderate Alzheimer's disease already receiving a cholinesterase inhibitor: a randomized, double-blind, placebo-controlled trial. *Curr Alzheimer Res.* 2008;5(1):83-9.
[37] Schneider LS, Dagerman KS, Higgins JP, McShane R. Lack of evidence for the efficacy of memantine in mild Alzheimer disease. Arch Neurol. 2011;68(8):991-8.
[38] Nyth AL, Gottfries CG. The clinical efficacy of citalopram in treatment of emotional disturbances in dementia disorders. A Nordic multicentre study. Br J Psychiatry. 1990;157:894-901.
[39] US Food and Drug Administration. August 24, 2011. FDA Drug Safety Communication: Aβnormal heart rhythms associated with high doses of Celexa (citalopram hydrobromide). Available at http://www.fda.gov/Drugs/DrugSafety/ucm269086.htm, 2011.
[40] Weintraub D, Rosenberg PB, Drye LT, et al. Sertraline for the treatment of depression in Alzheimer disease: week-24 outcomes. Am J Geriatr Psychiatry. 2010;18(4):332-40.
[41] Petracca GM, Chemerinski E, Starkstein SE. A double-blind, placebo-controlled study of fluoxetine in depressed patients with Alzheimer's disease. Int Psychogeriatr. 2001;13(2):233-40.
[42] Banerjee S, Hellier J, Dewey M, et al. Sertraline or mirtazapine for depression in dementia (HTA-SADD): a randomised, multicentre, double-blind, placebo-controlled trial. Lancet. 2011;378(9789):403-11.
[43] Pritchard SM, Dolan PJ, Vitkus A, Johnson GV. The toxicity of tau in Alzheimer disease: turnover, targets and potential therapeutics. J Cell Mol Med. 2011;15(8):1621-35.

[44] Sano M, Ernesto C, Thomas RG, et al. A controlled trial of selegiline, alpha-tocopherol, or both as treatment for Alzheimer's disease. The Alzheimer's Disease Cooperative Study. N Engl J Med. 1997;336(17):1216-22.

[45] Freitas C, Mondragón-Llorca H, Pascual-Leone A. Noninvasive brain stimulation in Alzheimer's disease: systematic review and perspectives for the future. Exp Gerontol. 2011;46(8):611-27.

[46] Bishop, M., Davis, A.P & Grimshaw, J. (2006). *Snowdrops: A Monograph of Cultivated Galanthus*. Griffin Press, Cheltenham.

[47] Davis, A.P. (1999). *The Genus Galanthus*. Royal Botanic Gardens, Kew in association with Timber Press, Oregon.

[48] Heinrich, M. & Teoh, H. L. Galanthamine from snowdrop – the development of a modern drug against Alzheimer's disease from local Caucasian knowledge. J. Ethnopharmacol. 2004; 92: 147-162.

[49] Ramirez et al. 2005. Prevention of Alzheimer's disease pathology by cannabinoids. The Journal of Neuroscience. 2005; 25: 1904-1913.

[50] Israel National News. December 16, 2010. "Israeli research shows cannabidiol may slow Alzheimer's disease."

[51] Eubanks et al. A molecular link between the active component of marijuana and Alzheimer's disease pathology. Molecular Pharmaceutics. 2006; 3: 773-777.

[52] Marchalant et al. Anti-inflammatory property of the cannabinoid agonist WIN-55212-2 in a rodent model of chronic brain inflammation. Neuroscience,2007; 144: 1516-1522.

[53] Hampson et al. 1998. Cannabidiol and delta-9-tetrahydrocannabinol are neuroprotective antioxidants.Proceedings of the National Academy of Sciences. 1998; 95: 8268-8273.

[54] Science News. 1998. "Marijuana chemical tapped to fight strokes."

[55] Campbell and Gowran. Alzheimer's disease; taking the edge off with cannabinoids? British Journal of Pharmacology. 2007; 152: 655-662.

[56] Walther et al. Delta-9-tetrahydrocannabinol for nighttime agitation in severe dementia.Physcopharmacology. 2006; 185: 524-528.

[57] BBC News. August 21, 2003. " Cannabis lifts Alzheimer's appetite."

[58] Volicer et al. Effects of dronabinol on anorexia and disturbed behavior in patients with Alzheimer's disease. International Journal of Geriatric Psychiatry. 1997; 12: 913-919.

[59] Ali, R. E. and Rattan, S. I. Curcumin's biphasic hormetic response on proteasome activity and heat-shock protein synthesis in human keratinocytes. Ann N Y Acad Sci. 2006;1067:394-399.

[60] Ji, M., Choi, J., Lee, J., and Lee, Y. Induction of apoptosis by ar-turmerone on various cell lines. Int J Mol Med. 2004;14(2):253-256.

[61] Shrikant Mishra and Kalpana Palanivelu. The effect of curcumin (turmeric) on Alzheimer's disease: An overview. Ann Indian Acad Neurol. 2008; 11(1): 13–19.

[62] Zhang L, Fiala M, Cashman J, Sayre J, Espinosa A, Mahanian M, et al. Curcuminoids enhance amyloid -beta uptake by macrophages of Alzheimer's disease patients. J Alzheimers Dis. 2006;10:1–7.

[63] Frautschy SA, Hu W. Phenolic anti inflammatory antioxidant reversal of b induced cognitive deficits and neuropathology. Neurobiol Aging. 2001;22:993–1005.

[64] Kim, D. S., Park, S. Y., and Kim, J. K. Curcuminoids from Curcuma longa L. (Zingiberaceae) that protect PC12 rat pheochromocytoma and normal human umbilical vein endothelial cells from betaA(1-42) insult. *Neurosci Lett* 4-27-2001;303(1):57-61.

[65] Baum, L. and Ng, A. Curcumin interaction with copper and iron suggests one possible mechanism of action in Alzheimer's disease animal models. *J Alzheimers Dis* 2004;6(4):367-377.

[66] Lim, G. P., Chu, T., Yang, F., Beech, W., Frautschy, S. A., and Cole, G. M. The curry spice curcumin reduces oxidative damage and amyloid pathology in an Alzheimer transgenic mouse. J Neurosci. 2001;21(21):8370-8377.

[67] Xu SS; Gao ZX; Weng Z; Du ZM; Xu WA; Yang JS; Zhang ML; Tong ZH; Fang YS;Chai XS; et al, Efficacy of tablet huperzine-A on memory' cognition' and behavior in Alzheimer`s disease. Chung Kuo Yao Li, Hsueh Pao16:391-5, 1995.

[68] Raves ML, Harel M, Pang YP, Silman I, Kozikowski AP, Sussman JL. Structure of acetylcholinesterase complexed with the nootropic alkaloid, (-)-huperzine A. Nat Struct Biol. 1997;4(1):57-63.

[69] Watkins PB, Zimmerman HJ, Knapp MJ. Hepatotoxic effects of tacrine administration in patients with Alzheimer's disease. JAMA. 1994; 271:992-8.

[70] Raves ML, Harel M, Pang YP, Silman I, Kozikowski AP, Sussman JL. Structure of acetylcholinesterase complexed with the nootropic alkaloid, (-)-huperzine A. Nat Struct Biol. 1997;4(1):57-63.

[71] Qian BC, Wang M, Zhou ZF, Chen K, Zhou RR, Chen GS. Pharmacokinetics of tablet huperzine A in six volunteers. Chung Kuo Yao Li Hsueh Pao. 1995;16(5):396-8.

[72] Mazurek, A. An open lAβel trial of Huperzine A in the treatment of Alzheimer's disease. Alternative Therapies. 1999; 5(2):97.

[73] Saxena A, Qian N, Kovach IM, Kozikowski AP, Pang YP, Vellom DC, Radic Z, Quinn D, Taylor P, Doctor BP. Identification of amino acid residues involved in the binding of Huperzine A to cholinesterases. Protein Sci. 1994;3(10):1770-8.

[74] Jimbo D, Kimura Y, Taniguchi M, Inoue M, Urakami K.Effect of aromatherapy on patients with Alzheimer's disease. Psychogeriatrics. 2009; 9(4):173-9.

Chapter 11

Distant Healing by the Supposed Vital Energy – Scientific Bases

Marcelo Saad and Roberta de Medeiros

Additional information is available at the end of the chapter

http://dx.doi.org/10.5772/50155

1. Introduction

Today in conventional medicine, electromagnetic energy is vastly used for diagnostic and curative purposes. For example, transcranial magnetic stimulation (the magnetic energy pulses through the skull), promotes modulation of neuronal activity in the limbic system for the treatment of depression. But some therapeutic practices encompass the manipulation of a supposed vital energy (SVE). This is a putative form of energy, hypothetic, yet to be detected, that is believed to be present in all living beings. According to these practices, living beings are infused with a subtle form of energy and the health would be modulated by the balance of this energy in the organism, achieved by natural exchange with the environment and harmonious distribution through the body. It is suggested that these energies may be accessed in various ways for therapeutic interventions

Distant healing (DH) includes a broad variety of complementary therapies. This chapter will discuss therapies whose effects could only be explained by an exchange of the SVE from the practitioner to the patient. In techniques based on those principles, the patient is not even touched by the practitioner, and they include Reiki, Johrei, QiGong, intercessory prayer, and other similar practices. This chapter will not approach energy therapies that may exert their effects through explainable elements such light touch, mind-body interaction (due to relationship with the therapist), or positive expectation. In these approaches, it is impossible to examine whether the effects distinguish themselves from a general relaxation effect that could be cognitive or somatic resulted. Therapies as acupuncture, for instance, have part of their theories based on alignment of subtle energy, but they involve also well known physiologic pathways that must be responsible for the major part of the therapeutic effect.

The terms related to these therapies are all borrowed by similarity from physics, in analogy to the knowledge of electromagnetic (EM) phenomena. Terms like bioenergy or biofield therapies has been used to encompass a set of techniques that may or may not belong in the same category. The biofield is defined as the endogenous, complex dynamic EM field that is proposed to be involved in self-organization and regulation of the living organism [1].

The concept of SVE and methods of its use for healing has been described for thousands of years, although known by different names. Approaches of DH for health purposes is maybe the oldest ancestral curative practice, practiced in all cultures over the entire world, throughout recorded history [2]. These vital energy concepts include the Indian term *Prana*, the Chinese *Ch'i*, the Japanese *Qi*, the Hawaiian *Mana*, and European terms as *animal magnetism* (from Anton Mesmer) or *bioplasma*. All refer to so-called subtle or nonphysical energies that permeate existence and have specific effects on the body-mind of all conscious beings.

Numerous schools and philosophies of healing exist, involving the engagement of the SVE of variant conceptions and descriptions. In an attempt to propose a classification, we would grossly refer a technique as:

a. performance-related systems (e.g., laying on of hands a few inches away from patient), or distant healing sent only by mental intention;
b. practitioner in proximity to the patient, or distant (either in other room or miles away);
c. techniques related to a religious tradition (as intercessory prayer, blessings), or not (as Reiki);
d. systems derived from ancient wisdom traditions, or modernly constituted systems;
e. self-healing systems (practitioner heals himself), or healing others (in a relation practitioner-patient).

2. Biophysics and physiology

For centuries, naturalists have noticed behavioral changes in plants and animals that seemed to be correlated with extremely small environmental influences such as variations in electrical, magnetic, and electromagnetic fields, including visible and near visible light. So, it is known for a long time ago that living organisms are extremely sensitive to energy fields. Energy fields are an important language of biocommunication; they go to the foundation of life [3].

An apparent paradox is that living organisms are more sensitive to tiny fields than they are to strong fields [3]. But this selectivity has arisen during evolution as part of survival mechanisms used to locate food, identify predators, and navigate. Moreover, organisms "tune-in" to the subtle variations in the earth's field to set their biological clocks. Geophysical and celestial rhythms influence plant and animal behavior. Living systems are very sensitive to bioinformation, often responding to energetic cues for survival or reproduction.

Cells maintain integrity by extremely subtle and minute shifts in molecular and sub-molecular balance. This involves continual inter- and intra-cellular communication in order to convey chemical and electromagnetic messages. The activity of living tissues and cells produces certain collective frequencies. Living structures and functions are orderly, and their biological oscillations are organized in meaningful ways. They contribute information to a dynamic vibratory network that extends throughout the body and into the space around it [4].

Organisms have energy fields around them, and these fields can produce meaningful interactions between organisms. One explanation is that subtle energy fields in the vicinity of an organism can produce or induce electrical and magnetic fields within the organism, and that these signals have potential to activate, enhance or suppress cellular and molecular processes. We may see these effects on cell surface receptors, enzymes, and reaction kinetics [3]. The exposure to low intensity, non-ionizing radiation can induce and/or modulate events within biological tissues.

It is hypothesized that the action of exogenous EM fields on biologic systems is mediated by endogenous energy fields resonating with and modulated by external fields. Experimental data also supports the theory that exogenous EM fields may either induce or perturb endogenous fields. There is an evidence to show EEG synchrony between bioenergy practitioners and client occurs during healing [4].

Cells can respond to extremely weak electromagnetic fields. Internal biochemical reactions can be accelerated by an extremely weak magnetic field, the order of millitesla. Some of these ranges are similar in intensity and frequency with the emissions in the human body. Extreme low frequency electromagnetic fields for example, could induce relatively rapid phosphorylation of specific receptor proteins in T-cell membranes. Hence a cascade of intra-cellular signals may be initiated, accelerated or inhibited [4].

Also enzymatic processes themselves are field-sensitive. Weak electric fields can change the probability that molecules of the reacting materials will encounter each other[3]. Ions are also highly sensitive to entrainment with external EM fields. Free radicals like nitric oxide are also involved in the coupling of EM fields to chemical events in the signal cascade.

Research showed that extremely low intensity, non-ionizing EM fields, having even less energy content than the physical thermal noise limit, can produce biologic effects. Some evidence suggests that molecular-level receptor proteins on cell membranes may be one locus where electromagnetic fields act on the cell, acting as interface between EM field and biomolecules. These processes also appear capable of acting on specific regions of DNA and regulate expression of several proteins in cultured cells.

At such extremely low levels, the energy content of the signal is irrelevant. Such extremely low-level fields cannot act energetically on organisms, because the energy content is negligible. Thus, it has been proposed that they are acting informationally. Fields carrying biologically relevant information have been called "electromagnetic bioinformation". It is proposed here that they interact directly with the biofield [1]. The human biologic field is an organizing field which hypothetically regulates the biochemistry and physiology of the body. There is no consensus among scientists regarding the nature of the biologic field (i.e., whether it is electromagnetic or not, or whether it consists of electromagnetic components together with other uncharacterized fields) [1].

DH therapies may be mediated by means of extremely low-level electromagnetic fields emitted from the healer, which are associated with psycho-physiologic states of the practitioner's intention. Regulatory interactions and the impact and mechanisms of self-organization and healing have a theoretic fit with energy balance and reported changes in the autonomic nervous system [1]. The biofield seem to interact with biological tissue at the cellular level, mimicking the response obtained when externally applied pulsed electromagnetic fields. The exchange of low-frequency energy could give up to 18 inches of the body, a distance that would include many therapies that do not involve touch [5]

One theory that could explain the effects of distant healing is that the energy field of one person can interact with that of another, producing or inducing specific beneficial energetic signals within a patient. Living systems are regarded as complex, nonlinear, dynamic, self-organizing systems at a global or holistic level according to the principles of non-equilibrium thermodynamics of open systems and chaos theory. Living systems are constantly exchanging energy-with-information at multiple levels of organization with their surroundings in order to maintain themselves. This biophysical view of life provides the rudiments of a scientific foundation for complementary therapies involving the transfer of bioinformation carried by a small energy signal [1].

3. Theories related to DH

No text provides a mechanistic model of how putative energy modalities might work. The explanation would attribute the beneficial effects of DH to "real" but currently unknown physical forces, which are "generated" by the therapists and "received" by patients. There may be mechanisms as yet not described by scientific laws. Many theoretical models postulate about human energy fields. None has been proven or validated conclusively by Western science. Efforts to make sense of energy healing typically have referenced the physical sciences to provide theories for understanding a putative therapeutic effect. Representative examples include information transport mechanisms, quantum entanglement, and transmission and reception of extremely low frequency electromagnetic energy.

Most scientists and funding agencies are unaware of the evidence or the relevant literature. The work of healers has elicited controversy and skepticism. The existence and transmission of potentially therapeutic healing energy seem to contravene the conventional worldview underlying modern biomedicine. Criticism and rejection of bioenergy healing by Western physicians is expected, in light of misunderstandings resulting from unfamiliarity with the topic. Due to prejudice and ignorance, suggestion or placebo effects are the most obvious alternative explanation of energy medicine. An element of suggestion is present in complementary therapies, as it is in conventional therapies. Randomized controlled trials suggest, however, that several complementary therapies are of significantly greater benefit than the effects of suggestion shown in the mock-therapy control groups [6].

Generally, any theory about DH systems based on the SVE must comprises [7]: a. a source which generates energy and modulates it in some manner such that it conveys information; b. a coupling mechanism connecting the bioenergy source to a transfer medium; c. a transfer medium through which the bioenergy flows; d. a coupling mechanism connecting the transfer medium bioenergy sink; e. a terminal sink which includes a mechanism for the perception of information. The input and output coupling depend on properties of the source and the transfer medium, likewise for the sink. Perception is used rather than reception to imply some active process which uses some form of perceptual reasoning in processing the information based on its content.

3.1. Classic systems visions

Various researchers and practitioners in the field have different understandings of the concept of bioenergy as a result of their diverse educational and experiential backgrounds. While the concept is broadly meant to describe the basis of healing in a varied set of practices, it does not identify a particular type of energy, per se [7].

Energy medicine practitioners state that, in addition to the physical body, an energy body exists that has a direct influence on health. Problems with the energy body can precede physical problems. Similarly, a positive change at the energetic level can lead to physical healing. The energy body is in constant flux according to individuals' emotional, physical, mental, and other states. It is held that energy follows the intentions of both the healer and the person receiving the healing.

According to existing theories of bioenergy, this biofield surrounding the body of all living beings constitutes a dynamic living matrix of information. This matrix communicates information to and among the human energy body, instructing or informing the physical, mental, emotional, and spiritual states of the individual. Correcting and maintaining this system of energy allows for a free flow of information, which in turn enables the biofield to self-regulate—that is, to automatically correct any imbalance that may be causing symptomatic or pre-symptomatic disease [8]

It is believed that an imbalance or attenuation of this energy leads to disease. This theory leads to the belief that vital energy can be redirected or strengthened to promote or restore health. When there is an imbalance of the SVE, allegedly the body would be prone to develop dysfunctional physiologic actions that may origin even physical diseases. The treatments based in distant healing intend to restore the amount and distribution of the SVE of the patient by the intervention of a practitioner. The practitioner seeks to facilitate the flow of bioenergy throughout the biofield.

Certain challenges present in the energy field are commonly encountered by energy practitioners. These include energy depletion, distortion, and congestion. A depletion in the energy field refers to a deficiency of energy in a particular region of the field. A distortion of the energy field is characterized by an area in which energy is present but not evenly distributed. Congestion in the energy field refers to an obvious excess of energy, or blockage in its flow. DH work is done to facilitate the balanced flow of energy and information throughout the client's energy field. The practitioner's clinical objective is not to treat a disease process, but rather to enable a client's energy to go where it needs to go—by rectifying depletions, smoothing out distortions, and removing congestion. The corrections or healings that occur in bioenergy practice are a result of the energy system rebalancing itself.

The suggested mechanism of action of biologic energies purportedly used by complementary therapies practitioners include activation or unblocking of patients' energies, projection of the practitioners' own energies, channeling of energies by the therapist from nature (e.g., the earth, cosmic energies), and interventions of spiritual agents. Many modalities have their own variations on these theories that are relevant to their particular approaches.

Therapists who are sensitive to bioenergies report they can feel or see an aura surrounding the body. It would reflect the physical, emotional, mental, relational, and spiritual conditions of the person. The energy fields are believed to be templates for what occurs within the body, being shaped by genetic, mental, emotional, and environmental factors. In addition to sensing people's conditions, healers can enhance people's states of health by interacting with the bioenergy field.

Many DH therapists hold that they can maneuver the energy body through various means. Some claim to do so simply by directing their intention; others use their hands. Stones, tuning forks, colors, visualization exercises, chanting, breathing practices, and many other approaches may also be used. Training in various modalities varies.

A practitioner can direct his bioenergy by intentionally redirecting the internal flow of biocurrent in his body. The underlying assumption is that an undirected practitioner s bioenergy is distributed throughout his body in a nonrandom (organized) manner but that the net biofield generated is either zero or radiating more or less uniformly in space (referred to as isotropic radiation). When healing, the practitioner does not have any more energy than normal but rather focuses his internal energy or focuses an external source of energy to a specific purpose. A common thread within these techniques is the use subtle energy to stimulate one's own healing process

There are at least three elements of the healing process [7]. The first is the physical transfer of energy through bioenergy fields at a distance (impedance matching). The second is the transmission of bioenergy at an appropriate carrier frequency of the electromagnetic radiation which carries the modulation or signal and the recipient to tune to this frequency (tuning a resonant circuit). The third, the ability of the recipient to decode this modulation (decoding phenomena).

The role of the recipient must not be neglected. The recipient must need or desire or be motivated to be healed; the recipient must be, at least to some degree, either actively or passively receptive. The recipient can increase the reception of this energy by focusing his attention (intention) to receive the energy with the minimal mismatch of impedance.

There are common components in all healing systems [9]. These include an essential role of consciousness, the perception of the etiology and meaning of the illness, an intention to change and improve, belief by the individual in the therapy and in the practitioner, and a mutual expectation for recovery. There are other components that are frequently described. One is the occurrence of emotional and physical healing, "vital energy," as well as a connectivity that often manifests as compassion.

These concepts can be often endorsed among healers [10]: (1) the idea that human beings possess an ability to facilitate healing for one another through use of the hands, either in contact with the body (touch healing) or proximal to it (noncontact healing); (2) a reliance upon an innate human capability to access inner guidance; and (3) assertion that the life force intrinsically "knows" where it is needed and that the healer's principal role is to dispassionately channel or facilitate this transmission.

3.2. The supposed vital energy

In physics, the term "energy" refers to "the capacity to do work and overcome resistance". Matter and energy are fundamentally interrelated, however, fields of force vary according to energy expressed, and information carried. The term "field" refers to "a force which can cause action at a distance". Though field effects may be weak in terms of power, they may have a measurable effect on matter.

The SVE would be a "subtle biofield", something not related to one of the four fundamental forces accepted by current physical knowledge (gravity, electromagnetism, the strong nuclear force and the weak nuclear force). In fact, it has been argued that several complementary practices appear to act in a manner described as nonlocal, non-temporal and non-mediated and thus do not conform to commonly accepted definitions of energy. Non-locality is the interactions between two entities that do not depend on spatial proximity, shielded from ordinary physical and psychological influences, excluding all known causal pathways of human interaction

So, the term energy does not make sense when referring to a distant therapeutic effect that pushes past the known limits of the transmission of any form of energy ever validated. Preferable terms are consciousness and nonlocal mind, since physical scientists have successfully validated and made sense of the sorts of operations at a distance for these constructs that experimental and theoretical work has yet to validate for energy healing [8].

Rather than an exchange of energies, there could be an exchange of information. Information is neither energy nor matter in itself, although energy or matter is its carrier. Information exists only in relationship, and always involves at least two entities, a sender and a receiver, and it depends on the context. Information for a living system conveys meaning, although the meaning to the organism may not always be conscious [1]. In Homeopathy, there may be information stored in the substrate of the remedy that the patient receives. Structured water, or water that has stored information of the original substance dissolved in it, may be the active agent in classic homeopathy.

Another form of passing information associated with bioenergy transfer is that due to resonance, or the inducing of a synchronizing effect in a recipient. In the process of radiated information transfer it is also conjectured that the information content transferred by the practitioner may create a resonance phenomena within the recipient such that the effect is essentially independent of the transferred energy level as long as the level exceeds a detection threshold of the recipient [7].

The phenomena are subject to external influence. The environment is cluttered with a multiplicity of confounding electric, magnetic, and electromagnetic signals. However it is not clear that this ambient radiation may not be the carrier of the information between a practitioner and a receiver and that the practitioner may simply modulate this already existing energy rather than radiate his own energy [7].

The concept of subtle energy may have some relation to a recent issue brought by physics, the concept of dark energy. It is so called because physicists don't know its exact nature. Even so, dark energy may account for 70% of the total mass-energy of the universe. Another bizarre issue, the dark matter, makes up about 25% of this sum. The rest - everything ever observed with all of our instruments, all normal matter - adds up to less than 5% of the Universe. An explanation for dark energy is that it is a new kind of dynamical energy fluid or field, something that fills all of space but whose characteristics are the opposite of that of matter and normal energy.

Some theorists have named this "quintessence," a name that comes from the classical elements of the ancient Greek philosophers. The ether, a pure "fifth element" (quinta essentia in Latin), was thought to fill the Universe beyond Earth. This quintessence would be a contribution to the overall mass-energy content of the Universe. In physics propose, the ether would be a space-filling substance or field, thought to be necessary as a transmission medium for the propagation of electromagnetic waves. The assorted ether theories embody the various conceptions of this "medium" and "substance". This early modern ether has little in common with the ether of classical elements from which the name was borrowed.

Albert Einstein was the first person to realize that empty space is not nothing. According to the general theory of relativity [11], space is endowed with physical qualities; in this sense, therefore, there exists an ether. But this ether may not be thought of as endowed with the quality characteristic of ponderable media, as consisting of parts which may be tracked. The special theory of relativity compel us to assume the existence of an ether. To deny the ether is ultimately to assume that empty space has no physical qualities whatever. Besides observable objects, another thing, which is not perceptible, must be looked upon as real. Since electromagnetic fields also occur in vacuum, the ether appears as bearer of such fields. The ether of the general theory of relativity is a medium which is itself devoid of all mechanical and kinematical qualities, but helps to determine mechanical (and electromagnetic) events. Ether determines the metrical relations in the space-time continuum, e.g. the configurative possibilities of solid bodies as well as the gravitational fields. Einstein stated that, if we could succeed in comprehending the gravitational field and the electromagnetic field together as one unified conformation, the contrast between ether and matter would fade away [11].

3.3. The role of the mind

DH techniques postulate that the intention of one person can influence the health of a distant person. Intentions of one or more persons can interact with the physiological, psychological and/or behavioral status of one or more distant living systems. Healers hold a mental intent, meditative focus, or prayer for the improvement of the healed, through mental focus.

There is evidence to suggest that mind and matter interact in a way that is consistent with the assumptions of distant healing [12]. Mental intention may have some limited effects on living systems. A review [13] of reports on energy medicine, spiritual healing, distant healing and prayer showed that there is evidence, though not conclusive, to suggest an interaction between mind and matter consistent with the claims of many DH modalities. Skin conductance and the autonomic nervous systems of living organisms are more strongly affected. More objective effects of various forms of DH are likely small.

Nonlocal consciousness, in which the awareness of the therapist may connect with the awareness of the patient, is an alternative explanation for some of the effects obtained with energy medicine. Energy medicine practitioners suggest that the mind, acting through biologic energies, can influence states of health and illness profoundly [14]. The therapist may reprogram in some way the patient's disease patterns of perception, behavior, or bioenergy states, promoting changes toward health.

Healing depends on conditions of the therapist such as intention, motivation, emotional engagement, mindfulness, commitment and trust. Communication, clinical method, caring, competence, and treatment characteristics are differentiated as mediating processes; expectancy and conditioning are positioned as antecedents of healing relationships [15]. So, maybe it is not the technique that matters, but rather characteristics of the practitioner and the context of its application in the healing encounter. Effective healing requires all three of these factors: focus, compassion, and intention. The elements of personality most important for healing success are empathy and warmth, sincerity or honesty—and the ability to enhance positive expectancy on the part of the patient.

We know very little about what qualifies a person to successfully express therapeutic intention as a healer. Most investigators believe that the sincerity and genuineness of prayer must surely make a difference, but in most prayer experiments these factors are merely assumed without being rigorously assessed [16]. Variability associated with healing interventions can be expected because of the reliance on human operators who are subject to psychological influences such as expectation and to physical influences such as fatigue.

The level of well-being of the therapist can affect treatment outcome. The practitioner must be in a good healing state. It is expected from practitioners maintaining a daily routine of compassionate practice that seeks to mobilize these states within themselves, as a way of life. It also should facilitate the kind of personal growth that is required to embody the states of wholeness and balance that healers seek to engender in their clients [8].

4. Problems associated with DH

There is much skepticism and negation by scientists about the validity of distant healing therapies. This is mainly due to the impossibility to detect and measure the SVE by the current available instruments. A barrier to taking such work seriously may be the belief that it is fundamentally incompatible with the scientific world view. Physics-based models are not presented as explanatory but rather as suggestive. In essence, DH postulates that mental intention alone can affect living systems at a distance, unbounded by the usual constraints of both space and time. This postulate challenges scientific assumptions that often go unexamined, including the nature of causality [17]

A principal impediment to the acceptance of healing as an established form of therapy has been its seeming resistance to rigorous, systematic empirical research. The reason for this perception is that published research has been largely (but not exclusively) unrigorous and unsystematic. The generally poor quality of current research with inadequate design, measurement, and analysis prevented this field of scientific inquiry from moving forward. There is a lack of an universal accepted theory that would constitute the base for the DH paradigm. Fundamental non-responded issues includes [10]: what is the source of healing and the pathway by which it is transmitted to the client; what it is precisely being transmitted or channeled or worked with; what exactly healers do when they perform healing; and what is required of the client in order to receive healing.

Other obstacle is the lack of objective standards to offer DH modalities as health treatment. There is no established protocol for any of the DH modalities. Appropriate dosage would be a critical element in assessing the efficacy of treatment. It is not well established how many sessions in a series the person should have to observe an effect. The amount of time is often determined by the healer's sense of adequacy or experience. Also, there may be variations that are seldom considered regarding the preparation, the innate characteristics or the state of consciousness required of healers. There are no universally accepted standards for training and certification of the therapist. Some licensed practices require years of training, with hundreds of hours of documented time with clients required for certification. Many healers describe what they do as a gift that they have cultivated without formal training. The professional training of healers needs a model of continuing education and credentialing. Most energy medicine practitioners are not familiar with conventional medical diagnoses or research methodology.

What is problematic in the study of these therapies is the lack of measurability of these healing energies using the instruments available. Unfortunately, most current tools of measurement is based on responses to electrical signal. These instruments cannot detect and characterize the putative healing energies or forces of life. We cannot observe the biofield directly, isolate it, or analyze it comprehensively. But there are many unobservable aspects of nature known only indirectly in physics by their effects. Since there is always noise associated with a transfer of energy, there is a limit to the amount of information which can be transferred from one system to another based on the signal (the desired information carrying power) to noise (undesired interfering power) ratio.

The effects of distant healing therapies are so many variable and unpredictable that is very difficult to be scientifically studied. Variables related to the patient, the practitioner and other elements of the environment can interfere on the observable outcomes. The unpredictability of the response to treatment contributed to skepticism about its benefits and increases the tendency to attribute the effects of these therapies to placebo effect or to spontaneous remission of diseases. This poses a challenge in establishing an appropriate time frame in which to determine the effect, because the time period may often be variable. For example, one person may experience some effects immediately, whereas others may not experience the effects for a day or more [18].

Ethical considerations must be established when offering DH. These modalities have no serious side effects, but an occasional undesirable effect is that symptoms such as pain may increase in the first few sessions. This effect is taken by experienced healers as a good sign, indicating that the energetic components that lie behind the symptom are being released. When treatment is continued, symptoms usually improve, but patient must be aware of these facts. DH can be given as a complement to any other allopathic approaches, with no dangerous interactions with other treatment [6]. However, delaying other treatments that are potentially beneficial is a conceivable problem. Problems may arise when patients defers biomedical interventions for an extended period of time to pursue energy modalities. If paradigm conflicts arise between conventional and complementary approaches, practitioners of DH must assume the commitment to not suggest to patient to abandon the conventional treatment. When clinical deterioration occurs due to lack of compliance with these principles, the prejudice against DH is reinforced.

5. Results of researches

Against the skeptic vision surges a quantity of researches about the effects of therapeutic uses of the SVE over simple animal, the biochemistry of bacteria and cells in culture, and over the growth of yeasts and seeds. There are dozens of randomized controlled studies in humans, animals, plants, bacteria, yeasts, and enzymes that suggest spiritual healing can be effective for pain, anxiety, depression, AIDS, hypertension, arthritis, wound healing, and other problems [6].

There are evidence of intentionality effects at the clinical level, as in healing studies involving whole persons; at the tissue level, as in studies involving populations of various types of cells; at the microbial level, as in studies involving growth rates of bacteria, yeasts, and fungi; at the molecular level, as in studies involving enzyme kinetics and biochemical reactions [12]. The fact that intentionality effects are demonstrated across this enormous spectrum of nature suggests that there is a general, pervasive principle in nature—the ability of intentionality to change matter. There are many studies on the effects in animals, plants, bacteria, yeasts, or cells in vitro, enzymes and DNA, many of which show highly significant effects [6]. Some studies indicate that the consciously focused intention can prevent the growth of tumor cells in vitro, and also influences both DNA replication and the conformation states of the DNA helix [5].

To determine if energy healers could affect the metabolism of geranium leaves, Creath et al [19] designed a study to test their effectiveness on the biophoton emission. They compared effects of treated leaves to untreated control leaves from a single geranium plant. Leaves from intervention sample were treated for 10–15 minutes with a healing intention using an energy healing technique. Leaves from the untreated sample were placed in similar conditions to act as a control. The treated leaf sections have noticeably less biophoton emission, and there are fewer clumps with less activity near the edges, showing a healthier state [19].

Studies of DH in humans are quite promising; however, the effects seem more marked in small animals or simple life forms. At this point, they can only suggest that these healing modalities have efficacy in reducing anxiety; improving muscle relaxation; aiding in stress reduction, relaxation, and sense of well-being; promoting wound healing; and reducing pain [20]. Although research findings show that such interventions are promising, more research is needed.

In human subjects, there are around two dozen major-controlled studies, approximately half of which show statistically significant results favoring the intervention group toward whom healing intentions were extended. Approximately eight systematic or meta-analyses of studies involving healing intentions and prayer have been published in peer-reviewed journals. All but one arrived at positive conclusions [12]. In a systematic review of randomized double-blind controlled trials about DH the positive and negative results were almost identical. A statistically significant effect was found in almost all categories of DH studied (16 papers). A limitation of this review was the heterogeneity and methodological limitations in many studies [21]. In another review of 191 randomized controlled trials of ADT, 124 showed statistically significant effects [6].

A systematic review [2] examined 66 clinical studies with a variety of biofield therapies in different patient populations. They conducted a quality assessment as well as a best evidence synthesis approach to examine evidence for biofield therapies in relevant outcomes for different clinical populations. Biofield therapies show strong evidence for reducing pain intensity in pain populations, and moderate evidence for reducing pain intensity hospitalized and cancer populations. There is moderate evidence for decreasing negative behavioral symptoms in dementia and moderate evidence for decreasing anxiety for hospitalized populations. There is equivocal evidence for biofield therapies' effects on fatigue and quality of life for cancer patients, as well as for comprehensive pain outcomes and affect in pain patients, and for decreasing anxiety in cardiovascular patients [2]

In University of Arizona, Tucson (USA), a study [22] described particularities of Reiki practitioners and the treatment scenario. To do it, wild type E.coli bacteria were heat shocked for 25 minutes at 49ºC just prior to Reiki treatment. Samples were then randomly assigned to the treatment and control groups. Those samples brought to the treatment room were given 15 minutes of Reiki. some practitioners took part in healing treatments on a real patient, prior to their sessions working with the bacteria. The results showed that the bacteria which were treated straight after a healing treatment was given grew significantly better than those which were given Reiki without a healing context, and that practitioner well-being, as measured by questionnaires before and after every session also had an influence on the success of the treatment. They also found that prior negative feelings by the practitioner correlated with low or even negative growth of the bacteria.

A study, using functional magnetic resonance imaging (fMRI) technology, demonstrated that distant intentionality (DI), defined as sending thoughts at a distance, is correlated with an activation of certain brain functions in the recipients [23]. Eleven healers at distance were recruited. The recipient was placed in the MRI scanner and isolated from all forms of sensory contact from the healer. The healers sent forms of DI that related to their own healing practices at random 2-minute intervals that were unknown to the recipient. Significant differences between experimental (send) and control (no send) procedures were found ($p = 0.000127$). Areas activated in the recipient brain during the experimental procedures included the anterior and middle cingulate area, precuneus, and frontal area. It was concluded that instructions to a healer to make an intentional connection with a sensory isolated person can be correlated to changes in brain function of that individual [23].

A promissory form to monitoring biofields around living organisms was presented by Creath et al. [19]. Experimental evidence indicates that biophotonic emission (light) plays an important role in certain biological functions and processes. Advances in low-noise, cooled, highly sensitive CCD (charge-coupled device) cameras able to count photons over thousands to millions of pixels have made it possible to image biophoton emission in completely darkened chambers. Images of biofields can now be recorded and changes can be monitored over time. The biophoton emission imaging provides information about metabolic functioning, state of health of the organism, and that BE appears to be able to be modulated by the intention of a healer [19].

6. Suggested solutions

Outcome of DH are often not disease specific. Biomedical research generally develops a specific treatment aimed at a specific problem based on an understanding of the mechanisms of action, which could be physical, biochemical, neurologic, or genetic. Understanding of the mechanism of disease or disorder is critical to matching an intervention to alter the progress of disease, restore function to an organ or system, or repair a malfunctioning aspect. DH therapies are not designed as treatments for specific diseases; appropriate outcomes, effective dosages, and time lines to detect efficacy are unknown. Therefore, it is challenging to design studies that can adequately control variables so that a causal relation can be detected [18]. The DH must be seen more as a complementary intervention than treatment for specific diseases. Many hospitals incorporate Reiki, therapeutic touch, or similar initiatives, particularly to help people before or after surgery or the discomfort related to cancer treatment.

DH practice emphasizes, as a clinical objective, the strengthening or reinforcement of the client's innate resources to enable one to withstand pathogenic exposures or threats, thus ameliorating susceptibility to disease and/or facilitating recovery. DH can be applied not just to correct a present pathological state and to restore balance, but also to prevent future pathology in a normal client and to elevate a healthy client to a state of high-level wellness. DH seeks to empower one's innate healing resources, and not to attack a disease process, as in Western biomedicine [24]. Also, DH must not be offered as a substitute to conventional medical treatment or without a clinical diagnosis by a doctor.

When considering therapies based purely on the putative manipulation of bioenergy fields, patients should be warned that the mechanism of action is not fully understood and that the benefits vary from individual to individual and take the financial implications into consideration. They may reduce stress and have a modest effect on pain relief but have no antitumor effects [25]. Patient must be aware that intense emotional experiences and memories may also surface. Therapies based on bioenergy fields are safe and may provide some benefit for reducing stress and enhancing quality of life [25].

Some patient-oriented practice recommendations are suggested by Rindfleisch [20]: Energy modalities can be useful when integrated with primary care medicine. Energy medicine is generally safe and may help to modestly decrease pain (roughly 1 point on the 10-point scale), and to reduce anxiety and to improve wellbeing measures. Consider energy medicine when: A biomedical diagnostic workup has not been revealing; Patients make it clear that such an approach would resonate with their belief systems. Adverse effects: as intense emotions may arise during sessions, it should be used with caution in people who have psychoses. Evaluation of healers' qualifications is also important: How much time have they spent in training? Are they licensed or certified? How is their acceptance to integrate their treatment with the conventional one?

Energy medicine interventions may complement conventional care and have minimal risks. Patients report high satisfaction with energy medicine interventions perhaps because complementary therapists often offer patients significant amounts of time to talk about their problems. Conventional medical wisdom can inform and enhance energy medicine practice by encouraging further research. It is hoped that the future will bring more collaboration, greater acceptance of integrative care, and greater appreciation of energy medicine

The evidence presented so far are sufficiently interesting to warrant further study. Recent research suggests that there is a sound basis for accepting DH as a legitimate intervention. It is essential to recruit multidisciplinary teams to investigate the biofield: physicists, biophysicists, chemists, engineers, biologists. Figure 1 presents key questions that must be answered by future researches in order to establish the ultimate paradigm which will make

DH fully acceptable by the current biomedical model. Below are also some directions for future research [26] to accelerate the progress of understanding the source and the biological effects of DH:

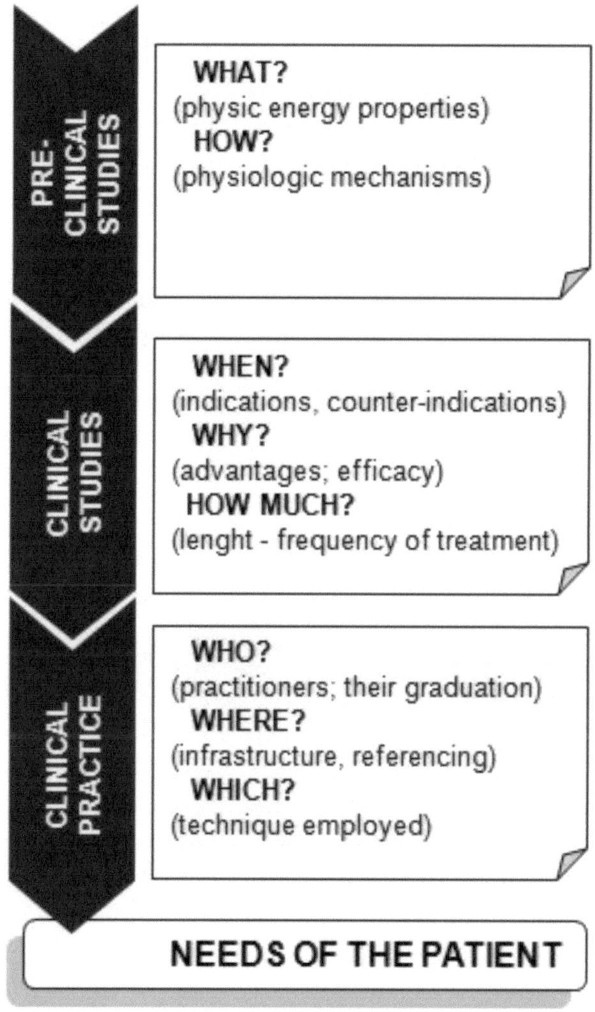

Figure 1. Key questions to establish the ultimate paradigm of distant healing>

- Clarify the scientific hypotheses. Develop further theories to resolve questions of mechanism of action. Researchers must seek whether ancient theories supposing subtle energetic effects of these therapies are supported by current data
- Develop pre-clinical models (cell, tissue, animal) to validate their biological effects and mechanisms of action.
- Validate markers attesting to the biological effects. Maybe specific biomarker associated with stress and relaxation response systems should be examined to determine impact of biofield over autonomic nervous system
- Investigate the ultra-weak electromagnetic components of the biofield. Although the purported subtle energy cannot be directly measured, bioelectric signal measurement can be examined at least as a shadow or a trace of this energy
- Clarify issues that are clues to DH: characteristics of the therapist; potential moderators or mediators of treatment (e.g., expectation, empathic resonance); the regime of ministration and dosage needed; etc.

7. Conclusion

Figure 2 (mostly based on information from Tiller [27] presents a proposal intended to summarize all the information presented in this chapter. This scheme starts with some external afferent EM energy (A), which source may be the organism of the practitioner or even EM waves from the environment. The focused intention of the practitioner (B) imprints information in this EM energy, modifying the waves (C) that arrive to the patient body (D). This would modulate the chemical reactions in cell, generating a new structure expression that would set a physiologic function (E).

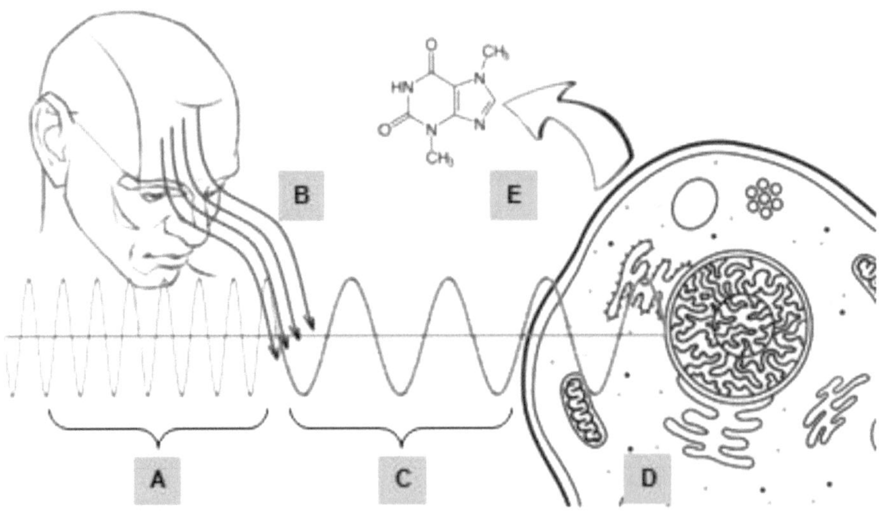

Figure 2. A proposal to summarize all presented information. A = external afferent EM energy, from the organism of the practitioner or waves from environment. B = focused intention of the practitioner imprinting information in this EM energy. C = afferent modified EM waves. D = a cell representing the patient body. E = a new set of some physiologic function>

"Subtle energy" effects are neither supernatural, nor do they require a revision of physics. One reason that a particular event cannot be explained by science might be due to human ignorance. Our science is constantly under revision. In fact, the known universe seems far too big for us to believe that we will ever fully comprehend all of its potentially knowable scientific laws. The effects could be due to factors beyond the current scientific understanding, which will be better understood with time. The failure of science to characterize the SVE does not confirm that it does not exist.

As Dossey posed [12], the key question is not how large the effects are, but whether they exist at all. In other words, what matters is whether human consciousness can act non-locally to affect the material world, beyond the reach of the senses. If only a single one of these studies is valid, then a nonlocal dimension of consciousness exists. In this case, the universe is different than we have supposed, and the game changes.

Author details

Marcelo Saad*
Hospital Israelita Albert Einstein, Brazil

Roberta de Medeiros
Centro Universitario S. Camilo S. Paulo - SP, Brazil

8. References

[1] Rubik B. The Biofield Hypothesis: Its Biophysical Basis and Role in Medicine. J Altern Complement Med 2002;8(6):703–717
[2] Jain S, Mills PJ. Biofield Therapies: Helpful or Full of Hype? A Best Evidence SynthesisInt. J. Behav. Med. (2010) 17:1–16
[3] Oschman JL. Energy and the healing response. Journal of Bodywork and Movement Therapies (2005) 9: 3–15
[4] Movaffaghi Z, Farsi M. Biofield therapies: Biophysical basis and biological regulations? Complementary Therapies in Clinical Practice (2009) 15: 35–37
[5] Denner SS. The Science of Energy Therapies and Contemplative Practice. Holist Nurs Pract 2009;23(6):315–334
[6] Benor DJ. Energy Medicine For The Internist. Medical Clinics Of North America. 2002;86(1):105-125
[7] Hintz KJ, Yount GL, Kadar I, Schwartz G, Hammerschlag R, Lin S. BioEnergy Definitions and Research Guidelines. Alternative Therapies in Health & Medicine. 2003,9:13-30.
[8] Levin J, Mead L. Bioenergy healing: a theoretical model and case series. Explore 2008, 4(3): 201-9
[9] Jonas WB, Chez RA. Recommendations Regarding Definitions and Standards in Healing Research. The Journal Of Alternative And Complementary Medicine. 2004, 10(1):171–181

* Corresponding Author

[10] Levin J. Energy Healers: Who They Are And What They Do. Explore 2011; 7:13-26
[11] Einstein A. Ether and the Theory of Relativity. Presentation delivered on May 5th, 1920, in the University of Leyden, the Netherlands
[12] Dossey L. Healing Research: What We Know and Don't Know. Explore 2008, 4(6): 341-52
[13] Jonas WB, Crawford C. Science and spiritual healing: a critical review of spiritual healing, "energy medicine," and intentionality. Altern Ther Health Med 2003;9(2):56–61
[14] Benor DJ. Spiritual Healing. In Shannon S (editor): Handbook of Complementary and Alternative Therapies in Mental Health. Academic Press, Inc. San Diego, USA, 2002.
[15] Miller WL, Crabtree BF, Duffy MB, Epstein RM, Stange KC. Research guidelines for assessing the impact of healing relationships in clinical medicine.Altern Ther Health Med. 2003;9(3 Suppl):A80-95.
[16] Schwartz SA, Dossey L. Nonlocality, Intention, And Observer Effects In Healing Studies: Laying A Foundation For The Future. Explore 2010; 6:295-307
[17] Schlitz M, Radin D, Malle BF, Schmidt S, Utts J, Yount GL. Distant healing intention: definitions and evolving guidelines for laboratory studies. Altern Ther Health Med. 2003;9(3 Suppl):A31-43.
[18] Engebretson J, Wardell DW. Energy-Based Modalities. Nurs Clin N Am 42 (2007) 243–259
[19] Creath K, Schwartz GE. What Biophoton Images of Plants Can Tell Us about Biofields and Healing. Journal of Scientific Exploration, 2005;19(4):531–550
[20] Rindfleisch JA. Biofield Therapies: Energy Medicine and Primary Care. Primary Care: Clinics in Office Practice 2010;37(1):165-179
[21] Astin JA, Harkness E, Ernst E. The Efficacy of "Distant Healing": A Systematic Review of Randomized Trials. Ann Intern Med. 2000;132:903-910
[22] Rubik, B., Brooks, A.J., Schwartz, G.E. In vitro effect of Reiki treatment on bacterial cultures: role of experimental context and practitioner wellbeing. Journal of Alternative and Complementary Medicine. 2006; 12(1); 7-13.
[23] Achterberg J, Cooke K, Richards T, Standish LJ, Kozak L, Lake J. Evidence for correlations between distant intentionality and brain function in recipients: a functional magnetic resonance imaging analysis. J Altern Complement Med. 2005;11(6):965-71.
[24] Levin J. Scientists and healers: toward collaborative research partnerships. Explore 2008; 4(5):302-310
[25] Deng GE et al. Evidence-Based Clinical Practice Guidelines for Integrative Oncology: Complementary Therapies and Botanicals. Journal of the Society for Integrative Oncology. 2009, 7(3):85–120
[26] Anonymous (National Center for Complementary and Alternative Medicine, National Institutes of Health, USA). Expanding Horizons of Health Care - Strategic Plan 2005-2009. NIH Publication number 04-5568 December 2004.
[27] Tiller WA. A Personal Perspective on Energies in Future Energy Medicine. The Journal Of Alternative And Complementary Medicine. 2004;10(5):867–877